# Pain Management
## in Nursing Practice

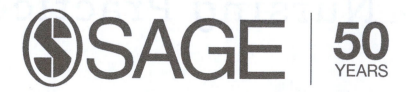

**SAGE** was founded in 1965 by Sara Miller McCune to support the dissemination of usable knowledge by publishing innovative and high-quality research and teaching content. Today, we publish more than 750 journals, including those of more than 300 learned societies, more than 800 new books per year, and a growing range of library products including archives, data, case studies, reports, conference highlights, and video. SAGE remains majority-owned by our founder, and after Sara's lifetime will become owned by a charitable trust that secures our continued independence.

Los Angeles | London | Washington DC | New Delhi | Singapore

# Pain Management
## in Nursing Practice

## Shelagh Wright

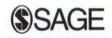

**IASP®**

**SAGE**

Los Angeles | London | New Delhi
Singapore | Washington DC

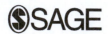

Los Angeles | London | New Delhi
Singapore | Washington DC

SAGE Publications Ltd
1 Oliver's Yard
55 City Road
London EC1Y 1SP

SAGE Publications Inc.
2455 Teller Road
Thousand Oaks, California 91320

SAGE Publications India Pvt Ltd
B 1/I 1 Mohan Cooperative Industrial Area
Mathura Road
New Delhi 110 044

SAGE Publications Asia-Pacific Pte Ltd
3 Church Street
#10-04 Samsung Hub
Singapore 049483

In association with

IASP®

International Association for the Study of Pain
1510 H Street N.W. Suite 600
Washington, D.C. 20005-1020

Editor: Alex Clabburn
Associate editor: Emma Milman
Production editor: Katie Forsythe
Proofreader: David Hensley
Indexer: David Rudeforth
Marketing manager: Camille Richmond
Cover design: Naomi Robinson
Typeset by: C&M Digitals (P) Ltd, Chennai, India
Printed in Great Britain by CPI Group (UK) Ltd,
Croydon, CR0 4YY

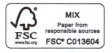

© Shelagh Wright 2015

First published 2015

**Library of Congress Control Number: 2014940396**

**British Library Cataloguing in Publication data**

A catalogue record for this book is available from
the British Library

ISBN 978-1-4462-8199-4
ISBN 978-1-4462-8200-7 (pbk)

This book is dedicated to the memory of my husband Tom,
brave endurer of rheumatic heart disease, proud father and loving grandfather

# Contents

# List of figures and tables

## Figures

# Tables

# About the author

Shelagh Wright trained as a State Registered Nurse at St George's Hospital, London (1970), and as a Registered Midwife at the Rotunda Hospital, Dublin (1973). She studied Single Honours Psychology, Trinity College Dublin (1988), undertook a PhD by research (Psycho-oncology) (NUI-Galway, 1999), and has an MA in Healthcare Management (IPA/UCD, 2004) and a Postgraduate Diploma in Statistics (TCD, 2010). Shelagh was Senior Health Promotion Officer for Older Persons (2002–2007), Health Services Executive, Dublin. More recently, Shelagh was instigator, coordinator and Programme Chair for the Dublin City University accredited MSc in Psycho-oncology and Co-Principal Investigator of a postdoctoral study 'Meaningful methods of identifying psychological distress in patients with advanced cancer' (Irish Cancer Society), which sought to validate the (NCCN) Distress Thermometer in an Irish context. She is a Registered Psychologist (Psychological Society of Ireland) and PRINCE2 Practitioner (APMG) and is recipient of several awards. An author of non-peer- and peer-reviewed papers, Shelagh has many years' experience teaching undergraduate and postgraduate students as well as substantial experience delivering lectures with video and digital technology. She has a particular interest in Autogenic Training, having completed certificate training under the mentorship of Dorothy Crowther, FRCN Chief Executive Officer, Centre for Autogenic Training, Wirral Holistic Care Services, UK.

# Preface

I am delighted to endorse *Pain Management in Nursing Practice* the first written format of the official nursing curriculum for the International Association for the Study of Pain (IASP) co-published by SAGE and IASP.

Undergraduate and newly qualified nurses need to develop their professional nursing knowledge and skills for competency in pain management in nursing practice which is a truly vital area of patient care in primary, secondary and tertiary settings.

Pain-related research-based knowledge, investigative technologies and range and types of pain treatments and interventions are advancing rapidly. Multidisciplinary team service delivery of pain prevention and management is a key aspect of population health. Nurses have a major influence on patients and their families and their health outcomes through patient education and support, promoting monitoring of and adherence to treatment regimens and modification of lifestyles.

In providing a readable and up-to-date synthesis of pain theories and models and their application to modern day, individualised, patient-centred pain management in nursing practice, this book will be an invaluable contribution to the continuing pain management education of undergraduate and newly qualified nurses in Ireland and internationally.

Finally I wish to acknowledge and recognise the valuable contribution Dr Wright has made to the development of a strong evidence base to guide safe practice.

Siobhan O'Halloran, PhD, Chief Nursing Officer, Department of Health,
Dublin, Ireland, 2014

# Acknowledgements

This book, first suggested in early 2011, is the product of a collaboration between the Editor in Chief of the International Association for the Study of Pain, Professor Maria Adele Giamberardino, and her team and the Senior Commissioning and Associate Editors of SAGE, London, Alex Clabburn and Emma Milman, and their team. I owe each a debt of gratitude for their expert guidance during the lengthy process of project development for this book.

I am exceptionally privileged to have been granted permission to write this book, the fruition of an idea based on my academic years of experience teaching pain management (based on the curriculum of the International Association for the Study of Pain (IASP)) to undergraduate nurses in several universities in Ireland. This book aims to provide undergraduate nursing students with easy access to the IASP nursing curriculum content and basic concepts and theories of pain required for entry-level qualified nurses. I hope this book will facilitate the continued promotion of quality patient care in pain management in nursing practice worldwide.

I am indebted to President Professor Brian MacCraith, colleagues in Senior Management, Dr Gerry Moore, Head of Department of the School of Nursing and Human Sciences, Dublin City University (DCU) and DCU Information Systems and Services for their kind support throughout the writing of this book. I am also indebted to DCU Nursing Librarian Amanda Halpin for her guidance in establishing excellent book and online library resources in pain management. This book was also made possible through the kind assistance of librarians in Trinity College Dublin.

My sincere gratitude is extended to President Professor Laserina O'Connor, officers and colleagues on the committee of the Irish Pain Society, Chapter of the International Association for the Study of Pain, for their truly invaluable support and encouragement during the writing of this book.

I would like to thank my family and my extensive support network for their kindness to me during the writing of this book. A special thank you to my current and former mentors globally who continue to inspire and encourage me. Latest research developments provide more hope for prevention, innovative treatments and educational interventions to improve quality of life for patients with pain – people working together to reduce pain and its associated evil.

---

Disclaimer: the reader is asked to note that this book is intended as a teaching and learning tool, with clinical and other examples included for illustrative purposes. All prescribing and/or medication administration is the reader's responsibility according to their scope of professional practice, with reference to guidelines, national legislation and drug formularies of their country.

# Publisher's acknowledgements

Every effort has been made to contact the copyright holders of third-party materials in the text. However, if any copyright owners have not been contacted, the publishers will be pleased to make the necessary arrangements at the first opportunity.

Figure 2.1: Loeser's Onion is from Loeser, J.D. (2005) Pain, suffering and the brain: a narrative of meanings. In D.B. Carr, J.D. Loeser and D.B. Morris (eds), *Narrative, Pain, and Suffering: Progress in Pain Research and Management* (Vol. 34). Seattle, WA: IASP. Copyright (2005). Republished with permission of IASP.

Figure 3.2: (Two-way) Pain pathway from periphery to brain is from D'Mello, R. and Dickenson, A.H. (2008) Spinal cord mechanisms of pain. *British Journal of Anaesthesia,* 101: 8–16. Copyright (2008). Republished with permission of Oxford University Press.

Figure 3.3: The Gate Control Theory is from Adams, N. (1997) *The Psychophysiology of Low Back Pain.* Churchill Livingstone, p.48. Republished with permission of Elsevier.

Figure 3.4: Top-down factors in pain is from Fields, H.L. (1992) Is there a facilitating component to central pain modulation? *American Pain Society Journal,* 1: 139–141, Figure 1. Republished with permission of Elsevier.

Figure 4.1: The psychobiological model of chronic pain is from Flor, H. and Turk, D.C. (2011) *Chronic Pain: An Integrated Biobehavioural Approach.* Seattle, WA: International Association of the Study of Pain (IASP). Copyright (2011). The figure has been reproduced with permission of the International Association for the Study of Pain® (IASP). The figure may NOT be reproduced for any other purpose without permission.

Figure 4.2: Mechanisms of normal sensitization and central sensitization is from Woolf, C.J. (2011) Central sensitization: implications for the diagnosis and treatment of pain. *Pain,* 152: S2-S15. Copyright (2011). The figure has been reproduced with permission of the International Association for the Study of Pain® (IASP). The figure may NOT be reproduced for any other purpose without permission.

Table 4.2: Prevalence rates by pain type in children and adolescents is from King, S., Chambers, C.T., Huguet, A., MacNevin, R.C., McGrath, P.J., Parker, L. and

MacDonald, A.J. (2011) The epidemiology of chronic pain in children and adolescents revisited: a systematic review. *Pain,* 152: 2729–2738. Copyright (2011). Republished with permission of Elsevier.

Table 5.1: Comparison of somatic and visceral nociceptive pain is from Griffin, R.S., Fink, E. and Brenner, G.J. (2010) Functional neuroanatomy of the nociceptive system. In S.M. Fishman, J.C. Ballantyne and J.P. Rathmell (eds), *Bonica's Management of Pain* (4th edn). Riverwoods, IL: Wolters Kluwer/Lippincott Williams and Wilkins. Copyright (2010). Republished with permission of Lippincott Williams and Wilkins.

Figure 5.1: Spinal nerves give rise to peripheral nerves which innervate dermatomes is from *Gray's Anatomy for Students* (2nd edn), by Drake, R.L., Vogl, A.W. and Mitchell, A.W.M. (2010). Copyright Elsevier (2010). Republished with permission of Elsevier Mosby.

Figure 5.2: Pain impacts the dimensions of quality of life. Copyright (1995). Republished with permission of Betty Ferrell and Marcia Grant, City of Hope Medical Center.

Figure 5.3: Initial Pain Assessment Tool is from Pasero, C. and McCaffery, M. (2011) *Pain Assessment and Pharmacologic Management.* St Louis, MO: Elsevier Mosby. Copyright (2011). Republished with permission of Elsevier.

Figure 5.4: Short-Form McGill Pain Questionnaire (SF-MPQ-2). Copyright (2009). SF-MPQ-2 © R. Melzack and the Initiative on Methods, Measurement, and Pain Assessment in Clinical Trials (IMMPACT), 2009. All Rights Reserved. Contact information and permission to use: Mapi Research Trust, Lyon, France. E-mail: PROinformation@mapi-trust.org – Internet: www.proqolid.org. Republished with permission of MAPI.

Figure 5.5: Wong-Baker FACES® Pain Rating Scale. Copyright (1983). © 1983 Wong-Baker FACES® Foundation, www.WongBakerFACES.org. Originally published in *Whaley and Wong's Nursing Care of Infants and Children.* © Elsevier Inc. Republished with permission of Wong-Baker FACES® Foundation (2014).

Figure 5.6: The Faces Pain Scale-Revised is from Hicks, C.L., von Baeyer, C.L., Spafford, P.A. van Korlaar, I. and Goodenough, B.L. (2001) The Faces Pain Scale-Revised: toward a common metric in pediatric pain measurement. *Pain,* 93: 173–183. Copyright (2001). Republished with permission of Elsevier.

Figure 5.7: The Premature Infant Pain Scale is from Stevens, B., Johnston, C., Pteryshen, P. et al. (1996) Premature Infant Pain Profile: development and initial validation. *Clinical Journal of Pain,* 1: 13–22. Republished with permission of Lippincott Williams and Wilkins. Copyright (1996). Republished with permission of Lippincott Williams and Wilkins.

Figure 6.1: The common and distinct components of the patient centred approach and biopsychosocial model is from Creed, F. (2005) Are the patient-centered and biopsychosocial approaches compatible? In P. White (ed.) *Biopsychosocial Medicine: An Integrated Approach to Understanding Illness.* Oxfrod: Oxford University Press. Copyright (2005). Republished with permission of Oxford University Press.

Table 6.2: Humanizing and dehumanizing communication attitudes is from Duldt, B.W. (1991). 'I-Thou': research supporting humanistic nursing communication theory. *Perspectives of Psychiatric Care,* 27 (3): 5–12. Copyright (1991). Republished with permission of John Wiley and Sons.

Table 6.3: Facilitative and blocking behaviours used by nurses when communicating with patients with cancer is from Wilkinson, S. (1991) Factors which influence how nurses communicate with cancer patients. *Journal of Advanced Nursing,* 16, 677–688. Copyright (1991). Republished with permission of John Wiley and Sons.

Figure 7.1 : Analgesia system of the brain and spinal cord. Copyright (2011). This figure was published in Hall, J.E. (2011) *Guyton and Hall Textbook of Medical Physiology* (12th edn). Copyright Elsevier. Republished with permission.

Figure 7.2: Caudal epidural block. Copyright (2014) This figure was published in O'Connor, T. and Abram, S. (2014) *Atlas of Pain Injection Techniques* (2nd edn). Copyright Elsevier. Republished with permission.

Figure 7.3: RestoreUltra® SureScan® MRI Neurostimulator. Copyright (2012) Republished with permission of Medtronic, Inc. © 2012.

Figure 7.4: A flexible, non-stepwise approach to chronic pain management is from *The Essence of Analgesia and Analgesics.* Sinatra, R.S., Jahr, J.S. and Watkins-Pitchford, J.M. (eds), p.70. Copyright (2011). Republished with permission of Cambridge University Press.

Table 8.1: Starting dose for patient-controlled analgesia is from Greco, C. and Berde, C.B. (2010) Acute pain management in children. In S.M. Fishman, J.C. Ballantyne and J.P. Rathmell (eds), *Bonica's Management of Pain* (4th edn). Riverwoods, IL: Wolters Kluwer/Lippincott Willliams and Wilkins. Copyright (2010). Republished with permission of Wolters Kluwer/Lippincott Williams and Wilkins.

Table 8.2: Harmful effects of unrelieved pain is from McCaffery, M. and Pasero, C: *Pain: Clinical Manual,* p. 24. Copyright 1999. Republished with permission of Elsevier Mosby.

Figure 8.1: Cardiac pain referral mechanism. Copyright (2014). Republished with permission of Bloomsbury Educational Ltd. Source: A. Syrimis, Cardiac Pain Referral Mechanism, www.clinicalexams.co.uk.

Figure 9.1: A model regarding brain circuitry involved in the transition of acute to chronic pain is from Apkarian, A.V., Hashmi, J.A., Baliki, M.N. (2011) Pain and the brain: specificity and plasticity of the brain in clinical chronic pain. *Pain,* 152: S49–S64. Copyright (2011). The figure has been reproduced with permission of the International Association for the Study of Pain® (IASP). The figure may NOT be reproduced for any other purpose without permission.

Figure 9.3: Relationship between musculoskeletal ageing and the development of osteoarthritis. Copyright (2009). Source: *Hazzard's Geriatric Medicine and Gerontology* (6th edn), Halter, J.B., Ouslander, J.G., Tinetti, M.E., Studenski, S., High, K.P. and Asthana, S. (eds), Chapter 112: Aging of the muscles and joints, Figure 112–5; p. 1360. McGraw Hill Medical. Copyright. Republished with permission of McGraw Hill (2009).

Figure 10.2: Screening tools for measuring distress. Reproduced with permission from the NCCN Clinical Practice Guidelines in Oncology (NCCN Guidelines®) for Distress Management V.2.2014. © 2014 National Comprehensive Cancer Network, Inc. All rights reserved. The NCCN Guidelines® and illustrations herein may not be reproduced in any form for any purpose without the express written permission of the NCCN. To view the most recent and complete version of the NCCN Guidelines, go online to NCCN.org.

Figure 11.1: Proposed model for integration of palliative care. Copyright. Source: S.M. Fishman, J.C. Ballantyne and J.P. Rathmell (eds), *Bonica's Management of Pain* (4th edn). Riverwoods, IL: Wolters Kluwer/Lippincott Williams and Wilkins. Republished with permission of Lippincott Williams and Wilkins.

Figure 11.2: Opioid conversion chart. Republished with permission of Our Lady's Hospice and Care Services Dublin.

Figure 12.1: Mechanism for regulation of glucocorticoid secretion. Copyright (2011). Source: *Guyton and Hall Textbook of Medical Physiology* (12th edn). J.E. Hall. Chapter 77: Adrenocortical hormones, p.932, Figure 77.7. Republished with permission of Elsevier.

Figure 13.1: Pain management domains and core competencies is from Fishman et al. (2013) Core competencies for pain management: results of an interprofessional consensus summit. *Pain Medicine,* 14: 971–981. Copyright (2013). Republished with permission of John Wiley and Sons.

Table 13.1: Patient education - essential topics. Copyright (2011). Source: Institute of Medicine (2011) *Relieving Pain in America: A Blue Print for Transforming Prevention, Care, Education and Research.* Washington, DC: The National Academies Press. Reprinted with permission from the National Academy of Sciences, courtesy of the National Academies Press.

Figure 13.2: Opioid Risk Tool is from Webster, L.R (2005) Predicting aberrant behaviours in opioid-treated patients: preliminary validation of the Opioid Risk Tool.

*Pain Medicine*, 6 (6): 432–442. Copyright (2005). Republished with permission of John Wiley and Sons.

The extract from The Declaration of Montréal is reprinted with permission of the International Association for the Study of Pain® (IASP). The Declaration may NOT be reproduced for any other purpose without permission.

The extract from the Desirable Characteristics of National Pain Strategies: Recommendations in Chapter 14 is reproduced with permission of the International Association for the Study of Pain® (IASP). The extract may NOT be reproduced for any other purpose without permission.

The extract from the Australian National Pain Strategy in Chapter 14 is from National Pain Strategy (Pain Australia) (2010), www.painaustralia.org.au/images/pain_australia/NPS/National%20Pain%20Strategy%202011.pdf. Republished with permission of Pain Australia.

The extract from the Prague Charter in Chapter 14 is from The Prague Charter (2010), www.eapcnet.eu/Themes/Policy/PragueCharter.aspx. Republished with permission of the European Association for Palliative Care.

The extract from the SIP Road Map in Chapter 14 is from Societal Impact of Pain (SIP) Societal Impact of Pain. Available at: www.sipplatfonn.eu/home.html. Republished with permission of Grünenthal Europe and Australia.

The extract from *Relieving Pain in America: A Blueprint for Transforming Prevention, Care, Education, and Research* (Institute of Medicine, USA) in Chapter 14 is republished with permission from the National Academies Press.

The extract from the World Medical Association resolution in Chapter 14 is republished with permission of the World Medical Association. Copyright, World Medical Association. All Rights Reserved.

The extract from the Canadian Pain Strategy in Chapter 14 is from Canadian Pain Summit (2012) *Rise Up Against Pain*. Available at: http://canadianpainstrategy.ca/en/home/about-the-2012-summit.aspx. Republished with permission of the Canadian Pain Society.

# 1

# Leaders in pain care: an historic overview

## Learning objectives

The learning objectives of this chapter are to:

- recognize the origins of understanding and treating pain
- be aware of how social practices across ages influenced cultural attitudes to pain
- be cognizant of some eminent leaders in pain treatment and management
- view a transition from a linear view of pain to a complex systems perspective

## Introduction

This chapter offers a brief overview of the important contributions of some eminent leaders in pain philosophy, medicine and nursing from ancient to modern times, describing the achievements of these leaders within their socio-political and cultural contexts. There was no linear development from ancient to modern times towards understanding mechanisms underpinning human pain experience. Multiple factors, at different times over very lengthy time spans, provided a context for discoveries which improved understanding of mechanisms underpinning pain experience, as well as pain diagnostics, treatment and management (Dormandy, 2006).

## A view of pain from antiquity

One of the few human constants between now and antiquity is the inherent anatomical structure and neurobiochemical function underpinning human physiology, with the human person living in a social and cultural context. It is now acknowledged and undisputed that pain is a subjective experience and that this experience always takes place in a context which impacts on both how the pain is experienced as well as the meaning of the pain for the person. Prehistoric man viewed pain relief as part of a package bestowed by the gods, which addressed sleep, happiness, hope and joy, and which was handed down and utilized by healers in early civilizations. The viewpoint began to change with the beginnings of Western civilization in ancient Greece, a context of frequent wars, resulting in serious injuries, without knowledge of a central nervous system and only the rudimentary beginnings of study of anatomy and physiology (Dormandy, 2006).

Records of the experience of pain in ancient Greece emphasize the experience of pain related to war and fighting, more than to long-term illness or death and dying. Homer, for example, in the *Iliad* (8th–4th-century BC), used a vocabulary which included descriptions of psychological experiences of mourning, grief and worry as well as acute pains of childbirth and pains related to wounds or stings caused by arrows and sharp objects. The pains caused by the latter gave rise to exhaustion, the pain being alleviated by the removal of the sharp object and 'remedies that relieve afflictions' (Rey, 1993). The word 'suffering' is used in the *Iliad* in the context of 'putting up with/working with' pain and acknowledging the recurrence of pain. Pain in those ancient times was described both in terms of its temporal nature, that is, how long the pain sensation lasted, and the type of pain, for example, 'sharp', 'cutting', often referring to the instrument which caused the pain (Rey, 1993). Homer's *Iliad* is a war record of the beginning of Western civilization. Death from injury was described in the context of the person dying, the weapon associated with death and pain, how the weapon entered the body of the person dying and the wound produced. This latter element described painful death as deconstruction of human life. The mortally wounding weapon not only accessed the body of the fighter, but also wounded his close social others. Homer's *Iliad* portrayed:

> the spear that cuts through the sinew of Pedaeus's head, passing through his teeth and severing his tongue, passes also through the work of goodly Theano, who 'reared him carefully even as her own children'; the Bronze point that enters Phereclus through the right buttock, pierces bladder and bone, and pierces as well the ship building and craftsmanship bodied forth in this son of Tecton, Harmon's son. (Scarry, 1985: 123)

# Hippocrates (*c.* 460–377 BC)

Living in a culture of war, **Hippocrates** was the first ancient Greek physician to change the concept of causes of disease from punishment by the gods to natural causes. Hippocratic medicine focused on observation, and especially the description of the pain experience provided by the patient to the doctor. Hippocrates took a new perspective of viewing pain as a symptom. With a philosophy that 'pain signifies', the elicited pain information formed an essential part of the overall patient examination, contributing to the patient's prognosis in a system of medicine which viewed illness as a process (Rey, 1993). Hippocrates, known as the 'Father of Medicine', taught physicians the guiding principle of 'first do no harm' (*primum non nocere*) and required physicians to take the Hippocratic Oath (Boring, 1957; NIH, 2012).

In the books of the Hippocratic collection, written from 430 BC to 380 BC, the various treatises emphasize that the doctor's duty was to alleviate suffering and to know when to intervene, through interpretation of the patient's case history. The verb 'to suffer' (*poneo*) was used to describe suffering and illness as an experienced state. Pain location, often defined in approximate terms: 'in the area of' or 'about', as well as playing a role in illness identification, was linked to the type of treatment prescribed. The Hippocratic understanding of the aetiology of pain varied and was without an empirical foundation. As one example, use of the principles of likes and opposites was invoked, with certain pains being considered to be brought on by heat in 'cold' people and by cold in 'warm' people. Ignorance of anatomy was due to the legal ban on the dissection of human bodies, so medical practice relied on knowledge obtained from animal dissection. Hippocrates, notwithstanding the limitations imposed by these conditions, aimed for objectivity in his medical teachings and practice, turning away particularly from the use of magic and magical potions (Dormandy, 2006; Rey, 1993).

Hippocratism spread to the entire known world. The fame of Alexandria from 331 BC spread as an advanced, intellectual and scientific Hellenistic culture in Egypt. The Egyptians had better knowledge of anatomy than the Greeks because embalming, with dissection, had been practised for thousands of years. In Alexandria, the great Alexandrian anatomists Herophilus (335–280 BC) and Erasistratus (310–250 BC) revealed the brain as part of the central nervous system (Keele, 1957).

## Influences on pain in the first and second centuries AD: Galen and Aristotle

Galen (*c.* 129–199 AD) was a physician to the Roman emperors. He published extensively in Greek and his works, subsequently translated into Arabic and Latin, were, for more than a millennium, considered the definitive medical references. Galen had a profound influence on the medical profession for longer than any other doctor in history (Dormandy, 2006). Also strongly influenced by the dissection work of the Alexandrian anatomists and localizing the mind in the brain (Boring, 1957), Galen placed considerable importance on pain in his work, which emphasized both sensation and perception. Galen devised a humeral system of pathology in which information characterized by pain, heat, redness and swelling contributed to a differential diagnosis of affliction in various organs. Pain, along with other symptoms, was responsible for identifying unhealthy organs. Galen was responsible for classifying different forms of pain, such as 'pulsing', 'throbbing', 'stretching' or 'lancinating', terms which are still used today (Rey, 1993). However, he was very reluctant to use pain-relief potions, especially 'carotic drugs', a term which referred, at that time, to medications which could produce stupor or sleep, particularly opium, although he did reluctantly recommend the latter for pain relief but only in older people (Dormandy, 2006).

Galen's particular contribution was to offer the first systemic thinking about pain, which up to that time in ancient Greek medicine was considered as a diagnostic and prognostic tool and was without a theoretical framework. Galen can also be considered as offering the first definition of pain as 'the sudden change of temperament (the balance of the four forces of blood, phlegm, choler and black bile) and the rupture of continuity' (Cohen, 2010: 88).

Another of Galen's great contributions to medicine was his re-establishing of the central nervous system as the organ for sensory perception, in contrast to the Greek philosopher Aristotle (384–322 BC), who put forward the concept of correlation of all sensory input by a 'sensorium commune' in the heart. While he advanced systemic thinking about pain, Galen had included unsupported anatomical errors and dogma in his writings which would later be refuted by modern scientific evidence. Though there were major differences in both viewpoints across the ages, both Aristotelian and Galenic physiology survived until the end of the eighteenth century. Galen disagreed with Aristotle's assertion allowing immortality to the intellectual part of the soul. The high importance placed on saving the soul may have been one factor which caused Galen's work to become obscured under the shadow of Aristotle's work from the time of the fall of the Roman Empire (Keele, 1957).

## The Middle Ages: Christian and Galenic cultures

Galenic medical tradition, largely published in Greek, was nearly lost to the Latin West after the decline and fall of the Roman Empire. At this time, the need to save the human soul took precedence over everything and determined attitudes to pain. Hospitals and hostels were established in the East and the West to look after the poor and sick and to help those in pain. In the sixth century AD one of the monastic rules composed for the original Benedictine monasteries was: 'the care of the sick is to be placed above every other duty as if indeed Christ were being directly served by waiting on them'.

By the eighth century, Islam had conquered the Arabian Peninsula and from this time Galen became the supreme medical authority. Galenic medicine was kept alive in the Greek-speaking Asian cultures and passionately translated into Arabic for Muslim cultures. However, it did not go unchallenged, especially regarding pharmacological preparations, at which Islamic chemists excelled (Dormandy, 2006).

# Renaissance and the refuting of Galen's ideas: Leonardo da Vinci and pain

Galenic medicine re-emerged in the West during the Renaissance, which began in Italy in the fourteenth century and spread throughout Europe. Marked by creativity in arts, music, architecture, literature and theology, the Renaissance culture provided the context for medical texts to be translated from their original Greek into Latin and the European languages (Dormandy, 2006). However, while Galenic medicine led the field, by offering a fact-fitting system and overall philosophy, Galen's ideas were now questioned in the light of new anatomical learning. From this time, the search for the truth of anatomy paved the way for the discoveries of the Renaissance; anatomy was a hugely exciting area at that time, and many artists performed dissections and autopsies of human bodies. While **Leonardo da Vinci** (1452–1519) contributed more than 600 anatomical drawings, his experience of human dissection is not known. Leonardo da Vinci attached major importance to pain, commenting:

> the chief good is wisdom, the chief evil is body pain. Seeing therefore that we are made up of two things, namely soul and body, of which the first is the better and the worse is the body, wisdom belongs to the better part and the chief evil belongs to the worst part and is the worst. The best thing in the soul is wisdom and even so the worse thing in the body is pain. (Keele, 1957: 61)

# Beginnings of modern science: Cartesian linear theory of pain

Modern science began in the seventeenth century and was accompanied by major contributions to scientific knowledge. For example, Harvey's discovery of the circulation of the blood in 1628 is regarded as the beginning of biological science, and Hooke's experiments with dogs established mechanisms of circulation and respiration. Scientific observations and medicine were breaking free from Galenic views as a consequence of investigations. However, scientific evolution was taking place at different rates in different countries. The nature of pain was reinterpreted at this time, primarily by French philosopher **René Descartes** (1596–1650), who is often referred to as the 'Father of Modern Philosophy'. He believed in a free, insubstantial soul and a mechanically operated body, solving any incompatibility with his theory of dualism. Descartes made an analogy of the human being with clocks and other automata, so that physiology could be seen in terms of matter in motion; using reductive mechanistic philosophy, the machine became the model to explain the living. Descartes equated the soul with the mind and, as only humans had souls, therefore only humans could have mind and consciousness. Mind and body were therefore almost separate.

A devout Catholic, living at a time of inquisitions and punishment for heresies, Descartes aimed to solve the conflict regarding the soul – between religion and science – through dualism (Boring, 1957). In his *Principles of Philosophy* (1644), Descartes explained sensation, and especially pain, as a way of understanding the union of soul and body (Rey, 1993). Descartes put forward the best description of the first theory of pain, known as 'specificity theory' (Melzack and Wall, 1982). In *Passions of the Soul* (1649), Descartes described how the soul 'linked with every part of the body all at once'. He located the soul in the pineal gland because it was a single gland and not replicated. Descartes stated: 'only one sensation is felt by the soul and there must therefore be only one place where the sensations come together and which permits the nature of the sensation to be well defined' (Rey, 1993: 75). As shown in Figure 1.1, in a working model used for centuries, Descartes described his linear concept of the mechanism of pain:

> If for example fire (A) comes near the foot (B) the minute particles of this fire, which as you know move with great velocity, have the power to set in motion the spot of the skin of the foot which they touch, and by this means pulling upon the delicate thread (cc), which is attached to the spot of the skin, they open up at the same instant the pore (de) against which the delicate thread ends, just as by pulling at one end of a rope one makes to strike at the same instant a bell which hangs at the other end. (Keele, 1957: 72)

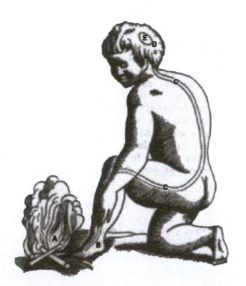

**Figure 1.1** Descartes' (1664) concept of the pain pathway

Source: Descartes, R. (1664) *L'homme*. Translated by M. Foster in *Lectures on the History of Physiology during the 16th, 17th and 18th Centuries*. Cambridge: Cambridge University Press, 1901. Cited in Keele, K. (1957) *Anatomies of Pain*. Oxford: Blackwell Scientific

# Anaesthetics and the transition to pain-free surgery

At the beginning of the nineteenth century, pain and suffering were viewed as inter-woven into the normal fabric of European and American life, across all socio-economic and occupational divides. Life was very harsh and pain was fre-quently considered normal; it was not something to be avoided, but rather it provided a foundation for social order. However, attitudes changed dramatically in the first three decades of the nineteenth century so that, by 1840, some doctors considered pain as an evil to be defeated at all costs (Dormandy, 2006).

**Anton Mesmer** (1734–1815) was an eighteenth-century doctor who introduced into his own clinical practice the hypnotic effect produced in patients known as 'mesmerism' or 'animal magnetism'. While there was no general scientific interest in this new phenomenon, successful mesmerism was the forerunner of anaesthesia. In 1837, **John Elliotson** (1791–1868), Professor of Medicine at University College Hospital, London, having personally witnessed an effective demonstration, tried to introduce mesmerism into clinical practice within the hospital. However, the University Council passed a resolution forbidding 'the practice of mesmerism or animal magnetism within the hospital' and Elliotson resigned (Boring, 1957).

In India, where there was governmental open-mindedness, **James Esdaile** (1808–1859), having heard of Elliotson's work, successfully induced analgesia with mesmerism. Between 1846 and 1847 in India, Esdaile demonstrated the effectiveness of mesmerism for anaesthesia and reducing peri-operative shock. He performed many major and minor operations (Boring, 1957). Esdaile had governmental, but not professional, support for his work. While finding mesmerism safer than ether or chloroform in terms of potential side-effects, there was insufficient scientific and medical interest, and too few trained mesmerists available to provide a service for the new norm of surgery under anaesthesia. This placed a burden on the mesmerists. In addition, inducing a trance in some patients required much time (Forrest, 1999). In a newly opened, small, experimental hospital in Calcutta, Esdaile undertook fur-ther research on the potential benefits of mesmerism. After carrying out a comparative trial between ether and mesmerism, Esdaile found that ether produced the more profound trance. Esdaile concluded that:

> Ether … will soon become a safe means of procuring sensibility for the most formidable surgical operations ever. … All Mesmerists … will rejoice at having a means of bringing to light one truth more, especially as it will free them from the drudgery required to induce Mesmeric insensibility to pain. (Robinson, 1947: 74)

# The first civilian operation under anaesthetic

Ether was the first general anaesthetic to be used to prevent pain in major surgery. The first procedural administration of ether can be attributed to **Crawford Williamson**

Long (1815–1878) in America. In March 1842, performing surgery for the first time under general anaesthesia by ether, Long removed a neck tumour from a patient who had delayed the procedure because of fear of pain. The brief operation required the patient to inhale ether throughout. The patient felt nothing and recovered from the operation, according to Long's records. However, while recognizing that discovering the mode of painless surgery would be a massive achievement, Long was extremely cautious about making any claims of the benefits of ether as a general anaesthetic. He could not rule out possible pain insensitivity or the role of suggestion in the operation's success. Although he kept detailed notes, continued to use ether and became a successful surgeon, Long's findings were not published and did not impact on the development of anaesthesia. Long was given recognition through a colleague's publication in 1877, a year before his own death in 1878 (Dormandy, 2006).

While 'gas frolics' were a Victorian social pastime, and were sometimes indulged in personally by medical and dental practitioners, inhalation administration of soporific substances was, in general, considered hazardous, unsafe and uncontrollable in the medical and surgical context. The claim for the discovery of general anaesthesia for surgery was to prove extremely contentious. (Dormandy (2006) provides a very readable account of the unpleasant controversies between experts and charlatans in the fight for recognition of the discovery.)

## General anaesthesia: Horace Wells and William Thomas Morton

At that time communication among pioneers was slow (usually by letter), so sometimes there were cross-communications about events. John Collins Warren, Chief of Surgery at the Massachusetts General Hospital, USA, operated under a glass dome on top of the Bullfinch Building, out of hearing distance from the rest of the hospital. In February 1845, against his better judgement, Warren was persuaded by qualified dental practitioner **Horace Wells** (1815–1848) to allow a demonstration of 'his discovery' of the potential of nitrous oxide for pain-free dental extraction. Wells had witnessed a successful demonstration and personally experienced a pain-free dental extraction in 1844 under nitrous oxide administration. However, on this occasion, the demonstration went badly wrong. Following Wells' administration of the anaesthetic, the patient cried out loudly at the beginning of the extraction and the demonstration had to be abandoned. Wells left the hospital theatre feeling very humiliated. The real triumph occurred for his former student and colleague **William Thomas Morton** (1819–1868) a year later. Morton successfully utilized ether in 1846 in a public demonstration, again at the Massachusetts General Hospital with Warren. This highly successful anaesthetic event and other similar events which followed very shortly, led to an ether revolution in surgical practice which rapidly spread internationally (Clark, 1938; Dormandy, 2006).

**James Young Simpson** (1811–1870), renowned Professor of Obstetrics at Edinburgh University, was fervent about finding a method of painless childbirth. While encountering massive opposition from conservative Kirk ministers, devout laypersons and doctors strongly opposed on religious grounds to relieving the pains of childbirth, Simpson very knowledgeably and successfully fought back and won his arguments (Clark, 1938; Dormandy, 2006).

**John Snow** (1813–1858), the first anaesthetist, became a role model for good practice, high standards and patient safety in surgical anaesthesia, for which he adopted a strong scientific orientation (Snow, 2006). As a trainee, Snow had witnessed the appalling suffering of patients undergoing surgical interventions. Snow's viewpoint, that surgical pain was life-threatening, adding to surgical risks and shock for patients, while serving no physiological purpose, went against the grain of current thinking.

At that time, surgeons considered the ethical imperative was to ensure that patients did not die as a consequence of surgery. Many considered that ether and chloroform increased the risk to patients' lives, although they did provide some benefits. However, patients were now aware that pain-free surgery was possible and they therefore more readily consented to operations. While it was recognized that ether and chloroform, although giving pain-free surgery, were very risky, patients were often willing to take the risk rather than experience the pain. Snow believed passionately that anaesthesia protected against shock and the risks of surgery, and that the pain of surgery posed a greater risk to patients' lives than correctly administered anaesthesia. To this end, Snow adopted a rigorous scientific approach to discover the properties and conditions required to enhance the safety of anaesthetics. Snow compared the physical, chemical and pharmacological characteristics of a group of volatile anaesthetic agents and identified their primary physiological characteristics.

Snow recommended that all fatalities should be investigated and insisted on the high-quality and purity of anaesthetic agents. Adherence to Snow's recommendations, with safety being a major element of anaesthesia practice, has had a long-term and continuing impact on the practice of anaesthetics. Snow kept three case books in which he detailed 4,500 anaesthetic administrations in London hospitals and his private practice between 1848 and his death in 1858. Acknowledged to be the most skilled administrator of his day, Snow recorded the anaesthetic used, the procedure, who administered the anaesthetic, the surgeon and the patient's views on the anaesthetic, providing invaluable and accurate accounts of surgical practice of surgery and dentistry in 1850s. While surgical mortality and post-operative infection remained unchanged until the 1870s, Snow's substantial addressing of the problem of pain in surgery led to radical changes in thinking and practice regarding surgery (Snow, 2006).

In 1853, Snow administered chloroform to Queen Victoria when she was delivered of Prince Leopold, and again two years later, when she gave birth to Princess Beatrice. In her diary, Queen Victoria described the effect of chloroform as 'soothing, quieting and delightful beyond measure'. Her affirmation of 'that blessed chloroform', as Queen Victoria described the gas, greatly helped to change attitudes in the medical profession and worldwide to painless childbirth (Dormandy, 2006).

## Anaesthesia, military wounds and pioneers at the Crimea

The horrendous injuries, infections and loss of life sustained by wounded soldiers in the Crimean War (October 1853–February 1856) provided the, albeit contentious, learning context for appropriate anaesthesia in military practice. Snow delivered a lecture to medical personnel of the United Services Institution in May 1847, on the benefits of ether for pain and shock prevention, less than a year after the arrival of anaesthesia to Britain. Snow stated that 'the pain of a surgical operation is greater than that of the wound itself ... a great part of the danger of an operation consists in the pain of it, which gives a shock to the system from which it is sometimes unable to recover'. Snow determined that 'the wounded man suffers two shocks together, that of his wound and that of the operation' (Connor, 1998: 161).

On the Russian side of the Crimean War, **Nikolai Pirogov** (1810–1881), now considered the Father of Field Surgery, having gained extensive experience using ether anaesthesia in the military field context from 1847, utilized his renowned surgical skills with great effectiveness in the Crimean War. British Army surgeons at the Crimea had little or no experience of the new technology, and consequently administration of both ether and chloroform at their military field hospitals was, initially, managerially and practically problematic (Connor, 1998). Graphic accounts from Constantinople, by the *Times* correspondent, of wounded soldiers suffering in appalling conditions, with gross lack of facilities, their even basic needs unaddressed, caused public outrage.

Sidney Herbert, as England's Secretary at War, personally asked **Florence Nightingale** (1820–1910) to go to the Crimea to improve the organization of the care of the severely suffering wounded soldiers, who were being denied even the barest necessities. Nightingale, having by then acquired experience as a volunteer nurse in Prussia, England and Paris, was assigned by Herbert to reorganize the British Army Medical Department supplies and improve nursing standards of care for the wounded. Regarded as the Founder of Modern Nursing, Nightingale adopted a highly strategic approach to gain the confidence and cooperation of the British Army, and successfully revolutionized the management of army, housekeeping and nutritional supplies and nursing care of the wounded soldiers. Countless operations took place on the battlefields, affording a massive learning experience for the effective use of ether and chloroform. Nightingale attended as many operations as she could to ease patient suffering and strengthen the patient by her presence.

# Safety concerns about the choice of anaesthetic for surgery

The experience provided by caring for extensive battle injuries added to the recognition for the need to address surgical pain (Harmelink, 1971; Pollard, 1891). By the 1860s surgeons recognized that it was a duty to their patients to reduce both the risk of fatalities and protect patients from surgical pain and the consequences of surgery in terms of shock and haemorrhage (Snow, 2006).

For the century following from 1846–1847, ether, nitrous oxide and chloroform were the most important of known anaesthetic agents (Clark, 1938). There were serious debates between American and British doctors over the choice of whether ether or chloroform was the safer anaesthesia. In 1871, the *British Medical Journal* decided that ether was preferable to chloroform as the latter was responsible for many deaths which were not effectively investigated. Progress in scientific accuracy depends on the availability of the appropriate technology. By the 1930s it was possible to demonstrate, in the laboratory context, that **cardiac syncope** was linked with chloroform administration (Clark, 1938). Nitrous oxide (laughing gas), discovered and developed by **Joseph Priestley** in the 1770s, was further experimented on by **Sir Humphry Davy** (1778–1829), who stated in research published in 1800 that: 'since nitrous oxide appears capable of totally destroying physical pain, it could probably be used with advantage during not unduly prolonged surgical operations in which no great effusion of blood takes place' (Dormandy, 2006: 165). While this recommendation was not acted upon for 50 years as doctors considered the potential for side-effects was too hazardous, nitrous oxide with oxygen as anaesthesia was in use in Great Britain by 1870, 70 years after Davy's research conclusions about the potential efficacy of this anaesthetic combination (Clark, 1938).

# Major shift to systems theory perspectives on pain

The **Second World War** provided the context for more intense learning of the consequences of severe wounds sustained by soldiers. In 1959, **Henry Knowles Beecher** (1904–1976) published accounts of his clinical experiences as a senior anaesthetist in the US Army working with soldiers who had been severely wounded in battle in North Africa and Italy. When the soldiers arrived into the combat hospitals, only one in three required immediate morphine analgesia for their pain. Beecher's work highlighted the importance of context and the subjective meaning of pain for pain perception. Beecher attributed the soldiers' lack of need for immediate analgesia to their relief at having escaped alive from the appalling conditions on the battlefield (Melzack and Wall, 1982/1988).

**John Bonica** (1917–1994), in his youth, assumed responsibility for his Sicilian family as immigrants in New York. Bonica paid his way through medical school as a professional exhibition wrestler, consequently suffering many chronic joint aches. In 1944 Bonica was appointed Chief Anaesthetist of a 7,000-bed Army hospital, caring for 10,000 wounded soldiers from Asia and Europe, whose suffering inspired his lifelong dedication to the management of pain. He published his ground-breaking book *The Management of Pain* in 1953, declaring 'war on pain'. Two beliefs sustained his determined ideology:

- first, that the pain deserved to be treated even when its cause was unknown or untreatable; and
- second, that such treatment could be effective only through the combined effort of doctors, nurses, psychologists, physiotherapists, and, when indicated, other health professionals (Dormandy, 2006).

Bonica's major contribution was the concept of the **multidisciplinary pain clinic**, which was revolutionary to conventional practice and met a recognized, unmet need of under-treated pain. Pain had never been part of the learning curriculum. The consequence for this was raised awareness of the growing problem of chronic pain, especially pain which had no apparent or certain origin. Bonica organized the first international symposium on the treatment and management of pain in Seattle in 1973, leading to the establishment of the **International Association for the Study of Pain (IASP)**. He published prolifically and had an immense influence on improving standards of care in pain management. In a letter to the editor, published in 1979 in the journal *Pain*, the peer-reviewed journal of the IASP, Bonica commented that, according to his extensive experience, most injuries are accompanied by pain shortly after injury. Bonica recognized the need for intensive pain research in all areas, especially in the growing area of **neuroscience**. In the same letter, Bonica commented:

> Pain is the net effect of incredibly complex interactions of ascending and descending neural systems, biochemical, physiologic, and psychologic mechanisms and neocortical processes that involve dynamic, constantly changing activities in most parts of the nervous system which occur simultaneously. By the time that pain is perceived, it has been submitted to the action of many of these neural systems. Consequently, it cannot be artificially dichotomized into sensory pain and pain associated with emotional components. (Bonica, 1979: 204; see also Cope, 2010; Meldrum, 2003)

**Dame Cicely Saunders** (1918–2005) who, because of chronic back pain, had left her career as a qualified nurse at St Thomas's Nightingale School of Nursing, London, to become a medical social worker, witnessed, as a hospice volunteer, the untreated pain of patients at end of life. Saunders decided to become a doctor to start a home for the dying to better fight the problem of pain, qualifying in 1957. Saunders, now considered as the 'Mother of Palliative Care', and known for her outstanding leadership and personal qualities, especially her tenacity and dogged determination, developed a modern strategy for hospice care and introduced a new philosophy and practice for care at end of life, particularly for patients with cancer pain. Saunders sought to convince the medical community that it was totally unnecessary for patients with cancer to die in pain. Her philosophy was founded on the principles of prevention rather than the alleviation of pain, combined with a thorough understanding of available pain relieving drugs (Clark, 2002).

Saunders was the first doctor to focus her work entirely on end-of-life care, based on the conviction that the then prevalent medical attitude to cancer pain of 'there is nothing more we can do' had to be changed to 'we must think of new possibilities of doing everything'. Saunders developed the concept of '**total pain**' by addressing the social, emotional-psychological and spiritual elements of the patient's quality of life and that of their close others, recognizing the interaction of mind and body and the link of mental distress to bodily pain. In 1963 Saunders stated: 'if physical symptoms are alleviated, then mental pain is lifted also'. Saunders' approach to the care of patients in pain required that healthcare professionals, especially doctors and nurses, listen to the meaning of the pain for the patient and try to understand their experience of suffering, recognizing that their pain was not separate in terms of mind and body, but linked to the person and their social context (Clark, 2002).

## Melzack and Wall's Gate Control Theory

Studies in the nineteenth and early twentieth centuries had recognized the possible existence of mechanisms of suppression and regulation of pain information input in different areas of the spinal column. These threads of information were linked by **Melzack and Wall's** (1965) highly influential **Gate Control Theory**. Psychologist Ronald Melzack met physiologist Patrick Wall when they both worked at the Massachusetts Institute of Technology in the 1950s. Their Gate Control Theory provided a strong rationale to move away from the Cartesian, linear view of pain physiology to a contemporary systems approach. It lead to an understanding of how the brain filters, selects and modulates inputs and recognized that social, emotional and psychological factors were an integral part of pain processing. From a systems perspective, the Gate Control Theory provides a mechanism to explain how the encoding system – the brain and spinal cord – can change its input-output function both up and down (Yaksh, 1999). Melzack and Wall's (1965) Gate Control Theory and the work of Saunders and Bonica were heavily influenced by the relevancy of systems theory in healthcare.

Together with major advances in knowledge of human and animal anatomy and physiology, and in technology, these salient contributors have changed how pain is now viewed. The person experiencing pain is now seen as being inseparable from their social and cultural context, and it is a person's human right to be believed and have their pain treated. Other contributors, who have not been included in this overview because of space constraints, have also helped to influence the change to a more humanitarian approach to the care of the patient in pain.

## Chapter summary

- The perspective of holism practised in early civilizations towards the care of sick people altered with the beginnings of Western civilization in ancient Greece, within the context of frequent wars and the rudimentary beginnings of the study of anatomy and physiology.
- Hippocrates changed the concept of the causes of disease from punishment by the gods to natural causes: Hippocratic medicine focused on the patient's subjective pain experience. The major philosophy was that 'pain signifies'.
- The long-time cultural practice of post-mortem human dissection and embalming in ancient Egypt gave third-century BC Alexandria a high status in terms of improved scientific knowledge and the anatomical basis for medical practice.
- Diverse Aristotelian and Galenic viewpoints survived until the end of the eighteenth century. Galenic medicine, obscured by Aristotelian viewpoints in the Western world, had supreme authority in Islamic, Asian and Muslim cultures.
- Galenic medicine re-emerged in the West at the Renaissance, with the rediscovery and translation of texts into European languages. Errors from former Greek knowledge were recognized and progress occurred at varying rates in different countries.
- French philosopher René Descartes located the soul in the pineal gland, offering an alternative to Aristotelian thinking (which had located the mind in the heart). He explained sensation, and pain, as a way of understanding the union of soul and body. Descartes described the best-known specificity theory of pain.
- In the nineteenth century, anaesthesia transformed surgery and childbirth. John Snow, the first anaesthetist, focused on improving patient safety, especially by reducing the shock of surgical pain, by keeping excellent records and by promoting quality and standards in patient care.
- The Crimean War and, later, the First World War provided an horrific and contentious learning context for treating the pain and suffering of wounded soldiers. Experiences during the Second World War influenced the declaration of war on pain. The post-war application of systems theory to pain prompted a biopsychosocial focus to patient care.

## Reflective exercise

Consider how a transition from a linear to a complex systems theory approach to pain may improve standards of care for patients with pain.

## Recommended reading

Cervero, F. (2014) *Understanding Pain: Exploring the Perception of Pain.* Cambridge, MA: MIT.

Dormandy, T. (2006) *The Worst of Evils: The Fight against Pain.* New Haven, CT: Yale University Press.

Melzack, R. and Wall, P.D. (1982/1988) *The Challenge of Pain.* London: Penguin.

Morris, D.B. (1993) *The Culture of Pain.* Berkeley, CA: University of California Press.

## Websites relevant to this chapter

Comprehensive overview of the history of pain:
   http://unitproj.library.ucla.edu/biomed/his/painexhibit/index.html
Ancient plays depicting psychological and physical wounds inflicted by war:
   www.philoctetesproject.org/
Greek Medicine, History of Medicine Division, National Institutes of Health (2012):
   www.nlm.nih.gov/hmd/greek/greek_oath.html

# References

Bonica, J.J. (1953) *The Management of Pain.* Philadelphia: Lea and Febiger.

Bonica, J.J. (1979) The relation of injury to pain. *Pain*, 7: 203–207.

Boring, E.G. (1957) *History of Experimental Psychology* (2nd edn). Upper Saddle River, NJ: Prentice-Hall.

Clark, A.J. (1938) Aspects of the history of anaesthetics. *The British Medical Journal*, 2 (4063): 1029–1034.

Clark, D. (2002) *Cicely Saunders: Founder of the Hospice Movement: Selected Letters 1959–1999.* Oxford: Oxford University Press.

Cohen, E. (2010) *The Modulated Scream: Pain in Late Mediaeval Culture.* Chicago, IL: University of Chicago Press.

Connor, H. (1998) The use of chloroform by British Army surgeons during the Crimean War. *Medical History*, 42: 161–193.

Cope, D.K. (2010) Intellectual milestones in our understanding and treatment of pain. In S.M. Fishman, J.C. Ballantyne and J.P. Rathmell (eds), *Bonica's Management of Pain* (4th edn). Riverwoods, IL: Wolters Kluwer/Lippincott Williams and Wilkins.

Descartes, R. (1644) *Principes de la philosophie, Part IV.* Cited in R. Rey (1993) *The History of Pain.* (Trans. L.E. Wallace, J.A. Cadden and S.W. Cadden). Cambridge, MA: Harvard University Press.

Descartes, R. (1649) *Les Passions de l'âme. Part 1*. Cited in R. Rey (1993) *The History of Pain*. (Trans. L.E. Wallace, J.A. Cadden and S.W. Cadden). Cambridge, MA: Harvard University Press.

Descartes, R. (1664) *L'homme*. Translated by M. Foster in *Lectures on the History of Physiology during the 16th, 17th and 18th Centuries*. Cambridge: Cambridge University Press, 1901.

Dormandy, T. (2006) *The Worst of Evils: The Fight against Pain*. New Haven, CT: Yale University Press.

Forrest, D. (1999) *Hypnotism: A History*. London: Penguin.

Harmelink, B. (1971) *Florence Nightingale: Founder of Modern Nursing*. London: F. Watts.

Keele, K. (1957) *Anatomies of Pain*. Oxford: Blackwell Scientific.

Meldrum, M. (2003) A capsule history of pain management. *Journal of the American Medical Association*, 290: 2470–2475.

Melzack, R. and Wall, P.D. (1965) Pain mechanisms: a new theory. *Science*, 150: 971–979.

Melzack, R. and Wall, P.D. (1982/1988) *The Challenge of Pain*. London: Penguin.

National Institutes of Health (2012) Greek Medicine. Available at: www.nlm.nih.gov/hmd/greek/greek_oath.html (accessed 6 July 2014).

Pollard, E.F. (1891) *Florence Nightingale: The Wounded Soldier's Friend*. London: S.W. Partridge & Co.

Rey, R. (1993) *The History of Pain*. Cambridge, MA: Harvard University Press.

Robinson, V. (1947) *Victory over Pain: A History of Anaesthesia*. London: Sigma.

Saunders, C. (1963) Distress in dying. Letter. *British Medical Journal*, ii: 746.

Scarry, E. (1985) *The Body in Pain: The Making and Unmaking of the World*. New York: Oxford University Press. Chapter 2: The juxtaposition of injured bodies and unanchored issues.

Snow, S. (2006) *Operations without Pain: The Practice and Science of Anaesthesia in Victorian Britain*. Basingstoke: Palgrave Macmillan.

Yaksh, T.L. (1999) Regulation of spinal nociceptive processing: where we went when we wandered onto the path marked by the gate. *Pain Supplement*, 6: S149–S152.

# 2

# The biopsychosocial model of pain: rehumanizing care

## Learning objectives

The learning objectives of this chapter are to:

- recognize the application of systems theory to biopsychosocial patient care
- be aware of the different types of pain and their implications for quality of life
- appreciate the contribution of literature to cultural awareness of pain and suffering
- understand the subjective experience of pain as a computational neural and mental event

## Introduction

This chapter explores the application of systems theory and the biopsychosocial model to the care of the person in pain, as well as the impact of pain and suffering on the person's quality of life and how this is depicted in the classic and clinical literature. The chapter will lead towards understanding pain as a composite of subjective mental experience and neuronal activity.

## The biopsychosocial model of patient care

From the 1960s, systems theory research applied to healthcare began to influence thinking about viewing health services as potentially adaptive systems which could change to improve healthcare delivery as well as the ways in which patients' subjective illness experience was influenced by social, psychological and cultural factors (Engel, 1977; von Bertanlanffy, 1968). The holistic care philosophy of nursing has been fundamentally influenced by this systems approach to patient care, which is known as the **biopsychosocial model**. From the perspective of patients' pain experience, it is now agreed that individual biological, genetic, gender and age (bio), emotional, cognitive and spiritual (psycho) cultural, environmental and ethnic/racial (social) factors all contribute to the subjective experience of pain (Fillingham, 2010). Two renowned medical leaders, psychiatrist George L. Engel and palliative care physician Dame Cicely Saunders, separately recognized the need to see patients as people inseparable from their psychological and social context, instead of as just physical bodies separated from minds. Both were influenced by the new systems thinking applied to healthcare. Saunders' and Engel's work fundamentally influenced the entire approach to patient care in various specialities. Saunders especially led major change in treating and managing pain in advanced cancer and at end of life, from the patient's perspective. Engel proposed a new model to challenge the dominant biomedical model of care, to recognize the psychological and social aspects of care of patients with mental illness. These changes to patient care were to rehumanize medicine, by including the patient as a person who had a voice in their own care, rather than being viewed as a depersonalized body with a disease, independent of social and psychological influences (Clark, 2002; Engel, 1977, 1980).

## An introduction to different types of pain

The International Association for the Study of Pain (IASP) defines pain as: 'An unpleasant sensory and emotional experience associated with *actual* or *potential* tissue damage, or described in terms of such damage' (Mersky and Bogduk, 1994: 210, emphasis added). This definition accepts the psychological impact of the pain experience, that pain is always (1) subjective, (2) unpleasant, and (3) influenced by cognitive, affective and environmental factors (Turk and Okifuji, 2010).

To effectively interpret the patient's pain experience it is necessary to classify different types of pain, which are each discussed in separate chapters.

The two major types of pain are nociceptive (physiological) and neuropathic (pathological). **Acute pain** can be nociceptive or visceral in origin. Nociceptive somatic pain arises from injury to the body's skin, subdermal layers, muscle, connective tissues, bones and joints. Superficial somatic pain arises from activation of cutaneous (body surface) nociceptors and is usually sharp, stabbing, and sometimes burning in quality. Deep somatic pain arises from nociceptors in muscles, bones, joints or connective tissue, and is often described as dull, crampy and aching. Both superficial and deep somatic pain are usually well localized and often involve local inflammation of injured tissues. Visceral pain arises from nociceptors in visceral organs such as the gastrointestinal tract or the pelvic region, giving rise to different types of pain according to organ involvement. Visceral acute pain may be vague and poorly defined.

Acute pain (see Chapter 8) results when injury prompts activation of primary nociceptive afferents (nerve fibres which respond to pain) and consequent stimulus transduction, action potential transmission and modulation (the mechanisms of pain information transfer are discussed in Chapter 4), leading to acute pain perception, which generally lasts for a limited time span, depending on the cause (which may be related to trauma, some disease processes and invasive interventions), injury consequence and treatment interventions. Acute pain often prompts and requires healthcare intervention (Turk and Okifuji, 2010).

## The transition from acute to chronic pain

Research has shown that acute pain leads within minutes to a sensitization of the central nervous system (see Chapter 3), which is a major cause of chronic non-malignant pain (used interchangeably with the term 'chronic pain' in this book, see Chapter 9). Undertreated and unrelieved severe acute pain is a major predictor for chronic pain following surgery or trauma and for associated reduction in quality of life (Latremoliere and Woolf, 2009; Schug, 2011).

**Chronic (non-malignant) pain** (see Chapter 9) is subjective pain experience linked to a previous, not very recent, injury or chronic disease, and is often made worse by factors removed from the original cause of the pain. The distinction between acute and chronic pain is marked by an arbitrary time interval, varying between three to six months (Turk and Okifuji, 2010).

**Neuropathic pain** (see Chapter 3) is less well understood. While the International Association for the Study of Pain (IASP) defines neuropathic pain as 'pain initiated or caused by a primary lesion or dysfunction in the nervous system', the IASP Special Interest Group for neuropathic pain, NeuPSIG, has proposed redefining neuropathic pain as 'pain arising as a direct consequence of a lesion or disease affecting the somatosensory system' (Treede et al., 2008). There are many types of disorder associated with neuropathic pain; phantom pain, trigeminal neuralgia, painful diabetic polyneuropathy, postherpetic neuralgia and central post stroke pain are in this pain category (Treede et al., 2008).

People with chronic pain frequently require more and frequent healthcare. The problem is extensive and there are now strong moves internationally to have chronic pain recognized as a disease in its own right. Australia was first to enact legislation to this end in 2010 (Chronic Pain Policy Coalition, 2013; National Pain Strategy, 2010).

Often, a combination of treatments is required for the patient with chronic pain, for whom pain control requires multidisciplinary team planning and interdisciplinary care delivery. Sometimes 'trial and error' time is required to find out what works best to alleviate the person's pain. Environmental, emotional and cognitive factors interact with the already sensitized nervous system, contributing to the persistence of pain and associated illness behaviours. A biomedical model which omits addressing the social and psychological aspects of the patient's pain experience has serious negative impacts on the patient's quality of life, as well as being economically wasteful. Patients with chronic pain therefore require an holistic, interdisciplinary care model which includes psychosocial care and structured cognitive behavioural therapies to help the patient to improve his or her coping skills. Care needs to be taken not to make people with chronic non-malignant pain feel that their pain experience is less serious or of less concern than that of patients with cancer pain (Turk and Okifuji, 2010).

**Cancer pain** (see Chapter 10) is highly complex, comprising elements of both acute and chronic pain, both nociceptive and neuropathic in origin. The cancer pain experience is a compounded subjective pain experience brought about by disease progression, and potentially compounded by treatment side-effects. The disease of cancer is invasive and mechanical. An advanced spreading cancer disease may move body organs out of place, as well as invade all types of body tissues, organs and structures, with highly painful consequences. Potential treatment consequences of chemotherapy, radiotherapy, surgery may compound the pain experience. Although experienced by people of all ages, cancer is more frequently a disease of older age. An older patient's subjective experience of cancer pain may worsen the pain they already experience from a pre-existing comorbid condition, for example pain from arthritis or osteoporosis. While a separate classification of cancer pain, as distinct from acute and chronic pain, may not be advocated by some clinicians, it is important to realize the potential severity of cancer-related pain, which is sometime referred to as pain of malignant origin (Fitzgibbon and Loeser, 2010; Turk and Okifuji, 2010). Chronic pain caused by cancer is best thought of as acute pain persisting over time caused by concurrent involvement of different anatomical structures, as well as a constantly evolving local tumour progression and metastatic spread (Shipton, 1999).

**CLINICAL EXAMPLE**

# Acute pain

Mr B, 68-year-old retired office worker, enrolled on his first walking holiday to raise funds for charity. He had been advised that the climate was 'warm to hot' and he would need to ensure a certain basic level of physical fitness to be able to comfortably walk a minimum of 20 miles each day in temperatures of around 75°F. As Mr B exercised regularly in the gym and enjoyed excellent health, and had no previous health problems, he considered his personal fitness adequate for the project and did not seek medical or physiotherapy advice prior to the holiday. On the fourth afternoon Mr B twisted his right ankle while walking on a rocky pathway. Mr B disregarded the mild injury and did not seek assistance to have it treated with an ice pack, strapping or anti-inflammatory medication. The following morning he woke to find his right foot very swollen, throbbing and aching. Mr B sought medical aid, had to admit defeat and returned home early, with assisted transfer. Mr B sought further medical aid at home.

- Q: What category of pain did Mr B experience?
- A: acute, somatic pain indicative of inflammatory, musculoskeletal damage.

# Pain and quality of life

**Quality of life** is defined as each person's perceptions of their position in life in the context of the culture and value systems in which they live and in relation to their goals, expectations, standards and concerns. Quality of life can be considered as a subjective and complex amalgam of satisfactory functioning in **psychological, social, occupational** and **physical** domains (Fallowfield, 1990; WHOQoL Group, 1998). In psychological quality of life, typical indicators are anxiety, depression and adjustment to illness. **Uncontrolled pain** is one of the most **feared consequences** for patients with cancer, potentially negatively and severely impacting on quality of life of the patient and his or her close others. Research shows that severe pain is a reality of many patients' cancer experience (Breivik et al., 2009). Approximately 70% of patients with cancer experience severe pain at some time during their illness, with up to 75% of patients with advanced cancer experiencing pain and 50% of patients who are terminally ill experiencing moderate to severe pain (Breitbart et al., 2010). **Fear of pain** also plays a major role in reducing quality of life and incurring disability for people with chronic non-malignant pain (Flor and Turk, 2011). Hence, there is a need for National Pain Strategies and improved pain services for people with chronic non-malignant pain.

Saunders' statement that 'if physical symptoms are alleviated then mental pain is lifted' (1963b: 746) prompted recognition that psychiatric symptoms in patients with cancer pain must be viewed initially as a consequence of poorly controlled pain (Breitbart, 1989), with biological, psychological, social and spiritual factors both influencing and influenced by pain (Somers et al., 2010). Longitudinal analysis of a study of a group of patients with cancer by Williamson and Schulz (1995) revealed that as pain increased over time, so did activity restriction, which, in turn, predicted increased depressed mood. **Avoidance of pain** is one of the most basic human drives and one of the primary reasons for seeking medical help. Chronic pain severely restricts a person's ability to function and enjoy life and poses considerable psychological, social and economic stresses. The aims of counselling and cognitive behaviour therapies are to attempt to help patients improve their ability to cope with anxiety and depression and to adjust to their illness more satisfactorily. Patients with chronic low back pain, similar to people with cancer pain, exemplify the need for an interdisciplinary treatment and care model. As well as cancer pain, chronic non-malignant pain, such as severe low back pain, impacts on the **psychological domain** of quality of life, potentially incurring depression, anxiety and other disorders (Zepinic, 2009).

Cancer pain and chronic non-malignant pain are associated with major problems in the **occupational domain** of quality of life. Studies also show that there is an association between previous low back injury and increasing severity of present low back pain. Past work-related back injury may be a risk factor for future episodes of low back pain, together with disability, as low back pain is currently a significant public health problem in all industrialized nations (see Chapter 4) (Hincapié et al., 2008).

In the **social domain** of quality of life, chronically ill people frequently express fears of abandonment. In the absence of any means of treating disease, avoiding sick people would have been an important evolutionary adaptive behaviour to promote survival (Foster and Anderson, 1978). The experience of chronic pain serves no useful warning function and instead is a hindrance to quality of life. In the **physical domain** of quality of life, both cancer pain and chronic non-malignant pain are often associated with severe disease and disability, forcing dependency on others for the routine necessities of life and activities of daily living, such as the daily routine of self care, mobility, shopping, cooking and care of living quarters, causing a fundamental role loss with a concomitant loss of self-esteem. A study of the emotional and social consequences of cancer pain highlighted the profound consequences of pain: physical suffering, emotional distress, social handicap and altered family roles (Strang, 1992). The physical limitations, debility and emotional reactions imposed by cancer are increased by pain and a serious consequence is a reduction in patients' social activities and contact with friends (Bonica, 1990). Reliable emotional, informational and practical support from family, friends and healthcare professionals, along with social participation, are vital components of quality of life (Fallowfield, 1990; Winefield and Neuling, 1987).

To understand the personal impact of the experience of chronic pain on the patient's quality of life requires a full measurement and assessment of the patient's pain behaviours in terms of disability and dysfunction. The World Health Organization has developed a classification of functioning, disability and health, so that disability is recognized as a universal human experience and the focus is shifted from cause to impact on quality of life (WHO, 2002). Individual differences in pain responses and pain experiences are recognized and accepted as valid in the clinical setting. Therefore, both quantitative measures (see Chapter 5) and skilled listening (see Chapter 6) are required to ascertain and understand the impact of the patient's pain experience on their quality of life (Carr et al., 2005).

## Undiagnosed, untreated osteoporosis

CLINICAL EXAMPLE

Mrs K, a 60-year-old widow and avid golfer, sustained a vertebral compression fracture following a fall at her home, and was subsequently diagnosed with osteoporosis (a weakening and thinning of the bones). Mrs K is now very limited in mobility and functionality, compared to pre-injury, and cannot currently play golf, drive her car or walk any distance in comfort or contribute socially to her community. Analgesics (paracetamol) give some relief for her pain but her lowered mobility and functionality are the cause of her real distress, and the main indicator of her drastically reduced quality of life. Mrs K feels especially angry that she was not advised to have a DexaScan or to take medications (bisphosphonates and calcium supplements which help to strengthen bones) to prevent osteoporosis, which 'ran in her family' on her mother's side, and she had always thought that her walking (associated with frequent golfing) would be adequate prevention. Her former GP had advised that she would not need screening until aged 65 years or unless she had a fracture. Mrs K feels very let down by her former GP and is regretful she did not take a more active role in insisting on DexaScan screening and preventative medication treatment for osteoporosis. Mrs K has now changed her GP, has purchased private health insurance, is prescribed bisphosphonates and calcium with Vitamin $D_3$ tablets, has purchased and is using a Juvent machine and is scheduled to attend a pain clinic, contemplating further active treatment in the hope of regaining full function and quality of life.

- Q: Can you name the emotions Mrs K is feeling?
- Q: Do you think Mrs K should have been given a choice about having DexaScan screening at an earlier age?
- Q: Do you think there is a role for public education through media coverage of various risk factors for early identification of diseases which cause chronic pain?
- Q: Do you think that media coverage and public awareness impact on national and local treatment policies?
- Q: Has this change in her health status impacted (a) Mrs K's finances and (b) the cost to government?

## Pain and suffering

The **suffering** associated with pain is a personal experience. Listening to the **patient's narrative** of their pain experience is a particularly important aspect of nursing care. The person's subjective pain experience must be seen as related to their particular individual, social and cultural context. Suffering of a serious extent is exacerbated by disease, pain and depression. John Loeser, Professor of Neurological Surgery and Anesthesiology at the University of Washington, Seattle, stated that:

> … suffering should be important to healthcare providers. Along with pain, it drives patients to seek professional assistance. However, to understand suffering one must listen to the patient and listening takes time. In the current health care system in most developed nations, few patients have adequate access to their primary care physicians to allow for an understanding of their suffering. (Loeser, 2005: 20)

Suffering leads to **pain behaviours** which can extend from physical changes like grimacing, limping and poor posture to requiring more frequent visits to the GP and/or pain clinic and not being well enough to work. From the healthcare professional's perspective, the patient's behaviours are real behaviours, influenced by the patient's internal and external environmental contexts and sometimes a result of learning and trying to cope. One aim of the multidisciplinary team is to understand the factors behind the patient's behaviour in order to alleviate the symptoms. For example, the experience of chronic back pain, leading to lowered mood, reduced mobility and activity, poor sleep and loss of good health, can exacerbate disability. Pain behaviours are the things that the person says and does, or avoids doing, and can be measured quantitatively. Pain behaviours differ from suffering, which is the qualitative subjective pain experience of the patient. Loeser (1982) identified the four components that are necessary and sufficient to describe the **phenomenon of pain** as nociception (activation by noxious stimuli of specialized nerve endings and transmission of pain information to the peripheral and central nervous system), pain, suffering and pain behaviour (see Figure 2.1). Nociception and the perception of pain, when experienced in an acute injury/prevention context, act as a warning. Untreated or inadequately treated acute pain can easily become chronic, with no warning or survival advantage, leading to suffering and pain behaviour.

**Suffering** is experienced by people. **Disease** can be defined as an 'objective biological event' that involves disruption of body structures or organ systems caused by pathological, anatomical or physiological changes (Mechanic, 1986) whereas **illness** is defined as a 'subjective experience or self-attribution' of the experienced disease with components of physical discomfort, emotional distress, behavioural limitation and psychosocial disruption, and is highly relevant to the experience of cancer and chronic non-malignant pain. The person in pain frequently reports suffering from pain when they feel out of control, when the source of the pain is unknown, when the meaning of the pain is dire or when the pain is chronic. This relationship of pain to suffering must be acknowledged because suffering can be relieved, in the presence of continual pain, by making the source of the pain known, by changing its meaning

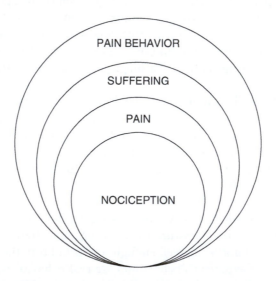

**Figure 2.1** Loeser's Onion: the four components that are necessary and sufficient to describe the phenomenon of pain

Source: Loeser, J.D. (2005) Pain, suffering and the brain: a narrative of meanings. In D.B. Carr, J.D. Loeser and D.B Morris (eds), *Narrative, Pain, and Suffering: Progress in Pain Research and Management* (Vol. 34). Seattle, WA: IASP. Copyright (2005). Republished with permission of IASP.

and by demonstrating that it can be controlled and that an end is in sight (Cassell, 1982, 1991/2004; Moon, 1985).

The **experience of suffering** involves an enduring or recurring experience or event perceived as negative or unpleasant, which may include, but is not limited to, physical pain and/or cognitive experiences or losses, resulting in some type or manner of distress. Pain, when present, is only one component of suffering. Suffering is an unpleasant mental state resulting from an event or situation that is perceived to be harmful, uncomfortable, unpleasant or psychologically or physically painful. While suffering is a broader concept than is pain, suffering brought about by enduring pain is well nigh impossible to alleviate (Benedict, 1981). Suffering is experienced by persons as a threat to their integrity as a complex social and psychological entity. Patients may tolerate severe pain without considering themselves to be suffering if they know that the pain has an identified cause, can be dealt with and will be relatively short-lived. On the other hand, relatively minor symptoms may cause suffering if they are believed or known to have a life-threatening cause, be intractable and reflect a hopeless prognosis (Cassell, 1982).

# Depictions of suffering and pain in fiction and non-fiction

Listening to the person's story is of major importance in caring for the person with pain. Both worlds of fiction and non-fiction have graphically outlined the very distressing consequences of suffering severe pain in isolation, when there is little or no hope of relief. High levels of fear, anxiety, loneliness, despair, uncertainty and sense of loss of hope are some of the psychological experiences portrayed. These psychological consequences cannot be separated from the person's experience of increased pain sensations, which are in turn exacerbated by their lowered pain threshold and tolerance to potentially eliminate a person's sense of control. It is no exaggeration to say that a person in pain can behave as a screaming animal driven mad with pain. The current author, 40 years ago, working as a nurse in a health system prior to the inception of the modern hospice movement, witnessed this pain behaviour several times in patients suffering from the pain of terminal cancer.

**Lawrence Le Shan** (1964) makes the analogy between the experience of chronic pain and that of a nightmare. In the terror dream: (1) terrible things are being done to the person; (2) others, or outside forces, are in control and the will is helpless; and (3) there is no time limit set, no ability to predict when the terror will end. People in pain are in the same terrible situation: terrible things are being done to them and they do not know if worse will happen; they have no control and are helpless to take effective action; and no time limit is given. This aspect of the psychic assault on the integrity of the ego that accompanies pain is a major one. The patient lives during the waking state in the cosmos of the nightmare, which is further emphasized by the meaninglessness and inexplicability of pain, which makes it extremely difficult to cope with. It is common, in the generalization from acute to chronic pain, to assign to pain the idea of a warning, a signal that something is wrong and that something should be done about it. Chronic pain, however, indicates only a state of existence. It does not warn or instruct and may be severe enough to disrupt potentially useful activities and habits. The adequate expression of thirst is to drink. The adequate expression of this kind of pain is only a scream (Le Shan, 1964, 1989/1994).

This situation is graphically illustrated in the novella by **Leo Tolstoy**, first published in 1886, *The Death of Ivan Ilych* (Tolstoy, 1960). The story centres on 45-year-old Ivan Ilych Golovin, a high court judge, who bruised his left side when he slipped from a step ladder, falling against the window frame knob, when showing a workman how to hang a curtain in a new apartment in St Petersburg. At first Ivan disregarded the continuing discomfort. However, soon the discomfort worsened. Inconclusive medical advice from expensive doctors increased Ivan's worry and concern. In the third month of his illness the pain took over Ivan's life and he became confined to bed, isolated at home physically and psychologically.

The theme of the Tolstoy's novella concentrates on issues of authenticity, honesty, purpose, suffering and meaning in life, reflecting Tolstoy's own personal and philosophical struggles with these issues. Ivan Ilyich felt he had lived a good life and did not deserve to suffer. The peasant Gerassim, who cared for Ivan in his sick room, and Ivan's own young son are the only two people in his household who showed kindness and sorrow to Ivan. Ivan found he could ask Gerassim to help him relieve his pain by temporarily changing his position and by staying with him for short lengths of time. Ivan's intense fear of death and pain is demonstrated in his protracted scream, which lasted for three days, and was alleviated at the last minutes of his life when his isolation was relieved by the presence of his family and his fear turned to joy at death being replaced by light, bringing an end to his suffering and, Ivan hoped, peace for his family.

The story is highly illustrative of pharmacological pain relief, which, while essential, is only one element in the comprehensive holistic care required to relieve pain and suffering at the end of life.

**C.S. Lewis**, in *The Problem of Pain* (2002/1940: 105), stated:

> When I think of pain – of anxiety that gnaws like fire and loneliness that spreads out like a desert … or sudden nauseating pains that knock a man's heart out at one blow, of pains that seem already intolerable and then are suddenly increased, of infuriating scorpion-stinging pains that startle into maniacal movement a man half dead with his previous tortures – it 'quite o'er crows my spirit' if I knew any way of escape I would crawl through sewers to find it …

Physician and musician **Albert Schweitzer**, having dedicated his life to the alleviation of the suffering of others, particular of the indigenous peoples of Lambaréné, Africa, in 1953, stated: 'We must all die. But that I can save [a person] from days of torture that is what I feel as my great and ever new privilege. Pain is a more terrible lord of mankind than even death itself.' Schweitzer was very concerned about how people relate to each other empathically – the person as a body relating to another person as a body – and how the shared condition of having a body impacts the empathic relations between living beings, described by Schweitzer (1921 (cited in Frank, 1995: 35)) as:

> Whoever among us has learned through personal experience what pain and anxiety really are must help to ensure that those out there who are in physical need obtain the same help that once came to him. He no longer belongs to himself alone; he has become the brother of all who suffer. It is this 'brotherhood of those who bear the mark of pain' that demands humane services.

Author and psychiatrist **Dr Viktor Frankl** (Holocaust and Auschwitz concentration camp survivor) stated:

> Suffering ceases to be suffering at the moment it finds a meaning. … Man's main concern … is to see a meaning in his life. … Meaning is possible even in spite of suffering, provided the suffering is unavoidable. If it were avoidable, the meaningful thing to do would be to remove its cause … be it psychologic, biologic or political. To suffer unnecessarily is masochistic rather than heroic. (Frankl, 2004/1959: 117)

**Dame Cicely Saunders** recognized that physical and mental suffering each influenced and shaped the other. In 1963, Saunders suggested that 'mental distress may be perhaps the most intractable pain of all', for which 'listening has to develop into real hearing' (1963a: 197). Saunders emphasized the need to understand the meaning of the pain for the patient, to understand the thoughts that contributed to and exacerbated the patient's suffering. One patient told Saunders that 'all of me is wrong' and another 'it was all pain', inspiring the phrase 'total pain', which was coined by Dame Cicely Saunders to emphasize the multidimensional ramifications of pain in advanced cancer (Saunders, 1967). The concept of 'total pain', which includes physical symptoms, mental distress, social problems and emotional difficulties, became and continues to be one of the most important and enduring concepts of care at end of life, reflecting the biopsychosocial orientation to care, seeing pain as indivisible from the body and the person (Clark, 2002).

A study which compared patient and family perceptions of cancer pain found that family members understood the patient's pain location about 75% of the time. However, family members rarely understood the patient's pain intensity, pain quality or pain pattern. The study suggested that discrepancies may exist between family members' and the patient's perceptions of their cancer pain experience (Madison and Wilkie, 1995). In *Cancer Ward* (1968), after Rusanov's hospitalization, **Aleksandr Solzhenitsyn** wrote: 'But, in a few days, this whole close-knit, ideal Rusanov family … had receded until it vanished on the other side of the tumour. … The tumour had divided him from them like a wall, and he remained alone on his side of it' (Abram, 1969; Solzhenitsyn, 1968).

# Pain as a neural and mental experience

The experience of pain is unquestionably a sensation in a part or parts of the body, but it is always unpleasant and is therefore an **emotional experience**. While acute pain usually has a physical cause and the experience of chronic pain is consequential to an original cause, pain is always a psychological state (Twycross, 1994). The word 'pain' can be used to refer to the total experience of both sensation and emotion (Moon, 1985). The perception of pain is modulated (changed, altered) by the patient's mood, morale and the meaning of the pain for the patient (Fields, 2007; Twycross, 1997).

Well-known studies by Wilder Penfield in the 1950s of electrical stimulation of the brain in awake patients undergoing surgery for epilepsy showed the process of projection, which is critical to understanding the pain experience. The experience of pain is a neural representation in the brain projected to the site of tissue damage. Pain is generated in the brain but experienced at the site of injury. Pain experience is both neural and mental; the neural component is the activity in nerve cells, while the subjective experience of pain takes place in the mind. Each person's nervous system is shaped by their unique sociocultural, linguistic and experiential background. Remembered representations of personal bodily and environmental factors inform and actively contribute to interpretation of ongoing experience in a two-way process. All pain is neural and mental, generated in the brain and perceived at a site distant from the injury due to projection. Projection is psychobiological, underpinning the metaphorical nature of neural activity – the human brain displaces subjective experience from intercranial representations to the body and environment. Projection explains the identical origins of emotional and physical pain. In accordance with the biopsychosocial model past history, expectation and contextual stimuli influence the neural representations of pain (Fields, 2007).

## Chapter summary

- Principles of systems theory applied to patient care consider each person as inseparable from his or her biological, psychological, social and cultural context. Multidisciplinary care is planned with and for the person.
- The biopsychosocial approach has rehumanized patient care, with nursing having a key role in pain treatment and management as part of the multidisciplinary team delivering interdisciplinary care.
- Acute, chronic (persistent) pain of non-malignant origin and cancer pain (a combination of acute pain and chronic pain) are different types of pain. Early treatment of acute pain is vital to prevent transition to chronic pain.
- Consideration of individual differences is essential in the care of the person with pain. Listening to their narrative helps to ascertain the impact of the patient's pain and suffering on his or her quality of life and the impact on close others.

- Loeser's Onion demonstrates nociception, pain perception and the suffering of the person in pain and elicited pain behaviours. Components interact with each other and the individual's environment, based on the biopsychosocial model.
- Altering illness and suffering perceptions may impact positively on the patient's health outcome. Suffering can be changed by changing the meaning of the pain, demonstrating that pain can be controlled and that an end is in sight, with improvement in quality of life.
- Le Shan, Tolstoy, C.S. Lewis and Solzhenitsyn described the mental suffering associated with untreated or undertreated pain on sufferers and their families. 'Mental distress may be perhaps the most intractable pain of all' (Saunders, 1963a: 197).
- Noxious information is conveyed by several pain pathways to the brain and spinal cord. The subjective experience of pain is a computational neural and mental event projected to, and experienced at, the site of tissue damage.

## Reflective exercise

Consider how pain is a subjective, emotional experience.

## Recommended reading

Cassell, E.J. (1991/2004) *The Nature of Suffering and The Goals of Medicine*. New York: Oxford University Press (2nd edn, 2004).
Frank, A.W. (1995) *The Wounded Storyteller: Body, Illness and Ethics*. Chicago, IL and London: University of Chicago Press.
Lewis, C.S. (2002/1940) *The Problem of Pain*. London: HarperCollins.
Livingston, W.K. (1998) *Pain and Suffering*. Edited by H.L. Fields. Seattle, WA: International Association for the Study of Pain.
Morris, D.B. (1991) *The Culture of Pain*. Berkeley, CA: University of California Press.

## Websites relevant to this chapter

International Association for the Study of Pain (IASP): www.iasp-pain.org
WHO International Classification of Functioning, Disability and Health: www.who.int/classifications/icf/en/
International Osteoporosis Foundation: www.iofbonehealth.org/
Juvent Machine: http://juventhealth.com/

# References

Abram, H.S. (1969) The psychology of terminal illness as portrayed in Solzhenitsyn's *Cancer Ward*. *Archives of Internal Medicine*, 124: 758–760.

Benedict, S. (1981) A linguistic analysis of the concept of suffering. Unpublished paper. University of Alabama at Birmingham School of Nursing, Alabama.

Bonica, J.J. (ed.) (1990) *The Management of Pain* (2nd edn). Philadelphia, PA: Lea and Febiger.

Breitbart, W. (1989) Psychiatric management of cancer pain. *Cancer*, 63: 2336–2342.

Breitbart, W.S., Park, J. and Katz, A.M. (2010) Pain. In J.C. Holland, W.S. Breitbart, P.B. Jacobsen, M.S. Lederberg, M.J. Loscalso and R.McCorkle (eds), *Psycho-Oncology* (2nd edn). Oxford: Oxford University Press.

Breivik, H., Cherny, N., Collett, B., de Conno, F., Filbet, M., Foubert, A.J., Cohen, R. and Dow, L. (2009) Cancer-related pain: a pan-European survey of prevalence, treatment, and patient attitudes. *Annals of Oncology*, 20: 1420–1433.

Carr, D.B., Loeser, J.D. and Morris, D.B. (2005) Why narrative? In D.B. Carr, J.D. Loeser and D.B. Morris (eds), *Narrative, Pain, and Suffering: Progress in Pain Research and Management* (Vol. 34). Seattle, WA: International Association for the Study of Pain (IASP).

Cassell, E.J. (1982) The nature of suffering and the goals of medicine. *New England Journal of Medicine*, 306: 639–645.

Cassell, E.J. (1991/2004) *The Nature of Suffering and the Goals of Medicine*. New York: Oxford University Press (2nd edn, 2004).

Chronic Pain Policy Coalition (2013), www.policyconnect.org.uk/cppc/ (accessed 9 February 2014).

Clark, D. (2002) *Cicely Saunders: Founder of the Hospice Movement: Selected Letters 1959–1999*. Oxford: Oxford University Press.

Engel, G.L. (1977) The need for a new medical model: a challenge for biomedicine. *Science*, 196: 129–136.

Engel, G.L. (1980) The clinical application of the biopsychosocial model. *American Journal of Psychiatry*, 137: 535–544.

Fallowfield, L. (1990) *The Quality of Life: The Missing Measurement in Health Care*. London: Souvenir Press.

Fields, H.L. (2007) Setting the stage for pain: allegorical tales from neuroscience. In S. Coakley and K. Kaufman Shelemay (eds), *Pain and Its Transformations: The Interface of Biology and Culture*. Cambridge, MA and London: Harvard University Press.

Fillingham, R.B. (2010) Individual differences in pain: the roles of gender, ethnicity and genetics. In S.M. Fishman, J.C. Ballantyne and J.P. Rathmell (eds), *Bonica's Management of Pain* (4th edn). Riverwoods, IL: Wolters Kluwer/Lippincott Williams and Wilkins.

Fitzgibbon, D.R. and Loeser, J.D. (2010) *Cancer Pain: Assessment, Diagnosis and Management*. Riverwoods, IL: Wolters Kluwer/Lippincott Williams and Wilkins.

Flor, H. and Turk, D.C. (2011) *Chronic Pain: An Integrated Biobehavioural Approach*. Seattle, WA: IASP.

Foster, G.M. and Anderson, B.G. (1978) *Medical Anthropology*. New York: Wiley.

Frank, A.W. (1995) *The Wounded Storyteller: Body, Illness and Ethics*. Chicago, IL and London: University of Chicago Press.

Frankl, V. (2004/1959) *Man's Search for Meaning: The Classic Tribute to Hope from the Holocaust*. London: Rider.

Hincapié, C.A., Cassidy, J.D. and Côté, P. (2008) Is a history of work-related low back injury associated with prevalent low back pain and depression in the general population? *BMC Musculoskeletal Disorders*, 9: 22.

Latremoliere, A. and Woolf, C.J. (2009) Central sensitization: a generator of pain hypersensitivity by central neural plasticity. *Journal of Pain*, 10: 895–926.

Le Shan, L. (1964) The world of the patient in severe pain of long duration. *Journal of Chronic Disease*, 17: 119–126.

Le Shan, L. (1989/1994) *Cancer as a Turning Point*. New York: Penguin.

Lewis, C.S. (2002/1940) *The Problem of Pain*. London: HarperCollins.

Loeser, J.D. (1982) Concepts of pain. In M. Stanton-Hicks and R.A. Boas (eds), *Chronic Low Back Pain*. New York: Raven Press, pp.145–148.

Loeser, J.D. (2005) Pain, suffering and the brain: a narrative of meanings. In D.B. Carr, J.D. Loeser and D.B. Morris (eds), *Narrative, Pain, and Suffering: Progress in Pain Research and Management* (Vol. 34). Seattle, WA: IASP.

Madison, J.L. and Wilkie, D.J. (1995) Family members' perceptions of cancer pain: comparisons with patient sensory report and by patient psychological status. *Nursing Clinics of North America*, 30: 625–645.

Mechanic, D. (1986) Illness behaviour: an overview. In S. McHugh and T.M. Vallis (eds), *Illness Behaviour: A Multidisciplinary Model*. New York: Plenum Press.

Merskey, H. and Bogduk, N. (1994) *Classification of Chronic Pain: Descriptions of Chronic Pain Syndromes and Definitions of Pain Terms*, 2nd edn. Seattle: IASP.

Moon, M.H. (1985) Psychological approaches to the treatment of chronic pain. In M.T. Hoskins (ed.), *Pain*. New York: Churchill Livingstone.

National Pain Strategy (Pain Australia) (2010), www.painaustralia.org.au/images/pain_australia/NPS/National%20Pain%20Strategy%202011.pdf (accessed 9 February 2014).

Saunders, C. (1963a) The treatment of intractable pain in terminal cancer. *Proceedings of the Royal Society of Medicine*, 56 (3): 195–7.

Saunders, C. (1963b) Distress in dying (Letter). *British Medical Journal*, ii: 746.

Saunders, C. (1967) *The Management of Terminal Illness*. London: Hospital Medicine Publications.

Schug, S.A. (2011) The Global Year against Acute Pain. *Anaesthesia and Intensive Care*, 39: 11–14.

Shipton, E.A. (1999) *Pain: Acute and Chronic*. London: Arnold.

Solzhenitsyn, A. (1968) *Cancer Ward*. London: The Bodley Head.

Somers, T.J., Keefe, F.J., Kothadia, S. and Pandiani, A. (2010) Dealing with cancer pain: coping, pain catastrophising and related outcomes. In J.A. Paice, R.F. Bell, E.A. Kalso and O.A. Soyannwo (eds), *Cancer Pain: From Molecules to Suffering*. Seattle, WA: IASP, p. 232.

Strang, P. (1992) Emotional and social aspects of cancer pain. *Acta Oncological*, 31: 323–326.

Tolstoy, L. (1960) *The Death of Ivan Ilych and Other Stories* (trans by R. Edmund. London: Penguin.

Treede, R.D., Jensen, T.S., Campbell, J.N., Gruccu, G., Dostrovsky, J.O., Griffin, J.W., Hansson, P., Hughes, R., Nurmikko, T. and Serra, J. (2008) Neuropathic pain: redefinition and a grading system for clinical and research purposes. *Neurology*, 70: 1630–1635.

Turk, C. and Okifuji, A. (2010) Pain terms and taxonomies of pain. In S. Fishman, J.C. Ballantyne and J.P. Rathmell (eds), *Bonica's Management of Pain* (4th edn). Riverwoods, IL: Wolters Kluwer/Lippincott Williams and Wilkins.

Twycross, R. (1994) *Pain Relief in Advanced Cancer*. Edinburgh: Churchill Livingstone.

Twycross, R. (1997) *Introducing Palliative Care* (2nd edn). Oxford: Radcliffe Medical Press.

von Bertanlanffy, L. (1968) *General Systems Theory*. New York: Braziller.

WHO (2002) *Towards a Common Language for Functioning, Disability and Health*. Geneva: World Health Organisation.

WHOQoL Group (1998) The World Health Organization Quality of Life Assessment (WHOQOL): development and general psychometric properties. *Social Science and Medicine*, 46 (12): 1569–1585.

Williamson, G.M. and Schulz, R. (1995) Activity restriction mediates the association between pain and depressed affect: a study of younger and older adult cancer patients. *Psychology of Aging*, 10: 369–378.

Winefield, H.R. and Neuling, S.J. (1987) Social support, counselling and cancer. *British Journal of Guidance Counselling*, 15: 6–16.

Zepinic, V. (2009) Post injury chronic low back pain and depression: comparative study between early and late-post injury sufferers show significant difference. *International Journal of Health Science*, 3.

# 3

# The neuropsychophysiology of pain

## Learning objectives

The learning objectives of this chapter are to:

- understand the mechanisms of pain information transfer from the periphery to the central nervous system
- be aware of how the progress of pain theories from linear to more complex systems models revolutionized pain treatments and patient care
- recognize that the complex systems models of pain include the two-way transfer of information and that socio-cultural factors impact on pain experience
- recognize the link between the biopsychosocial model of pain and the neuropsychophysiology of pain

## Introduction

This chapter assumes knowledge of the anatomy and physiology of the nervous system, particularly the neuron and synapse, processes involved in completing an action potential, and the function of neurotransmitters. It outlines the structures and processes of how pain information is conveyed via neuronal pathways to the central nervous system, ultimately leading to the experience of pain. The chapter:

(a)  outlines the structure and functions of the pain pathways;
(b)  links microstructure functions to structures and locations of the central nervous system; and
(c)  looks at the most recent pain theories.

## Microstructures of the central nervous system: basic definitions of the neuron and synapse

A major function of the central nervous system is to provide information about the occurrence or potential for threat or for injury. This is achieved through neurons and synapses.

The **neuron** (also known as a nerve fibre; 'neuron' and 'nerve fibre' will be used interchangeably in this text) is the basic unit of the nervous system and is composed of a cell body, dendrites and an axon. An afferent neuronal axon carries nerve impulses from a sensory organ to the central nervous system; an efferent neuronal axon carries information from the nervous system to body organs or the periphery.

Information is conveyed from neuron to neuron across minute gaps, or cellular locations, discovered and named the **synapse** by Sherrington (1857–1957) (Breedlove et al., 2010).

## Structure and function of nerve fibres

As shown in Table 3.1, nerve fibres are classified according to their diameter and conduction velocity. The thickness of the myelin sheath on each nerve fibre determines the conduction speed. Of the three types of nerve fibres which respond to stimuli leading to readily perceived sensations (Aβ: touch and pressure, Aδ: mechanical and thermal, C: mechanical, chemical and thermal stimuli), thickly myelinated Aβ fibres, which respond to touch and pressure stimulation, are the fastest nerve fibres, conducting at rapid speeds of 40–70+ metres per second. Junctures about 2–3 micrometres long, called Nodes of Ranvier, are dispersed along the myelinated axon about every 1–3 millimetres. In myelinated fibres, action potentials take place only at the nodes. This is called saltatory conduction. Only the nodes depolarize in salutatory conduction, thereby reducing the energy and metabolic requirements for re-establishing sodium and potassium concentration differences across the membrane. Thus, in myelinated nerve fibres the nerve impulse jumps along the fibre, allowing conduction speeds of up to 100 metres per second (the length of a football field in one second) (Hall, 2011).

Table 3.1 shows the different types of peripheral afferent nerve fibres, identified using electrophysiological and immunohistochemical methods. Knowledge to date should be viewed in the context of current technological limitations of studying minute neurological structures (Germann and Stanfield, 2005; Hall, 2011; Ness and Randich, 2010).

**Table 3.1**  Different types of nerve fibres, diameters, speed and response function

| Fibre group | Diameter (μm) | Response function | Conduction velocity (m/s) |
| --- | --- | --- | --- |
| Aα | 12–20 | Somatic motor/proprioception | 70–120 |
| Aβ | 5–15 | Touch and pressure | 30–70 |
| Aγ | 3–6 | Motor to muscle spindles | 15–30 |
| Aδ | 2–5 | Mechanical, thermal | 6–30 |
| B | 1–3 | Autonomic/sympathetic preganglionic | 3–15 |
| C | 0.3–1.3 | Autonomic/sympathetic postganglionic; chemical, mechanical, thermal | 0.5–2.3 |

# Structure and function of nerve fibres (nociceptors) which respond to noxious stimuli

The term 'nociceptor' refers to (a) the free nerve ending of a primary afferent neuron that responds preferentially to noxious (painful) stimuli as well as to (b) the entire sensory neuron capable of transducing and transmitting noxious (painful) stimuli. Nociceptors are sub-classified into three criteria:

1. An unmyelinated C-fibre afferent and a myelinated Aδ-fibre afferent.
2. Types of noxious stimulation that evoke a response by nociceptors.
3. Nociceptive response characteristics to noxious stimuli (Brenner, 2006; Gold and Gebhart, 2010; Raja et al., 1999).

Aδ nociceptors are thinly myelinated, while C-fibre nociceptors are unmyelinated. Aδ nociceptors conduct at velocities of 6–30 metres per second compared with slower C-fibre nociceptors, which have velocities of less than 2.5 metres per second. Aδ nociceptors respond to mechanical ($AM_{(mechano)}$) and thermal stimuli, producing fast, sharp pain. C-fibre nociceptors have 'free' nerve endings, that is, their peripheral terminals are not associated with any specific cell type. C-fibre nociceptors are polymodal ($CM_{(mechano)}H_{(heat)}$), which means they respond to mechanical, chemical or thermal stimuli or combinations of stimuli, often producing dull, burning pain. C-fibre pain is slow pain which becomes greater over time (Brenner, 2006; Germann and Stanfield, 2005; Gold and Gebhart, 2010; Hall, 2011). More recent study findings using microneurography techniques have identified some highly complex groupings of both Aδ and C nociceptors.

The International Association for the Study of Pain (IASP) has defined pain as 'an unpleasant sensory and emotional experience associated with actual or potential tissue damage, or described in terms of such damage' (Merskey and Bogduk, 1994). Under normal circumstances acute pain has a survival function, with noxious (painful) information being transmitted to the brain via action potentials along neuronal axons in complex pain pathways, giving a warning signal to remove the organism from the damaging stimulus. The ability to feel and respond appropriately to a painful stimulus is clearly a prerequisite for survival. Acute pain is an essential sense which has evolved in complex organisms to prevent and minimize physical damage to the organism and increase the possibility of prolonged survival. Humans learn from a young age, through personal experience of pain experienced by cuts, grazes, sports injuries and falls, as well as through vicarious learning of others' injuries, those situations and risk behaviours with potentially harmful and painful consequences (Raja et al., 1999).

## The reflex response

A reflex is the basic unit of motor behaviour (Sherrington, 1947/1906). Simple reflexes are involuntary, unlearned responses to painful mechanical, thermal and

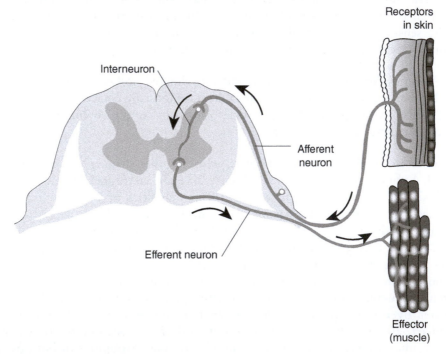

**Figure 3.1**    Basic reflex arc

Source: Sherrington (1947/1906)

chemical stimuli. Most simple reflexes are subcortical, taking place in the brain stem or spinal cord, and many are flexor (withdrawal) reflexes to remove the body area away from a painful stimulus. Most reflexes have a warning function to protect against potentially damaging stimuli. An example of a nociceptive reflex is when a person touches something very hot, thereby stimulating pain receptors in the skin and bringing about an action potential which is then conducted along an afferent nociceptive neuron to the spinal cord. As shown in Figure 3.1, the afferent nociceptive neuron synapses with the interneuron, which, in turn, synapses with an efferent motor neuron to flexor muscles in upper limbs which contract the muscles for limb or other body area withdrawal. This action does not require conscious thought (Raja et al., 1999; Seeley et al., 2007).

## Stimulus transduction of mechanical, thermal or chemical noxious stimuli

Pain perception requires information to be transmitted from the periphery to the central nervous system via afferent nerve fibres according to a sequence of transduction, conduction and transmission. In the first event, transduction, the energy of the mechanical, thermal or chemical noxious stimulus is converted into an electrical signal, resulting in depolarization of the peripheral terminals. Proteins responsible for transduction are considered to be intrinsic to nociceptors and vary according to the type of stimulus the nociceptor is sensitive to. Some nociceptors, stimulated by thermal or chemical stimuli, require on their surface membranes one or more molecules known as 'transient receptor potential' or TRP receptor molecules. Studies show that four different TRP receptor molecules respond to different gradations of temperature increases as well as to noxious stimuli. TRPV2 is activated by intense noxious heat, while TRPV3 and TRPV4 are both activated by warm temperatures. While the mechanisms are not yet fully understood, TRPV4, acid sensing ion channel type 3 (ASIC-3) and voltage-gated calcium channel (VGCC) CaV3.2 are proteins that are likely to play a role in the transduction of mechanical stimuli (Brenner, 2006; Dubin and Patapoutian, 2010; Gold and Gebhart, 2010; Willis, 2009; Woolf, 2004).

## The 'capsaicin molecule' TRPV1

Activation of the TRPV1 receptor molecule is specifically associated with pain sensation, particularly burning pain or itching. Widely researched studies show that the TRPV1 receptor molecule is a polymodal receptor, activated by capsaicin, the active substance in chilli peppers (8-methyl-N-vanillyl-6-nonenamide) and its agonist, resiniferatoxin, as well as tissue acidosis and a variety of endogenous compounds (Gold and Gebhart, 2010; Venkatachalam and Montell, 2007; Willis, 2009).

## TRPV1 'capsaicin molecule': potential for pharmacological interventions for pain

Capsaicin is a TRPV1 agonist. Animal studies in the 1990s showed that high doses of capsaicin applied to animals produced 'capsaicin desensitization', whereby the animals did not react with protective reflexes and inflammation to noxious chemicals, although they still responded to physical stimuli (Immke and Gavva, 2006). Topical capsaicin produces a period of increased burning sensation followed by reversible loss of function in nociceptive afferent neurons (Nickel et al., 2012).

In humans, TRPV1 is highly expressed in both Aδ and C-fibres, and is increased in certain pain states. After nerve injury, TRPV1 is decreased in injured nerve fibres but increased in uninjured C-fibres. Studies are strongly focused on the potential for targeting the TRPV1 molecule for pharmacological interventions for different types of pain, especially pain associated with nerve injury (neuropathic pain). Recent studies have found evidence for the safety and effectiveness of a high concentration capsaicin patch (capsaicin 8%) over a year in controlled trials for patients with postherpetic neuralgia following shingles (PHN: nerve pain) and for human immunodeficiency sensory polyneuropathy (HIV-DSP: abnormal sensations, usually burning pain and numbness, especially in the feet), both very difficult pains to treat, lasting for years, severely reducing quality of life (Baron et al., 2010; Simpson et al., 2010; Stemkowski et al., 2013). The 8% capsaicin patch has now been approved for neuropathic pain associated with postherpetic neuralgia by the US Food and Drug Administration (FDA) and the Medicines Boards of some countries, in accordance with clinical guidelines.

. . . . . . . . . . . . . . . . . . . . . . . . . . . . . . . . . . . . . . . . . . . . . . . . . . . . . . . . . . . . . . . . . . . . . . . . .

**CLINICAL EXAMPLE**

## The 8% capsaicin patch

Mrs G, a 65-year-old married lady with three adult, independent children, lives with her disabled husband. She presented at the General Practitioner's primary care unit with burning pain at the level of the intercostal nerve on her right side and a pain score of 7 on a number rating scale, worsening from 4 over the previous few days. Her sleep pattern was disrupted and she felt distressed and frightened by the increasing, unremitting pain. Mrs G was first diagnosed with Herpes Zoster (shingles) six weeks previously, following the appearance of a blistery rash just below her right breast spreading around to her back (along the intercostal nerve pathway). It was her first episode of shingles disease (which was accompanied by a temperature of 38.3°C (101°F) and general malaise), for which the GP had prescribed an antiviral medication for a week and antiepileptic medication to prevent the onset of neuropathic pain (gabapentin).

On this return visit by Mrs G, accompanied by her adult daughter, the GP checked her past and recent medical history, re-examined Mrs G and diagnosed postherpetic neuralgia (PHN). The GP, a trained pain specialist, discussed with Mrs G and her daughter the 8% capsaicin patch as a potential treatment. The GP explained that the application of the capsaicin patch required the prior application of a local topical anaesthetic to reduce an initial burning sensation produced when the capsaicin came into contact with the skin, and that the application would take one hour and would be carried out by the Primary Care Practice Nurse. Mrs G agreed to try the capsaicin patch and to take a weak opioid agonist Tramadol, which was immediately administered by injection by the GP, and then twice daily in tablet form for the next two weeks. This would keep her pain under control until the capsaicin patch took effect and help her to rest and recover her health with help from her family. The GP discontinued gabapentin which can interact with opioid medication. Following the patch application procedure, the Primary Care Practice Nurse advised Mrs G and her daughter on possible capsaicin patch side-effects, such as raised blood pressure and site redness, pain and itching, and how to care for herself in terms of avoiding showering the affected/ treated skin area for a few days. The nurse discussed weekly follow-up care visits to the Primary Care Practice Nurse in the short term to check her pain scores to see if further medication for neuropathic pain (SNRI venlafaxine which is safer for older people) was required and to see if another capsaicin patch session would benefit Mrs G – up to four patches in total can be administered for any single treatment cycle.

Mrs G was asked to keep a daily pain diary, which was supplied, and the Primary Care Practice Nurse explained to Mrs G and her daughter how to complete a daily number and verbal pain rating scale. Mrs G was instructed to contact the Primary Care Practice Nurse or GP immediately if she was concerned about any side-effects of the capsaicin patch or Tramadol treatments, especially if she experienced any breathing difficulties, palpitations, urinary retention, nausea, vomiting or dizziness. Mrs G was advised to take special care to monitor her balance and prevent possible risk of falls whilst taking Tramadol medication. She was asked to monitor and note the regularity of her bowel movements while taking Tramadol (slow release 50 mgs twice daily), to take a stimulant laxative (Senna) every day and to drink adequate water to guard against opioid associated constipation. Medications were written out in full with reason, dosages and times, and possible side-effects. Long-term monthly follow-ups with Mrs G by the Primary Care Practice Nurse, with referral to the GP when required, found that her postherpetic pain was well controlled with the application of one capsaicin patch every three months, together with regular use of a weak topical capsaicin cream and a daily regular 'at the clock' low dose of non-opioid medication for neuropathic pain (SNRI). Mrs G also found the regular use of TENS effective for mild pain episodes. Mrs G found that she required more rest, paced her activities of daily living carefully and took care to ensure her driving was not impaired by medication side-effects (Bennett, 2010). In a nonspecialist setting the capsaicin patch is not usually first line treatment and should only be used when advised and applied by a pain specialist (Dworkin et al., 2010; NICE, 2013).

- Q: Reflect on the impact of pain associated with postherpetic neuralgia on Mrs G's quality of life.
- Q: How can postherpetic neuralgia in older people be prevented?
- Q: Should the anti-shingles vaccine be readily available to all older people for whom it is suitable (contraindicated in people with weakened immune systems and certain diseases)?
- Q: Do you think national campaigns should encourage anti-shingles vaccination uptake by older people, with appropriate education about the consequences of shingles, postherpetic neuralgia and the vaccine benefits and risks in terms of precautions and warnings about possible side-effects?

# Stimulus conduction and transmission of nociceptive action potentials

Action potentials begin with a change from the resting negative potential, when the membrane is polarized, to a positive potential called depolarization, following influx of sodium ions through the membrane to the axonal interior. Within milliseconds, sodium channels close and the negative resting potential is restored through diffusion of potassium ions to the exterior, repolarizing the membrane. Voltage-gated sodium channels (VGSCs) cause both depolarization and repolarization during the action potential (Hall, 2011).

Tissue injury facilitates increased sensitivity to noxious stimuli and membrane depolarization. Reduced threshold of activation brings about increased channel activity and/or sensitivity, driving changes enhanced by pro-inflammatory mediators released by non-neuronal and neuronal cells such as epithelial, mast, endothelial and immune cells, Schwann cells, platelets, macrophages, fibroblasts and keratinocytes (see Table 3.2) (Ringkamp et al., 2013).

**Table 3.2** Most frequent pro-inflammatory mediators following injury

| | | | |
|---|---|---|---|
| Substance P | SP | Nerve growth factor | NGF |
| E-type prostaglandins | $E_2(PGE_2)$ | Leukemia inhibiting | LIF |
| Bradykinin | B | factor | |
| Serotonin | 5HT | Cytokines: e.g. | TNF-$\alpha$; interleukin |
| Tyrosine receptor kinases | TRK | Adenosine triphosphate | ATP |
| Protons | $H^+$ | Histamine | $H_1$ & $H_3$ |
| Platelet activating factor | PAF | Endothelin | |

# Voltage-gated sodium channels and the nociceptive action potential

In all excitable tissue the voltage-gated sodium channels (VGSCs) NaV1.7 and NaV1.8, working together, cause depolarization and repolarization during the action potential, through changes in membrane potential, which open and close their gates. VGSC NaV1.8 is primarily responsible for nociceptive action potential initiation. VGSC NaV1.8 has a number of unique properties. NaV1.8:

- is primarily expressed in nociceptors;
- has a high threshold for activation, through depolarization of -30mV or greater;
- is relatively resistant to steady-state inactivation, so continues to contribute to the upstroke;
- recovers rapidly from inactivation to allow sustained activation;
- is resistant to cooling-induced inactivation, being still functional at a low temperature of 4°C, facilitating noxiously-induced burning pain (Gold and Gebhart, 2010).

# The synapse in pain transmission

Release of neurotransmitters across the synaptic space is essential for transmission of nociceptive information to the central nervous system. This stage of nociceptive information transmission requires high threshold, voltage-gated calcium channels. The neurochemistry in the dorsal horn is very complex and dependent on pain type. The major excitatory neurotransmitters at the dorsal horn are excitatory amino-acids glutamate and aspartate, as well as neuropeptide substance P. Additionally, calcitonin gene-related peptides (CGRP), growth factors, bradykinin and other augmentors of excitatory amino-acids are released (Brenner, 2006; Gold and Gebhart, 2010; Hall, 2011).

# The structure and function of peripheral and central nervous system locations involved in pain processing

The current major challenge is understanding brain function, as this knowledge really helps to improve accurate pain diagnoses, treatment and management (Melzack, 1999). The following is a brief overview of how the neuropsychophysiology of pain is underpinned by nociceptive transfer of pain information via pain pathways to different peripheral and central nervous system structural locations, with cohesive functions involved in the processing of pain information.

## The ascending pain system

Pain information is conducted by fast Aδ and slower C-fibres to the dorsal horn of the spinal cord, where connections to nerve fibre tracts facilitate information transfer to different brain regions. Figure 3.2 shows the ascending and descending routes of the pain pathways beginning and ending with the dorsal horn.

Pain information is conducted from the periphery, through the dorsal root ganglion (DRG), by:

- fast Aδ pain nerve fibres which terminate in lamina I of the dorsal horn in the spinal cord, where the excitatory neurotransmitter glutamate is secreted by Aδ fibre nerve endings. 'Fast pricking' pain information is then transmitted across the synapse to second-order neurons of the neospinothalamic tract. The neoSTT fibres cross over (the term 'decussate' is often used) to the opposite side of the spinal cord and then travel upward to the brain in the anterolateral columns. Most fibres in the neoSTT go to the thalamus, from where signals are transmitted to basal brain areas and the somatosensory cortex.
- slow C-pain nerve fibres, nerve ending of which terminate in lamina II (known as the substantia gelatinosa) of the dorsal horn of the spinal cord, where the nerve endings secrete glutamate and substance P. Substance P is thought to subserve 'slow

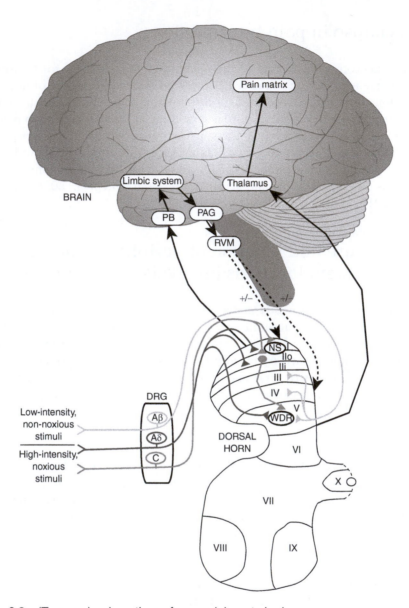

**Figure 3.2**   (Two-way) pain pathway from periphery to brain

Source: D' Mello, R. and Dickenson, A.H. (2008) Spinal cord mechanisms of pain. *British Journal of Anaesthesia*, 101: 8–16. Copyright (2008). Republished with permission of Oxford University Press.

Figure 3.2 (Ascending and descending) pain pathways from periphery to brain. Primary nociceptor fibres transmit impulses through the dorsal root ganglion (DRG) to the dorsal horn of the spinal cord. Nociceptive specific (NS) cells are located mainly in laminae I–II; most wide dynamic range (WDRs) are located in lamina V. The parabrachial area (PB) and periaqueductal grey (PAG), innervated by lamina 1 neurons are influenced by limbic system areas. Descending pathways from brainstem nuclei such as the rostral ventromedia medulla (RVM) modulate spinal processing. Lamina V neurons mainly project to the thalamus (spinothalamic tract) from where various cortical regions forming the 'pain matrix' (primary and secondary somatosensory, insular, anterior cingulate, and prefrontal cortices) are activated.

burning' pain information, signals of which are then transmitted via interneurons (very small connecting nerve fibres in the dorsal horn) to lamina V in the dorsal horn, where the interneurons give rise to fibres of the paleospinothalamic tract, paleoSTT which, like the neoSTT fibres, cross over to the other side of the spinal cord. Also travelling in the anterolateral columns of the spinal cord, paleoSTT fibres travel to the brain stem. Short fibres transmit information primarily to the medulla and pons, and some fibres go to the thalamus, hypothalamus and basal regions (Hall, 2011).

The **spinal cord and dorsal horn**: the spinal cord is segregated into gray matter (cell bodies) and white matter (predominately myelinated nerve fibre tracts). Gray matter layers have been classified by Rexed (1954) as **laminae** from 1 to 10, according to the topographical histology of cell bodies and dendrites. The dorsal horn of the spinal cord is composed of laminae I–VI. Most nociceptive input converges to laminae I–II (D'Mello and Dickenson, 2008; Hall, 2011; Ness and Randich, 2010; Todd, 2010).

The **brainstem** comprises the medulla oblongata (myelencephalon), pons (metencephalon) and midbrain (mesencephalon) and has connections to the hypothalamus and thalamus (diencephalon) located just above it (Drake et al., 2010; Lorenz and Hauck, 2010).

The **thalamus**: having synapsed with primary afferent nociceptive neurons in the dorsal horn, nociceptive second-order neurons cross over in the spinal cord to the anterolateral portions of the contralateral hemisphere and travel in the spinothalamic tract (STT) to the thalamus to target mostly lateral nuclei.

**Lateral thalamic nuclei** represent nociceptive-specific types of cells, while their synapsing fibres contribute to the encoding of thermal and pain sensation. It is thought that the **sensory-discriminative** components of pain experience are identified in this location and this information is further relayed by the STT afferent pathway onto the contralateral primary (SI) and bilateral secondary (SII) somatosensory cortices and insula.

The **medial thalamus** also receives major nociceptive input indirectly from spino-reticular, spinomesencephalic and spino-parabrachial tracts via the brainstem from the dorsal horn. Dense quantities of medial thalamic nuclei project to the complex limbic system structures which play a major role in the evaluation of emotional and fear (**affective-motivational**) components and **pain intensity**.

The **hypothalamus** is located below the thalamus on either side of the third ventricle just above the pituitary gland. As currently understood, the hypothalamus has an indirect role in nociception, with inputs from the midbrain, medulla and dorsal horn, along with convergence of autonomic and visceral information, with a major role in the stress response and control of homeostasis (Lorenz and Hauck, 2010).

The **reticular formation** (rhombencephalic) is a network of small and large fibres extending from the medulla up to the thalamus, with multiple connections in both ascending and descending systems within the brain stem and with many cortical and subcortical structures. The reticular formation plays a role in pain modulation, mediates motor, respiratory and cardiovascular functions, and is highly involved in conscious perception and behaviour. The reticular formation may have a role in pain experience impacting negatively on sleep because pain perception as well as arousal and alertness are linked to the reticular formation (Lorenz and Hauck, 2010).

The **limbic system**: located within the cerebral hemispheres, the limbic system comprises a widespread network of structures involved in learning and emotion. In the limbic system, a ring of cortical and subcortical areas from the frontal, parietal and temporal lobes form a reverberating circuit around the upper brainstem, hypothalamus and thalamus, called the circuit of Papez (Papez, 1937). Structures within the limbic system of importance for pain are the anterior cingulate gyrus, amygdala, hippocampus, insular cortex (referred to as the insula). Limbic areas are linked to the **emotional content and aversive quality of noxious stimuli** and are involved in motivating escape and avoidance behaviour.

The **primary somatosensory cortex (SI)**: the SI is located in the parietal lobe. Single cell recordings in awake monkeys have shown a strong correlation between SI firing rate and stimulus intensity and duration of painful stimuli. Studies in awake humans have shown that the SI processes nociceptive input, which is insufficient to cause pain sensation. The SI is considered to contribute to the **discriminative analysis** of painful stimuli.

The **secondary somatosensory cortex (SII)**: the SII is located lateral and posterior to SI. The SII receives input from the thalamus, sends output to the adjacent insula and links nociceptive information to the limbic system. While the role of SII is undefined, it appears to be associated with recognition and learning of painful events and in linking primordial sense representations with further **cognitive and affective evaluation** (Lorenz and Hauck, 2010).

The **basal ganglia**: consists of different groups of nerve cells which form a feedback loop with the somatosensory cortex and thalamus. Recent neuroimaging studies have highlighted the role of the basal ganglia in pain processing. Studies also indicate an important role for the basal ganglia in **sensory-discriminative, emotional/affective, cognitive aspects** and **modulation of pain experience** (Borsook et al., 2010).

## The descending pain system

Nociceptive processing by the descending pain pathway can be both inhibitory and facilitatory (pronociceptive), with substantial processing by the dorsal horn, to influence the subjective perception of pain. While key structures in this process are outlined in this section, it is essential to recognize that pain processing is highly dynamic, with information signals travelling up and down the pain pathways, consistent with the concept of a feedback loop. Figure 3.2 shows the descending pain pathways.

**Descending modulation** (change, alteration in signals) involves a number of brain regions, particularly the following:

- frontal lobe;
- limbic system structures: anterior cingulated cortex (ACC) insula and amygdala;
- hypothalamus;
- midbrain periaqueductal gray (PAG) and a midbrain group of neurons, the nucleus cuneiformis (NCF);
- in the pons, groups of nuclei in the dorsolateral pontine tegmentum (DLPT);
- groups of neurons in the rostral ventromedial medulla (RVM) (see Figure 3.2).

**Descending inhibition** involves the release of norepinephrine (NE) (noradrenaline) from brainstem nuclei, which inhibits transmitter release from primary afferent pain fibres and limits firing by dorsal horn projection neurons while activation of excitatory serotonin (5HT) appears to enhance spinal processing. One treatment for neuropathic pain is a combination antidepressant drug that blocks the re-uptake of both serotonin and norepinephrine (noradrenaline). This is called a serotonin-NE re-uptake inhibitor (SNRI) because it is as important to increase levels of norepinephrine (noradrenaline) as it is to block the re-uptake of serotonin levels in treating pain. Some drugs for treating pain (e.g. SNRIs, gabapentin) are dependent on activation of the serotonin molecule (D'Mello and Dickenson, 2008).

The **periaqueductal gray (PAG)**: the midbrain PAG plays a critical role in pain expression and emotional-related behaviours, and has a key role in descending pain modulation via projections to the medullary nucleus raphe magnus (NRM) and rostral ventromedial medulla (RVM). The PAG was the initial site for endogenous pain control research studies, which demonstrated that electrostimulation of the PAG produced analgesia, suggesting the existence of endogenous systems for pain modulation.

# From Descartes (1664) to the Gate Control Theory (1965)

It is very important to remember the context of Descartes' time, when discussing his mechanistic theory of pain perception. His theory was built on the concept of viewing the human body as a machine, separating the body from the soul (and thereby solving an increasing problem of territorial arguments between church and developing science). Descartes' view of specificity theory considered the possibility of: (a) pain sensors at the periphery being capable of detecting noxious stimuli, and (b) sensory-motor transformations, so that pain signals arriving at the pineal gland were reflected in a mirror-like brain to activate motor nerves to remove the body part from the stimulus.

Cervero (2005) and Keele (1957) both credit Descartes with the first rudimentary description of the reflex arc. A few years less than 250 years later, Charles Sherrington, who is often described as the 'Father of Pain Physiology', received the Nobel Prize for Medicine for his development of the concept of the reflex arc (1947/1906). The 1940s and 1950s were a time when the specificity theory was emphasized in all major textbooks and research. It rested on the assertion that the pain experience was proportional to the extent of the injury and that the only way to treat pain was to block the nerves and pathways by cutting. William K. Livingston, a Naval Commander and surgeon during the Second World War, who specialized in missile-induced peripheral nerve injuries, adamantly believed that pain is determined by interactions of inputs at all levels of the central nervous system and should be treated by modulating input rather than cutting nerves (Livingston, 1998). The Gate Control Theory (Melzack and Wall, 1965) addressed this new thinking.

## The principles of the original Gate Control Theory

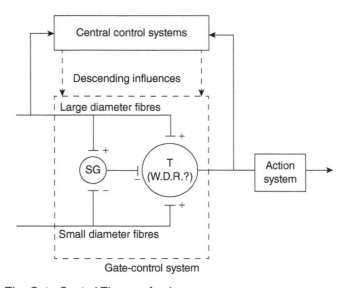

**Figure 3.3**   The Gate Control Theory of pain

Key: SG = substantia gelatinosa; T = transmitter cell; WDR = wide dynamic range cells; + = excitation; − = inhibition

Source: Adams, N. *The Psychophysiology of Low Back Pain*. Churchill Livingstone, p.48. Republished with permission of Elsevier.

As shown in Figure 3.3, large-diameter Aβ fibres convey non-noxious information and small-diameter Aδ and C-fibres convey noxious information to lamina II in the substantia gelatinosa of the dorsal horn, where the second-order inhibitory transmission interneurons (T-cells) increase their inhibition of noxious information transfer if greater input from the non-noxious Aβ fibres overrides the noxious input from smaller Aδ and C-fibres. The theory was updated to allow both excitatory and inhibitory links from the substantia gelatinosa to the transmission (T) cells, as well as descending inhibitory control for the brain stem systems, the latter being the vital and lasting legacy of the Gate Control Theory (Adams, 1997; Melzack and Wall, 1965, 1982/1988).

The Gate Control Theory maintained that pain is a complex experience involving different components. Sensory discriminative components select and modulate sensory input; affective-motivational components underpin the experiencing person's motivation to avoid the pain stimulus; cognitive components interact with previous learning and contextual factors to regulate the person's pain experience – 'simple' reflexes are now considered to have a cognitive component, as the experiencing person will usually regulate their pain behaviour according to their social context. The Gate Control Theory replaced the linear theory of pain with a systems theory perspective, with the integrated firing of the dorsal horn T-Cell as a response to neuronal input. The major element of the Gate Control Theory was the role of the dorsal horn in pain modulation (Keefe et al., 2005; Melzack and Wall, 1965, 1982/1988). While the original concept of inhibition of incoming sensory information by inhibitory interneurons in the substantia gelatinosa in lamina II of the dorsal horn has not been supported by updated research, studies show that the role of the dorsal horn in pain modulation is vital. Subsequent research from the 1970s through to the 1990s showed the importance of both inhibitory and excitatory pain-gating mechanisms in the dorsal horn, with implication for pharmacological interventions, including, but not limited to, μ-opioid agonists and NMDA antagonists at the level of the spinal cord (D'Mello and Dickenson, 2008; Fields and Basbaum, 1978; Yaksh, 1999). More recent studies show that the perception of pain is strongly influenced by noxious input to the spinal cord and that there are bi-directional effects on the dorsal horn input-output mediated by spinal and supraspinal systems, in line with the core of the original Gate Control Theory (Heinricher and Fields, 2013; Melzack and Wall, 1965; Sorkin and Yaksh, 2013; Yaksh, 1999).

The Gate Control Theory cannot be overestimated for bringing major change to how pain is viewed and treated. The Gate Control Theory revolutionized the approach to thinking about all aspects of pain perception, superceding previous linear-type pain theories with a systemic, multifactorial, individualized approach to understanding pain experience. This resulted in an explosion of pain research studies and new therapeutic approaches. The Gate Control Theory radically changed pain specialists' view of their patients' pain perceptions by emphasizing the interaction between psychological factors and pain physiology in subjective pain experience. Before the publication of the Gate Control Theory, psychological factors in the person's life were not considered relevant to their pain experience. The Gate Control Theory included psychological factors such as thoughts, beliefs and emotions as potentially painful stimuli impacting on the subjective pain experience (Cope, 2010; Turk et al., 2010; Yaksh, 1999).

# Recent models and theories of pain strongly influenced by the Gate Control Theory

**Cognitive behavioural models** of pain emphasize the influence of cognitions, emotions and behaviours on pain experience. Cognitive behavioural therapies help patients to learn adaptive coping skills through cognitive behavioural training to alter maladaptive cognitions and behaviours and help them regain sense of control and mastery. Cognitive behavioural training programmes are an essential component of chronic pain management (Keefe et al., 2005; Turk et al., 1983).

**The neuromatrix theory** highlights the role of psychological processes in the pain experience. According to the neuromatrix theory, a neural network in the brain integrates information from multiple sources. The neuromatrix theory integrates new findings from brain imaging studies and research about stress and cognitive behavioural factors and pain. Pain is a conscious experience where the type and duration of nociceptive input are influenced by a combination of factors which include the person's previous experience and pathology, along with cognitive, emotional, genetic and contextual factors to bring about a subjective complex multifactorial experience. The term 'pain matrix', while currently used to broadly describe a set of brain regions in human nociceptive processing, will be more accurately defined when technology allows specific neuroimaging of correlates of pain perception (Keefe et al., 2005; Melzack, 1999; Tracey, 2005).

**The pain transmission system** (1992), a theory put forward by neuroscientist Howard Fields, highlights the relevancy of the person's cultural and social context in subjective pain experience. As shown in Figure 3.4, cultural factors influence the T neuron in the dorsal horn. According to this model, bottom-up and top-down systems can be either inhibitory or excitatory, illustrating the interface between biology and culture (Fields, 2007).

# Genetics and pain

While recent genetic research has successfully identified particular genes associated with some very rare syndromes of pain insensitivity, studies show that genetic inheritance plays a vital role in some conditions associated with severe pain (Lötsch and Geisslinger, 2007).

When, very rarely, a person does not possess the ability to sense pain the consequences for them are potentially lethal. One of the foundations utilized by Melzack and Casey (1968) for distinguishing between sensory and affective pain components was the study of people with congenital insensitivity to pain. People born without the ability to feel pain are testimony to the essential survival value of the acute pain sensation. While, throughout history, there have been reports of

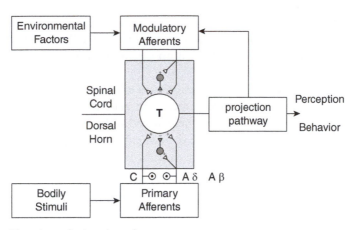

**Figure 3.4**  Top-down factors in pain

Source: Fields, H.L. (1992) Is there a facilitating component to central pain modulation? *American Pain Society Journal*, 1: 139–141, Figure 1. Republished with permission of Elsevier.

people with congenital insensitivity to pain, medical interest in the phenomenon became evident in the 1930s through published studies attempting to differentiate between different abnormal responses to pain. These studies, although infrequent, demonstrate the early mortality associated with, and extensive physical injuries sustained by, people with congenital insensitivity to pain through cuts, burns lacerations, falls and infections. Therefore, the ability to experience the acute pain sensation contributes to survival by protecting humans and other species from the effects of potentially damaging noxious stimuli (Melzack and Casey, 1968; Nagasako et al., 2003).

Recent advances in human genome research have contributed to understanding individual differences in nociception and the physiological substrates of the pain experience. Genes which cause very rare syndromes of insensitivity to pain have been identified. One of these is a mutation of the genes encoding the alpha-subunit of the voltage-gated sodium channel NaV1.7 (SCN9A) (Lötsch and Geisslinger, 2007). Cox et al. (2006) studied six children, ages ranging from 3 to 14 years, from three consanguineous families in northern Pakistan, none of whom had ever experienced pain of any type in any part of their body. All six children had sustained injuries of oral damage (some requiring plastic surgery), bruises, cuts and fractures. Neurologic examination showed that the children were all able to perceive touch, warmth and cold, tickle and pressure, but were unable to perceive painful stimuli. All six children were otherwise healthy, with full vision, hearing and normal appearance and development. Their parents and other siblings reported normal pain perception. Bioinformatics analysis mapped their congenital ability to experience pain as an autosomal-recessive trait to chromosome 2, in a region containing the gene SCN9A. Further analysis showed three distinct homozygous nonsense mutations of gene SCN9A, leading to mutant NaV1.7. These mutations caused loss of function of the voltage-gated sodium channel in NaV1.7. This study supported previous findings that the gene SCN9A is an essential requirement for nociception in humans (Cox et al., 2006).

Neuropsychophysiological substrates of pain are highly complex, underpinned by the potential for molecular, biochemical and genetic adaptations. The biopsychosocial model of pain links with the neuropsychophysiology of pain, facilitating an holistic approach to understanding the patient's pain experience and deciding appropriate patient care.

## Chapter summary

- The term 'nociceptor' refers to the free nerve endings of primary afferent fibres that respond to painful stimuli as well as to the entire sensory neuron capable of transducing and transmitting noxious information.
- Critically, all nociceptors are known to (1) encode stimulus intensity into the noxious range and to (2) sensitize. These properties are of major significance in enhancing blockage of peripheral nociception activity, aiming to remove the physiological substrates of pain experience.
- Mechanisms of transduction, transformation and transmission of pain information are dependent on action potentials initiated and sustained by voltage-gated sodium channels. Conduction speeds of noxious information depend on axonal myelination, with myelinated fibres conducting more rapidly.
- The synapse is the location of functional interaction between neurons with the release of neurotransmitters across the synapses being essential for transmission of nociceptive information to the central nervous system. This activity is dependent on high threshold voltage-gated calcium channels.
- Pain theories have evolved from Descartes' single pathway from body periphery to a pain centre in the brain to highly complex systems based on models exemplified by the Gate Control Theory (Melzack and Wall, 1965).
- The ascending pain pathways transmit information to various complex brain regions via the neo- and paleospinothalamic and other tracts. The descending pain pathways also involve a number of complex regions, particularly the midbrain periaqueductal gray (PAG), which plays a critical role in pain expression.
- The thalamus and adjacent structures appear important for evaluation of emotive and intensity aspects of the pain experience, interacting with the limbic system and reticular formation. The midbrain basal ganglia may also have a role in sensory-discriminative, emotional-affective and cognitive aspects of pain experience.
- Pain genetics is an important area of study and research, and a vital component of pain medicine. Specific genes, such as mutations of gene SCN9A, have been identified in conditions associated with (a) loss of ability to feel pain or (b) the experience of severe pain.

## Reflective exercise

Consider your understanding of the neuropsychophysiological mechanisms of pain perception and how this information links with the biopsychosocial model of pain.

## Recommended reading

Coakley, S. and Kaufman Shelemay, K. (2007) *Pain and its Transformations: The Interface of Biology and Culture.* Cambridge, MA: Harvard University Press.

Livingston, W.K. (1998) *Pain and Suffering.* Edited by H.L. Fields. Seattle, WA: International Association for the Study of Pain (IASP).

Merskey, H., Loeser, J.D. and Dubner, R. (2005) *The Paths of Pain, 1975–2005.* Seattle, WA: IASP.

## Websites relevant to this chapter

NCBI Gene Tests: www.ncbi.nlm.nih.gov/sites/GeneTests/lab/gene/SCN9A

National Human Genome Research Institute (use search term: pain): www.genome.gov/gwastudies/

Genetics/Genomics Competency Center for Education: www.g-2-c-2.org/start_search_map.php

International Society of Nurses in Genetics: www.isong.org/

National Institute for Health and Care Excellence: www.nice.org.uk

# References

Adams, N. (1997) *The Psychophysiology of Low Back Pain.* New York: Churchill Livingstone.

Baron, R., Binder, A. and Wasner, G. (2010) Neuropathic pain: diagnosis, pathophysiological mechanisms, and treatment. *Lancet Neurology*, 9: 807–819.

Borsook, D., Upadhyay, J., Chudler, E.H. and Becerra, L. (2010) A key role of the basal ganglia in pain and analgesia: insights gained through human functional imaging. *Molecular Pain*, 6: 27.

Breedlove, S.M., Watson, N.V. and Rosenzweig, M.R. (eds) (2010) *Biological Psychology: An Introduction to Behavioural, Cognitive and Clinical Neuroscience* (6th edn). Sunderland, MA: Sinauer.

Brenner, G.J. (2006) Neurophysiological basis of pain. In J.C. Ballantyne (ed.), *The Massachusetts General Hospital Handbook of Pain Management* (3rd edn). Riverwoods, IL: Lippincott Williams and Wilkins.

Cervero, F. (2005) The gate theory, then and now. In H. Merskey, J.D. Loeser and R. Dubner (eds), *The Paths of Pain, 1975–2005*. Seattle, WA: International Association for the Study of Pain (IASP).

Cope, D.K. (2010) Intellectual milestones in our understanding and treatment of pain. In S.M. Fishman, J.C. Ballantyne and J.P. Rathmell (eds), *Bonica's Management of Pain* (4th edn). Riverwoods, IL: Wolters Kluwer/Lippincott Williams and Wilkins.

Cox, J.J., Reimann, F., Nicholas, A.K.,Thornton, G., Roberts, E., Springell, K., Karbani, G., Jafri, H., Mannan, J., Raashid, Y., Al-Gazali, L., Hamamy, H., Valente, E.M., Gorman, S., Williams, R., McHale, D.P., Wood, J.N., Gribble, F.M. and Woods, C.G. (2006) An SCN9A channelopathy causes congenital inability to experience pain. *Nature*, 444: 894–898.

Drake, R.L., Vogl, A.W. and Mitchell, A.W.M. (2010) *Gray's Anatomy for Students. Head and Neck: Regional Anatomy,* (2nd edn). Edinburgh: Churchill Livingstone Elsevier

D'Mello, R. and Dickenson, A.H. (2008) Spinal cord mechanisms of pain. *British Journal of Anaesthesia*, 101: 8–16.

Dubin, A.E. and Patapoutian, A. (2010) Nociceptors: the senses of the pain pathway. *The Journal of Clinical Investigation*, 120 (11): 3760–3772.

Dworkin, R.H., O'Connor, A.B., Audette, J., et al. (2010) Recommendations for the pharmacological management of neuropathic pain: an overview and literature update. *Mayo Clin Proc*, 85(3 Suppl): S3-S14.

Fields, H.L. (2007) Setting the stage for pain: allegorical tales from neuroscience. In S. Coakley and K. Kaufman Shelemay (eds), *Pain and Its Transformations: The Interface of Biology and Culture*. Cambridge, MA: Harvard University Press.

Fields, H.W. (1992) Is there a facilitating component to central pain modulation? *American Pain Society Journal*: 139–141.

Fields, H.L. and Basbaum, A.I. (1978) Brainstem control of spinal pain transmission neurons. *Annual Review of Physiology*, 40: 217–248.

Germann, W.J. and Stanfield, C.L. (2005) *Principles of Human Physiology*. Reading, MA: Pearson/Benjamin Cummings.

Gold, M.S. and Gebhart, G.F. (2010) Peripheral pain mechanisms and nociceptor sensitisation. In S.M. Fishman, J.C. Ballantyne and J.P. Rathmell (eds), *Bonica's Management of Pain* (4th edn). Riverwoods, IL: Wolters Kluwer/Lippincott Williams and Wilkins.

Hall, J.E. (2011) Membrane potentials and action potentials. In *Guyton and Hall Textbook of Medical Physiology* (12th edn). Philadelphia, PA: Saunders Elsevier.

Heinricher, M.M. and Fields, H.L. (2013) Central nervous system mechanisms of pain modulation. In S.B. McMahon, M. Koltenburg, I. Tracey and D.C. Turk, *Wall and Melzack's Textbook of Pain* (6th edn). Philadephia, PA: Elsevier Saunders.

Immke, D.C. and Gavva, N.R. (2006) The TRPV1 receptor and nociception. *Seminars in Cell and Developmental Biology*, 17: 582–591.

Keefe, F.J., Dixon, K.E. and Pryor, R.W. (2005) Psychological contributions to the understanding and treatment of pain. In H. Merskey, J.D. Loeser and R. Dubner (eds), *The Paths of Pain, 1975–2005*. Seattle, WA: IASP.

Keele, K. (1957) *Anatomies of Pain*. Oxford: Blackwell Scientific.

Livingston, W.K. (1998) *Pain and Suffering*. Edited by H.L. Fields. Seattle, WA: IASP.

Lorenz, J. and Hauck, M. (2010) Supraspinal mechanisms of pain and nociception. In S.M. Fishman, J.C. Ballantyne and J.P. Rathmell (eds), *Bonica's Management of Pain* (4th edn). Riverwoods, IL: Wolters Kluwer/Lippincott Williams and Wilkins.

Lötsch, J. and Geisslinger, G. (2007) Current evidence for modulation of nociception by human genetic polymorphisms. *Pain*, 132: 18–22.

Melzack, R. (1999) From the gate to the neuromatrix. *Pain Supplement*, S121–S126.

Melzack, R. and Casey, K.L. (1968) Sensory, motivational and central control determinants of pain: a new conceptual model. In D. Kenshalo (ed.), *The Skin Senses*. Springfield, IL: Charles C. Thomas. pp. 423–433.

Melzack, R. and Wall, P.D. (1965) Pain mechanisms: a new theory. *Science*, 150: 971–979.

Melzack, R. and Wall, P.D. (1982/1988) *The Challenge of Pain* (2nd edn). London: Penguin.

Nagasako, E.M., Oaklander, A.L. and Dworkin, R.H. (2003) Congenital insensitivity to pain: an update, *Pain*, 101 (3): 213–219.

Ness, T. and Randich, A. (2010) Substrates of spinal cord nociceptive processing. In S.M. Fishman, J.C. Ballantyne and J.P. Rathmell (eds), *Bonica's Management of Pain* (4th edn). Riverwoods, IL: Wolters Kluwer/Lippincott Williams and Wilkins.

NICE (2013) *Neuropathic Pain-pharmacological Management. The Pharmcological Management of Neuropathic Pain in Adults in Non-specialist Settings*. Guideline CG173. London: NICE.

Nickel, F.T., Seifert, F., Lanz, S. and Maihöfner, C. (2012) Mechanisms of neuropathic pain. *European Neuropsychopharmacology*, 12: 81–91.

Papez, J.W. (1937) A proposed mechanism of emotion. *Archives of Neurology and Psychiatry*, 38: 725–743.

Raja, S.N., Meyer, R.A., Ringkamp, M. and Campbell, J.N. (1999) Peripheral neural mechanisms of nociception. In P.D. Wall and R. Melzack (eds), *Textbook of Pain* (4th edn). Edinburgh: Churchill Livingstone.

Rexed, B. (1954) A cyloarchitectonic atlas of the spinal cord in the cat. *Journal of Comparative Neurology*, 100 (2): 297–379.

Ringkamp, M., Rwaja, S.N., Campbell, J.N. and Meyer, R.A. (2013) Peripheral mechanisms of cutaneous nociception. In S.B. McMahon, M. Koltenburg, I. Tracey and D.C. Turk, *Wall and Melzack's Textbook of Pain* (6th edn). Philadephia, PA: Elsevier Saunders.

Seeley, R.R., Stephens, T.D. and Tate, P. (2007) *Essentials of Anatomy and Physiology* (6th edn). New York: McGraw-Hill International.

Sherrington, C. (1947/1906) *The Integrative Action of the Nervous System*. Cambridge: Cambridge University Press.

Simpson, D.M., Gazda, S., Brown, S., Webster, L.R., Lu, S.P., Tobias, J.K. and Vanhove, G.F. (2010) Long-term safety of NGX-4010 a high-concentration capsaicin patch in patients with peripheral neuropathic pain. *Journal of Pain and Symptom Management*, 39: 1503–64

Sorkin, L.S. and Yaksh, T.L. (2013) Spinal pharmacology of nociceptive transmission. In S.B. McMahon, M. Koltenburg, I. Tracey and D.C. Turk, *Wall and Melzack's Textbook of Pain* (6th edn). Philadelphia, PA: Elsevier Saunders.

Stemkowski, P.L., Biggs, J.E., Chen, Y., Bukhanova, N., Kumar, N. and Smith, P.A. (2013) Understanding and treating neuropathic pain. *Neurophysiology*, 45: 67–78.

Todd, A.J. (2010) Neuronal circuitry for pain processing in the dorsal horn. *Nature Reviews: Neuroscience*, 11: 823–836.

Tracey, I. (2005) Nociceptive processing in the human brain. *Current Opinion in Neurobiology*, 15: 478–487.

Turk, D.C., Meichenbaum, D. and Genest, M. (1983) *Pain and Behavioural Medicine: A Cognitive Behavioural Perspective*. New York: Guilford Press.

Turk, D.C., Swanson, K.S. and Wilson, H.D. (2010) Psychological aspects of pain. In S.M. Fishman, J.C. Ballantyne and J.P. Rathmell (eds), *Bonica's Management of Pain* (4th edn). Riverwoods, IL: Wolters Kluwer/Lippincott Williams and Wilkins.

Venkatachalam, K. and Montell, C. (2007) TPR channels. *Annual Review of Biochemistry*, 76: 387–417.

Willis, W.D. (2009) The role of TRPV1 receptors in pain evoked by noxious thermal and chemical stimuli. *Experimental Brain Research*, 196: 5–11.

Woolf, C.J. (2004) Pain: moving from symptom control towards mechanism-specific pharmacological management. *Annals of Internal Medicine*, 140: 441–451.

Yaksh, T.L. (1999) Regulation of spinal nociceptive processing: where we went when we wandered onto the path marked by the gate. *Pain Supplement*, 6: S149–S152.

# 4

# Epidemiology of chronic pain

## Learning objectives

The learning objectives of this chapter are to:

- recognize the prevalence of types of chronic pain for population age groups
- recognize the increased risk factors for chronic pain imposed by ageing
- know that low back pain is a major problem and a public health problem for nurses
- know the components of the biopsychosocial model and sensitivity of chronic pain

## Introduction

The **descriptive epidemiology** of chronic pain looks at the incidence, prevalence and patterns of chronic pain across different age groups, geographical locations and societies. **Analytic epidemiology** aims to identify most likely causes and risk factors for chronic pain in different age groups and geographical populations. As many sectors of the global population have increasing life expectancy, chronic pain, associated with syndromes common to ageing, especially cancer (discussed in Chapter 10), degenerative conditions (such as osteoporosis) and painful, inflammatory musculoskeletal conditions is set to become a major international health problem. This chapter:

- outlines the prevalence and impact of chronic pain types in different countries;
- outlines the prevalence of varying types of chronic pain in different population age groups;

- explores psychobiological mechanisms in chronic musculoskeletal pain;
- defines peripheral and central sensitization and discusses how these processes may underpin the development of chronic neuropathic pain.

## Prevalence and impact of chronic pain in adults

Of the world's current population of over 7.2 billion people, 841 million are aged 60 years or over, and numbers of people in this age group are projected to rise to 2 billion by 2050. It is estimated that there are currently 120 million people aged 80 years or over worldwide, and this number will triple to 392 million by 2050 (United Nations Department of Economic and Social Affairs, 2012; US Census Bureau, 2012).

While nociceptive processes related to reflex withdrawal and acute pain perception are protective of injury and survival for humans and animals, chronic – sometimes called persistent – pain does not provide any protective or survival advantage. Chronic pain severely impacts the quality of life of the chronic pain sufferer and his or her close others, and imposes high costs for society.

Prevalence studies of different types of chronic pain have been carried out in many developed countries and across Europe and the USA (Breivik et al., 2006; Johannes et al., 2010). These studies show highest chronic pain prevalence in the back, joints and neck, reflecting findings in studies in individual countries. In the **Health Survey for England (2011)** more women than men reported chronic pain across the life span. Pain prevalence was associated with lower income groups and increased with age (Health Survey for England, 2011). Findings from surveys show a strong tendency towards increased pain being associated with older age, with higher costs and with levels of depression. Greater pain prevalence is associated with lower socio-economic status, where the interference with work has a greater impact. Pain intensity, depression and illness are identified as predictors of disability (Azevedo et al., 2012; Johannes et al., 2010; Raftery et al., 2011; Raftery et al., 2012).

Two market surveys were carried out across Europe in 2010 – (a) the **Pain Proposal Patient Survey** and (b) the **Primary Care Physician Survey** – on behalf of the Pain Proposal Initiative. The Pain Proposal Steering Committee (a group of people with chronic pain, clinicians from different medical specialties, health economists, health policy specialists and industry representatives) asked 2,019 people with chronic pain and 1,472 primary care physicians across 15 European countries about chronic pain. Respondents surveyed included:

(a) people with chronic pain, which was defined as pain lasting more than three months;
(b) physicians working in primary care having at least three years' experience and treating at least 10 patients with chronic pain each month.

Findings from this survey indicate that about one in five people in Europe is suffering from chronic pain. This societal prevalence of chronic pain represents a significant burden to individuals in their capacity to lead a normal working and productive lives and severely impacts on their family and their social lives. The very high cost to European society is about €300 billion, about 1.5–3% GDP, annually (Baker et al., 2010).

Table 4.1 shows the most common perceived causes of chronic pain experienced by patient respondents of the Pain Proposal Patient Survey (2010) across Europe (Baker et al., 2010), with 55% stating back problems as the most common cause of their chronic pain, followed by joint pain (46%) and neck pain (34%).

**Table 4.1** The Pain Proposal Patient Survey (ECR, 2010) findings across 15 European countries

| Of patients with chronic pain surveyed | Patients' most common causes of chronic pain | Other causes of patients' chronic pain |
| --- | --- | --- |
| 55% | Back problems | |
| 46% | Joint pain | |
| 34% | Neck pain | |
| 22% | | Headache |
| 18% | | Arthritis |
| 16% | | Migraine |
| 13% | | Fibromyalgia |
| 11% | | Neuropathic pain |
| 10% | | Surgery/medical procedures |
| 7% | | Visceral (from internal organs) |
| 4% | | Diabetes |
| 2% | | Cancer |
| 1% | | Shingles (post herpetic neuralgia) |

In a **Survey of Chronic Pain in Europe** (of 15 European countries and Israel), by Breivik et al. (2006), 19% of 46,394 respondents reported having chronic pain, and many reported having chronic pain for more than five years and some for over 20 years. Constant chronic pain was experienced by 46% of respondents, most frequently in the 41–60 years age group. The study found that the chronic pain of moderate to severe intensity experienced by 19% of adult Europeans seriously impacted on their quality of life. While there were differences between the 16 countries surveyed by Breivik et al. (2006), the researchers concluded that chronic pain is a major public health problem in Europe. Nearly 50% of respondents had back pain, and more than 40% had joint pain, with arthritis and osteoarthritis being the most common cause of pain.

In a **Kantar National Health and Wellness** pain study across five European countries (Kantar, 2010), back pain accounted for 70% of cases of severe pain, 65% of cases of moderate pain and more than 50% of cases of mild pain.

A US **Community-Based Diary Survey** (conducted by telephone) (Krueger and Stone, 2008) of 3,980 individuals showed that 28.8% of men and 26.6% of women reported feeling some pain at sampled times during the day. The average pain rating increased with age, although there was little difference between men and women. Less income and/or less education equated with higher pain. Satisfaction with life or health was inversely related to pain. While this study did not identify the causes of pain, findings are in line with other studies in general, finding that socio-economic status predicts health and longevity. This study also strongly suggested that pain should be viewed as an economic and social burden which requires urgent attention. People who reported fairly high pain spent their day differently from those reporting less or no pain (Krueger and Stone, 2008).

In 2010 a **cross-sectional internet-based study** surveyed **the prevalence of chronic pain** in a US population representative sample of 9,326 respondents. The study showed that, for periods of at least six months, 8.1% of respondents experienced chronic low back pain, 3.9% experienced osteoarthritis and 18% experienced other types of pain (Johannes et al., 2010). The overall prevalence of self-reported chronic pain lasting at least six months was 34.5%.

A higher prevalence of pain was observed in females compared with males. In this survey, the most commonly reported body locations of chronic pain overall were: the lower back (48%), knee joints (38%), shoulder joint (27%), legs or feet other than joint pain (27%) and hip and feet joints (25% each). The age distribution increased through 55–64 years for chronic low back pain, increased steadily by age for osteoarthritic pain and peaked in the middle years for the other pain types (Johannes et al., 2010).

A survey by the **Centers for Disease Control and Prevention** in the USA of the percentage of adults aged ≥18 years who often had pain in the past three months, by sex and age group, during 2010–2011, found that during this period women (20.7%) were more likely than men (16.9%) to have pain overall and in all age groups except those aged ≥75 years. Among both men and women, those aged 18–44 years were likely to have pain less often than adults in older age groups (Centers for Disease Control and Prevention (USA), 2010–2011).

A **population-based survey of pain** by Portenoy et al. (2004) of differences among 1,592 white, African-American and Hispanic respondents showed that one-third of respondents in each group reported frequent or persistent pain for three months or longer during the previous year. Highly distressing perceptions were associated with disabling pain. Younger age, male gender, higher income and educational attainment and not being divorced predicted a low likelihood of disabling pain. Neither race nor ethnicity was associated with disabling pain. However, minority groups showed more pain-associated characteristics. Perception of control over pain experience was strongly associated with lower likelihood of disabling pain.

A **systematic review of the global prevalence of low back pain** by Hoy et al. (2012) identified 165 studies from 54 countries. The review concluded that low back pain was a major problem throughout the world, with highest prevalence in females aged between 40 and 80 years. This age group represents middle age, the most productive years of a person's life, so loss of work related to low back pain at this stage in life has a major impact on the person, their family, the work organization and society. A higher prevalence was found among females compared to males across all age groups, possibly associated with osteoporosis, pregnancy, sex and socio-cultural reporting differences in pain experience and high pain prevalence in adolescence. This review found that low back pain was less prevalent in lower-income compared with higher-income countries and that low back pain prevalence was high in adolescents. It is important to note that low back pain often has a contrasting socio-economic profile to most other types of pain.

## Low back pain in nurses

Low back pain is a serious workplace and public health problem for nurses. A study by Mitchell et al. (2009) found that of 170 female undergraduate nursing students, more than 30% reported significant back pain in the previous 12 months. Stress, coping, physical activity levels, age and lifting techniques associated with poor spinal posture were associated with low back pain in the student nurse cohort. This study found that among other biopsychoscial factors associated with low back pain, the risk factors common to all the nurses with significant low back pain group were: (a) older age; (b) more hours of weekly vigorous activity (which with incorrect posture could worsen a musculoskeletal problem); (c) a higher stress score; (d) more use of the coping strategy 'I get sick'; and (d) holding the lower spine in a more extended posture during transfers at bed height than other nurses in the study cohort.

These risk factors are modifiable and could form the basis of a biopsychosocial prevention approach, focusing on increasing coping strategies (learning problem-solving techniques, increasing optimism, social interaction and support), learning stress reduction and relaxation techniques, including adopting healthy lifestyles and engaging in adequate and appropriate physical activity and exercise to correct posture and strengthen the back, abdominal and leg muscles, and with advice from physiotherapy (including, but not limited to, Yoga, Pilates and T'ai Chi exercises, as advised).

Low back pain in nurses may be strongly associated with poor and incorrect spinal postures and movements during heavy-lifting, patient-related tasks and maintaining poor postures through tiredness and inappropriate coping with discomfort. It is very important to take instruction in correct bending and lifting in nursing. The Physiotherapist and Manual Handling Tutor can advise on correct spinal postures and muscle alignments for lifting heavy patients. In addition, factors such as poor: (a) cardiovascular, (b) back muscle endurance, (c) posture, and (d) motor control contribute to the onset of low back pain, all of which are modifiable through a preventative approach (Mitchell et al., 2009).

The approach to management of low back pain typifies the developments over the past 25 years. It has changed from a completely 'disease-focus' orientation (often advocating

CLINICAL EXAMPLE

*(Continued)*

*(Continued)*

prolonged bed rest, which resulted in a substantial loss of function and increased disability) to a biopsychosocial focus, in which the patient's report of disability, based on the restriction of activities of daily living, may be regarded as avoidance learning based on past experience of pain and the meaning of the pain (Waddell, 1992). Current knowledge about chronic pain syndromes recognizes the validity of sex and genetic factors interacting with the person's environment, and these contribute to individual differences in the etiology of chronic pain syndromes. Nurses frequently have to do heavy lifting and moving tasks, which are serious workplace risk factors for experiencing of low back pain. Studies suggest that there is a connection between menstrual issues and low back pain in nurses. One study of 816 Japanese nurses who were actively menstruating found that nurses who reported breast tenderness prior to menstruation were twice as likely to suffer low back pain, while those who reported breast tenderness during menstruation were almost twice as likely to suffer low back pain which interfered with daily activities (Smith et al., 2009). Increasing body weight was positively associated with the likelihood of low back pain interfering with daily activities and dysmenorrhoea pain was substantially associated with more likelihood of suffering low back pain in the previous year. Nurses in this study mostly treated their low back pain themselves, with either cold or hot compress, medication or professional treatments (Shiatsu massage, chiropractic care, physical therapy and acupuncture) (Smith et al., 2009).

These studies are set in the light of (a) women being over-represented in the numbers of patients with a range of chronic pain syndromes, and (b) experiments with laboratory mice showing sex differences in sensitivity to environmental issues (Mogil, 2003). They illustrate the need for a comprehensive occupational health focus on the prevention of low back pain in nurses, the recognition of workplace needs of nurses with menstrual disorders, the establishment of a health-promoting workplace culture encouraging nutritious diet, the correct type and level of exercise, smoking cessation, stress management, which is an often over looked yet vital factor, and sleep hygiene. Nurses' active management of their personal physical and psychological health and well-being may benefit from medical advice and checking progesterone and other hormone levels. Early diagnosis and treatment is essential to prevent low back pain from becoming chronic.

...................................................................................................

**A systematic review of the epidemiology of chronic pain in children and adolescents** by King et al. (2011) found a negative association between lower socio-economic status and higher pain prevalence, with a higher pain prevalence of all pain types in girls. This trend tends to increase with age, apart from abdominal pain, where results overall indicate no age and sex differences.

Table 4.2 shows the prevalence of different pain types associated with age and sex in children and adolescents in the review by King et al. (2011). The varying prevalence of headache was repeated across many studies. Different studies show similar trends of higher prevalence of headaches in girls at both primary and secondary school grade levels. Sometimes this is associated with lower socio-economic status, a family history of headaches (possibly indicating a genetic predisposition), and can be linked with symptoms of anxiety, depression and, for girls, low self-esteem. Studies indicate the prevalence of recurrent abdominal pain (RAP) (i.e. at least three

**Table 4.2** Prevalence rates by pain type in children and adolescents

| Pain type | Prevalence range | Age differences (among children) | Sex differences | Psychosocial/ demographic factors associated with ↑ prevalence |
|---|---|---|---|---|
| Headache | 8–82.9% | Older child> younger child | Girls>boys | Presence of anxiety and depression; low self-esteem (girls only); family history of headache; low SES* |
| Abdominal pain | 3.8–53.4% | Younger>older | Girls>boys | SES*; emotional symptoms; school stress |
| Back pain | 13.5–24% | Older>younger | Girls>boys | Emotional symptoms*; unclear link between back pain and sociodemographic factors |
| Musculoskeletal/ limb pain | 3.9–40% | Older>younger | Girls>boys | Feeling sad (girls only) |
| Multiple pains | 3.6–48.8% | Unclear | Girls>boys | Chronic health problems; frequent change of residence and TV watching; fewer interactions with peers |
| Other/general pain | 5–88% | Unclear; possible age and sex interaction | Girls>boys | Poor self-rated health; feeling low or irritable, bad temper, feeling nervous |

SES = socioeconomic status; * = conflicting findings
Source: King, S., Chambers, C.T., Huguet, A., MacNevin, R.C., McGrath, P.J., Parker, L. and MacDonald, A.J. (2011) The epidemiology of chronic pain in children and adolescents revisited: a systematic review. *Pain*, 152: 2729–2738. Copyright (2011). Republished with permission of Elsevier.

episodes of abdominal pain, severe enough to limit functioning, over a three-month period) is higher in girls overall, with findings varying regarding age. Recurrent abdominal pain is associated with maternal anxiety, anxiety and depression in the child, as well as school stress. Studies differ in findings regarding back pain. Some studies have found higher prevalence in girls while other studies have found no sex differences in back pain between children and adolescents. Musculoskeletal pains of the head, neck, shoulders, back and abdomen generally have a higher prevalence in girls compared with boys (King et al., 2011).

## Prevalence of pain in older persons

Older age is associated with increased risk of suffering chronic diseases, many of which are painful. The **United States 2011 National Health and Aging Trends Study** (Patel et al., 2013), which examined a large, nationally representative population sample aged 65 years or older, found that overall prevalence of bothersome pain in the last month was 52.9%, afflicting 18.7 million older adults. Pain did not vary across age groups and the majority (74.9%) of older adults with pain endorsed multiple pain sites (Patel et al., 2013; see also Arnstein and Herr, 2010). This level of reporting of pain prevalence is similar to the **2001 UK National Census** finding of 50% of people aged over 65 years experiencing pain or discomfort (José Closs, 2008). Other epidemiological studies suggest that the high pain prevalence in 55–65 years olds continues into older age at about the same prevalence rates. Also, persistent pain associated with degenerative joint disease is very prevalent in the older population and increases with age (Gibson and Lussier, 2012). The most common pain sites in older people are the back, leg, knee or hip and other joints, due variously to degenerative and inflammatory conditions (Abdulla et al., 2013). The common prevalence of pain in older people is likely to overlap with depression and/or dementia (José Closs, 2008).

Adaptation to chronic pain may involve the older person accepting the gap between his or her personal desired level of physical functioning and his or her personal experiential level of physical functioning. An already reduced level of activity and functionality may be worsened by attitudes of 'hurt' equating with 'harm', which may be reinforced by healthcare professionals or family, so that the person further avoids movement or activity, leading to further reduced functionality and a concomitant loss of muscle tone and physical strength. For an older person, this physical deconditioning may result in a major lifestyle alteration, for example, moving from a house to a bungalow, changing former busy daily routines to using 'pacing' – a word with a connotation of physically slowing down in order to be able to complete daily tasks, and using practical aids to assist limited mobility (Sofaer et al., 2005).

## Falls, fractures and painful conditions in older people

Falls in older people are a major public health problem, and it is estimated that approximately one in three people aged 65 years or more fall each year. Hip and other fractures are a serious and potentially lethal consequence. Falls are known to result from an interaction of the person with his or her environment. Personal physiological risk factors include, but are not limited to, poor gait and balance, foot pain, poor vision, osteoporosis, poor skeletal architecture and foot deformity, and reduced muscle strength and frailty. Disabling foot pain and associated problems are risk factors for fall injuries in older people. Multifaceted podiatry interventions, which include exercises for feet and ankles, advice on footwear and orthotics, and falls prevention education have been shown to reduce the incidence of falls in older people living in the community (Mickle et al., 2010; Spink et al., 2011). Chronic knee pain, usually attributed to osteoarthritis and suffered by both men and women, is associated with the loss of lower limb muscle strength, and increases the risk of falls and hip fracture (Fransen et al., 2014). Older people who are residents in long-term care, or who are hospitalized, are at particular risk of falls-related injuries. A falls risk assessment should be part of the overall assessment for this population group. Polypharmacy (multiple medication intake), poor mobility levels, the use of assistive devices and mood are all factors which contribute to the risk of falls for older persons. When the older, frail person is removed from their familiar environment through illness or reduced cognitive ability, the likelihood of their sustaining falls-related injuries increases. Studies show that carefully designed multifactorial interventions to reduce the incidence of falls are effective. In residential care homes, training and the involvement of all staff is essential (Neyens et al., 2009). Studies show convincing evidence of the benefits of T'ai Chi, which combines deep breathing with relaxation and slow, gentle movements, for falls prevention and improving the psychological health of older people (Lee and Ernst, 2014).

Osteoporosis, the thinning of the bone resulting in loss of bone density and deterioration of bone tissue, frequently results in acute and chronic pain in older people. Osteoporosis-related acute pain results from hip and spinal fractures, and both have serious consequences for the older person's quality of life, especially hip fractures, which frequently result in mortality or permanently reduced functionality. Over time, osteoporosis impacts on the skeletal structure to cause skeletal architectural mis-shaping (the Dowager's hump, with bent-over upper spine and extended neck, is a well-recognized consequence), and is a frequent cause of chronic pain in older people, particularly women. The disease is associated with possible reduced lung capacity, muscle spasm, heartburn, abdominal pain and bladder and bowel dysfunction. The altered spinal architecture may result in the misplacement of ribs impinging on the pelvis. Physical function, activity and muscle strength may decline, inducing frailty and increasing the person's risk of sustaining more falls and fractures, with the increased likelihood of early death or loss of mobility and independence. Prevention of osteoporosis in the older, frail or at-risk general population worldwide is a major, vital public health issue, as osteoporosis risk factors can be identified with careful biopsychosocial and family history and bone scanning. Osteoporosis onset in older age can be prevented, or certainly significantly delayed, with appropriate screening, diet, exercise and pharmacological and nonpharmacological management of selected risk factors. Treatment of osteoporosis-associated pain requires careful assessment to exclude other causes and a multidisciplinary care approach (Dore et al., 2013; Dowson, 2008; Rolland et al., 2008). Other painful conditions more commonly associated with ageing, and which lead to disability, are stroke, angina and arthritis, all of which can have a drastically negative impact on quality of life (Wu et al., 2013).

Figure 4.1 shows the biopsychosocial model of typical musculoskeletal pain. Flor and Turk (2011) suggest that preconditions for chronic pain and pain-related disability associated with typical musculoskeletal syndromes include:

- predisposing factors;
- eliciting stimuli;
- eliciting responses;
- maintaining processes.

**Predisposing factors:** Each person has their own unique life experience, which has contributed to the body's wear and tear. For genetic reasons, a person may have a predisposition towards developing a chronic pain syndrome in one body system, such as acute tension headache. Another person may have chronic low back pain from a previous injury or failed back surgery, a spinal architecture anomaly, arthritic degeneration of joints and cartilage, or ongoing muscle strain. The latter is often associated with poor posture, workplace issues and lifting heavy weights (Flor and Turk, 2011; Merskey and Bogduk, 1994).

**Eliciting stimuli:** As outlined in Figure 4.1, an event that is perceived as threatening, because it is associated with pain-related feelings due to memories and experience, has a negative meaning for the person. The brain associates the

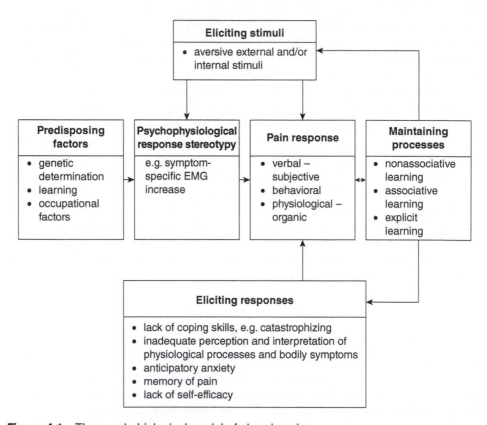

**Figure 4.1**   The psychobiological model of chronic pain

meaningful event with the perception of pain. These events may be unconditioned or conditioned stimuli, and the pain perception is accompanied by an avoidance stress response, where the body's flight reaction aims to remove the self from the aversive stressor (Flor and Turk, 2011).

**Eliciting responses:** Both the perception of pain (which is real for the patient) and the stress response can stay elevated until a sense of control is restored and the person feels the event is no longer of direct threatening significance to them. They can then successfully cope with or avoid the stressor.

**Maintaining processes:** When a person has developed a neural network of pain memories, even minor pain associated stimuli may trigger pain responses. If a person shows an avoidance response of movement reduction or reduction in any physical, social or cognitive activity, fearing that minor discomfort will lead to major pain sensation, their avoidance pain behaviour can soon lead to reduced activity on all levels followed rapidly by loss of muscle tone, strength and overall functionality (Flor and Turk, 2011).

# The development of chronic pain: the two phases of modulation of the pain system

When a person's body is repeatedly exposed to the same noxious stimulus, their nociceptive responses become amplified (enhanced). This amplification leads to modulation of the pain system, which is represented by reversible changes in the excitability of primary sensory and central neurons, known as sensitization. Sensitization has two phases, the peripheral and central phases (Latremoliere and Woolf, 2009).

**Peripheral sensitization:** The first phase in modulation is an increase in neuronal excitability of the peripheral terminals of nociceptors from changes in glutamate receptor and ion channel properties, following exposure of nerve fibre terminals to the sensitizing agents (e.g. PGE2, 5HT, bradykinin, epinephrine, adenosine, NGFs) (Latremoliere and Woolf, 2009; Woolf and Salter, 2000).

**Central sensitization:** With the induction of central sensitization in somatosensory pathways, a central amplification occurs, enhancing the pain response to noxious stimuli in amplitude, duration and spatial extent, while the strengthening of normally ineffective synapses recruits low-threshold sensory inputs to activate the pain circuit (as shown in Figure 4.2).

The most recent definition of central sensitization by the International Association for the Study of Pain is 'the increased responsiveness of nociceptive neurons in the central nervous system to the normal or subthreshold afferent input' (IASP, 2011). Central sensitization has been described as a manifestation of the remarkable plasticity of the somatosensory nervous system in response to activity, inflammation and neural injury (Latremoliere and Woolf, 2009).

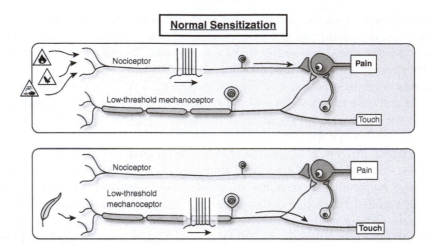

Normal sensation. The somatosensory system is organized such that the highly specialized primarily sensory neurons that encode low intensity stimuli only activate those central pathway that lead to innocuous sensations, while high intensity stimuli that activate nociceptors only activate the central pathways that lead to pain and the two parallel pathways do not functionally intersect. This is mediated by the strong synaptic inputs between the particular sensory inputs and pathways and inhibitory neurons that focus activity to these dedicated circuits.

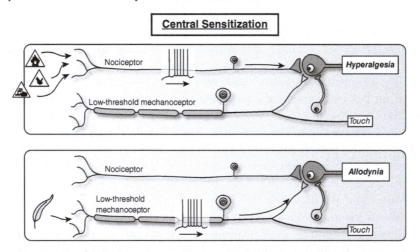

Central sensitization. With the induction of central sensitization in somatosensory pathways with increases in synaptic efficacy and reductions in inhibition, a central amplification occurs enhancing the pain response to noxious stimuli in amplitude, duraion and spatial extent, while the strengthening of normally ineffective synapses recruits subliminal inputs such that inputs in low threshold sensory inputs can now activate the pain circuit. The two parallel sensory pathways converge.

**Figure 4.2**   Mechanisms of normal sensitization and central sensitization

Source: Woolf, C.J. (2011) Central sensitization: implications for the diagnosis and treatment of pain. *Pain*, 152: S2–S15. Copyright (2011). The figure has been reproduced with permission of the International Association for the Study of Pain® (IASP). The figure may NOT be reproduced for any other purpose without permission.

# Central sensitization and chronic pain states

Studies suggest that central sensitization underpins the pain sensitivity experienced by patients suffering from any one of a number of chronic pain conditions, particularly musculoskeletal disorders with generalized pain hypersensitivity, fibromyalgia, osteo-arthritis, headache, temporomandibular joint disorders, dental pain, neuropathic pain, visceral pain hypersensitivity disorders and postsurgical pain (Woolf, 2011).

## Spontaneous pain

In many chronic pain syndromes, pain arises spontaneously, sometimes elicited by:

(a) increased pain from a stimulus that normally provokes pain, known as hyperalgesia;

(b) pain due to a stimulus that does not normally provoke pain, known as allodynia;

(c) these types of response can occur across many tissue and pain types and as a feature of peripheral and central sensitization. (IASP, 2011)

## 'Wind-up' as a form of sensitization

A third type of neuron, called Wide Dynamic Range (WDR), fires action potentials of graded intensity in response to stimulus intensity from each of the three types of sensory fibres. WDRs exhibit 'wind-up', which is a slow, temporal summation of pain due to rapid and repeated noxious stimulation of peripheral nerves or tissues. It is considered to be a form of sensitization. Interneurons in the spinal cord dorsal horn are, variously, excitatory (glutamatergic) and inhibitory (GABAergic), impacting the responses of both nociceptive cells and WDRs and, consequently, dorsal horn output (Bleakman et al., 2006; D'Mello and Dickenson, 2008; Turk and Okifuji, 2010).

# Chronic pain as a neurodegenerative disorder

Recent functional brain imaging studies suggest that severe chronic pain may be a neurodegenerative disorder, particularly affecting the prefrontal cortex, with implications for the descending inhibitory system and overall chronic pain experience. Functional imaging studies have confirmed the role of the thalamus in chronic pain, particularly in terms of deficits in thalamic blood flow (hypoperfusion). Insula and prefrontal cortical inactivation, which are common to studies of different clinical pain conditions, indicate an important role for the anterior insula with regard to subjective feelings of anxiety, depression, fatigue and fear (Tracey and Mantyh, 2007).

## Neuropathic pain

Neuropathic pain is highly complex and individualized. Biological factors interact with psychosocio-environmental factors to bring about individual pathophysiology. Neuropathic pain syndromes are named in accordance with the associated pathology. For example, neuropathic pain associated with diabetes is called diabetic neuropathy, neuropathic pain associated with the aftermath of shingles is called postherpetic neuralgia, and the neuropathic pain associated with HIV is called HIV neuropathy. Other neuropathies are central post-stroke pain, vitamin deficiency-induced pain, alcohol-induced pain, traumatic nerve injury, and neuropathy associated with phantom pain and dorsal root compression. Chemotherapy-induced neuropathy is a serious side-effect associated with certain chemotherapy treatments for cancer (Treede et al., 2008).

Factors in both the peripheral and central nervous system play a role in the experience of phantom pain, which is experienced by most people who have lost a limb. Causes of amputation include war injuries, and the clinical requirement for amputation includes diabetes complications, peripheral vascular disease and cancer. Mechanisms for phantom pain are not yet fully understood. However, studies show that nerve injury precipitates changes in the peripheral and central nervous system (in addition to peripheral and central sensitization), which play a role in the experience of phantom pain. Most people with amputations feel that the limb is still there and up to 80% have intermittent painful sensations referred to the missing limb, which to some extent diminish over time, so that the number of patients with severe pain is about 5–10%.

Phantom pain is often described as 'shooting', 'pricking' and 'burning'. Amputees with phantom pain are more likely to experience stump pain, the latter being associated with hyperalgesia and allodynia. Medications are used in line with other neuropathic conditions as there have been few large-scale studies specifically for the treatment of phantom pain. Amputation is a very traumatic experience and amputees often experience depression, anxiety and isolation.

## Chapter summary

- Chronic pain has a major detrimental impact on the quality of life of sufferers and is an economic and societal burden. Prevalence of chronic pain tends to increase with age. Some studies indicate that there is little difference between men and women, whereas others reveal a higher prevalence of chronic pain in women overall.
- Chronic pain in children shows a varying prevalence of headache in girls at primary and secondary school grade. Prevalence of abdominal pain is higher in girls overall, with musculoskeletal pains of the head, neck, shoulders, back and abdomen more prevalent in girls compared with boys.

- Older age is associated with a high prevalence of pain and multiple pain sites. Pain associated with degenerative disease increases with age, with the most common pain sites in older people being the back, leg, knee, hip and other joints. Fall-related injuries are a major problem.
- Osteoporosis risk factors can be identified with biopsychosocial and family history and bone scanning. The onset of osteoporosis can be prevented, or significantly delayed, with appropriate screening, diet, exercise and pharmacological and non-pharmacological management.
- Studies of the prevalence of chronic pain across Europe and the USA show that about one in five people is suffering chronic pain. Back pain, joint and neck pain are most common in Europe, and lower back and joint pain are most common in the USA. Low back pain is a major problem worldwide.
- Low back pain has the highest prevalence in females aged 40–80 years. It is a serious workplace and public health problem for nurses. Low back pain is associated with such factors as older age, stress, inadequate coping, incorrect posture, poor muscle tone, menstrual issues, and heavy lifting and moving tasks.
- Typical musculoskeletal pain, including low back pain, has changed from a 'disease-focus' orientation to a biopsychosocial focus. Preconditions and disability are comprised of predisposing factors, eliciting stimuli and responses and maintaining processes.
- Chronic pain involves phases of peripheral and central sensitization, the latter of which is described as a manifestation of the remarkable plasticity of the somatosensory nervous system in response to activity, inflammation and neural injury. Hyperalgesia and allodynia are key features of central sensitization. They possibly underpin the sensitivity of many chronic pain conditions.

## Reflective exercise

In the reference section for this chapter read:

(a) an article on the prevalence of chronic pain for a specific patient population, either in the USA or Europe, and consider the implications for the quality of life of the person and for society;
(b) the articles on low back pain in nurses and consider how you may take personal preventative action: for example, learning correct manual handling techniques, obtaining advice regarding back, abdominal and lower body muscles strengthening exercises, taking regular exercise, getting adequate rest, relaxation and sleep, maintaining a healthy lifestyle and, if required, seeking advice regarding menstrual disorders. Do you consider an occupation health focus on prevention of low back pain in nurses in the workplace to be important?

## Recommended reading

Adams, N. (1996 *The Psychophysiology of Low Back Pain.* New York: Churchill Livingstone.
Dowson, C. (2008) Osteoporosis. In P. Crome, C.J. Main and F. Lally (eds), *Pain in Older People*. Oxford: Pain Management Library.
Flor, H. and Turk, D.C. (2011) *Chronic Pain: An Integrated Biobehavioural Approach.* Seattle, WA: International Association of the Study of Pain.

# References

Abdulla, A., Adams, N., Bone, M., Elliott, A.M., Gaffin, J., Jones, D., Knaggs, R., Martin, D., Sampson, L. and Schofield, P. (2013) Guidance on the management of pain in older people. *Age and Ageing*, 42: i1–i57.

Arnstein, P. and Herr, K. (2010) Pain in the older person. In S.M. Fishman, J.C. Ballantyne and J.P. Rathmell (eds), *Bonica's Management of Pain* (4th edn). Riverwoods, IL: Wolters Kluwer/Lippincott Williams and Wilkins.

Azevedo, L.F., Costa-Pereira, A., Mendonça, L., Dias, C.C. and Castro-Lopes, J.M. (2012) Epidemiology of chronic pain: a population-based nationwide study on its prevalence, characteristics and associated disability in Portugal. *The Journal of Pain*, 13: 773–783.

Baker, M., Collett, B., Fischer, A., Hermann, V., Huygen, F.J.P.M., Tölle., T., Trueman, P., Varrassi, G., Vázquez, P. and Vos, K. C.J. (2010) *Pain Proposal: Improving the Current and Future Management of Chronic Pain: A European Consensus Report*. Available at: www.pfizer.pt/Files/Billeder/Pfizer%20P%C3%BAblico/Not%C3%ADcias/Pain%20Proposal%20-%20European%20Consensus%20Report%20final.pdf.

Bleakman, D., Alt, A. and Nisenbaum, E.S. (2006) Glutamate receptors and pain. *Seminars in Cell and Developmental Biology*, 17: 592–604.

Breivik, H., Collett, B., Ventafridda, V., Cohen, R. and Gallagher, D. (2006) Survey of chronic pain in Europe: prevalence, impact on daily life, and treatment. *European Journal of Pain*, 10: 287–333.

Centers for Disease Control and Prevention (USA) (2010–2011) QuickStats: Percentage of adults aged ≥18 years who often had pain in the past 3 months, by sex and age group, National Health Interview Survey, USA.

D'Mello, R. and Dickenson, A.H. (2008) Spinal cord mechanisms of pain. *British Journal of Anaesthesia*, 101 (1): 8–16.

Dore, N., Kennedy, C., Fisher, P., Dolovich, L., Farrauto, L. and Papaioannou, A. (2013) Improving care after hip fracture: the fracture? Think osteoporosis (FTOP) program. *BMC Geriatrics*, 13: 130.

Dowson, C. (2008) Osteoporosis. In P. Crome, C.J. Main and F. Lally (eds), *Pain in Older People*. Oxford: Pain Management Library.

Flor, H. and Turk, D.C. (2011) *Chronic Pain: An Integrated Biobehavioural Approach*. Seattle, WA: International Association of the Study of Pain (IASP).

Fransen, M., Su, S., Harmer, A., Blyth, F.M., Naganathan, V., Sambrook, P., Le Couteur, D. and Cumming, R.G. (2014) A longitudinal study of knee pain in older men: Concord Health and Ageing in Men Project. *Age and Ageing*, 43: 206–212.

Gibson, S.J. and Lussier, D. (2012) Prevalence and relevance of pain in older persons. *Pain Medicine*, 13: S23–S26.

Health Survey for England (2011) *Health, Social Care and Lifestyles*. Leeds: Health and Social Care Information Centre. Available at: www.hscic.gov.uk/catalogue/PUB09300 (accessed 23 January 2014).

Hoy, D., Bain, C., Williams, G., March, L., Brooks, P., Blyth, F. Woolf, A., Vos, T. and Buchbinder, R. (2012) A systematic review of the global prevalence of low back pain. *Arthritis & Rheumatism*, 64(6): 2028–2037.

IASP (2011) *IASP Taxonomy*. Seattle, WA: International Association for the Study of Pain, www.iasp-pain.org (accessed 5 January 2014).

Johannes, C.B., Le, T.K., Zhou, X., Johnston, J.A. and Dworkin, R.H. (2010) The prevalence of chronic pain in United States adults: results of an internet-based survey. *The Journal of Pain*, 11: 1230–1239.

José Closs, S. (2008) Assessment of pain, mood and quality of life. In P. Crome, C.J. Main and F. Lally (eds), *Pain in Older People*. Oxford: Pain Management Library.

Kantar (2010) *Kantar National Health and Wellness Survey*. www.kantarhealth.com.

King, S., Chambers, C.T., Huguet, A., MacNevin, R.C., McGrath, P.J., Parker, L. and MacDonald, A.J. (2011) The epidemiology of chronic pain in children and adolescents revisited: a systematic review. *Pain*, 152: 2729–2738.

Krueger, A.B. and Stone, A.A. (2008) Assessment of pain: a community-based diary survey in the USA. *Lancet*, 371: 1519–1525.

Latremoliere, A. and Woolf, C.J. (2009) Central sensitization: a generator of pain hypersensitivity by central neural plasticity. *Journal of Pain*, 10 (9): 895–926.

Lee, M.S. and Ernst, E. (2014) Systematic reviews of T'ai Chi: an overview. *British Journal of Sports Medicine*, 46: 713–718.

Merskey, H. and Bogduk, N. (1994) *Classification of Chronic Pain: Descriptions of Chronic Pain Syndromes and Definitions of Pain Terms* (2nd edn). Seattle, WA: IASP.

Mickle, K.J., Munro, B.J., Lord, S.R., Menz, H.B. and Steel, J.R. (2010) Foot pain, plantar pressures and falls in older people: a prospective study. *Journal of the American Geriatric Society*, 58: 1936–1940.

Mitchell, T., O'Sullivan, P.B., Smith, A., Burnett, A.F. Straker, L. Thornton, J. and Rudd, C.J. (2009) Biopsychosocial factors are associated with low back pain in female nursing students: a cross-sectional study. *International Journal of Nursing Studies*, 46: 678–688.

Mogil, J.S. (2003) Interaction between sex and genotype in the mediation of pain and pain inhibition. *Seminars in Pain Medicine*, 1 (4): 197–205.

Neyens, J.C.L., Dijcks, B.P.J., Twisk, J., Schols, J.M.G.A., van Haastregt, J.C.M., van den Heuvel, W.J.A. and de Witte, L.P. (2009) A multifactorial intervention for the prevention of falls in psychogeriatric nursing home patients: a randomised controlled trial. *Age and Ageing*, 38: 194–199.

Patel, K.V., Guralnik, J.M., Dansie, E.J. and Turk, D.C. (2013) Prevalence and impact of pain among older adults in the United States: findings from the 2011 National Health and Aging Trends Study. *Pain*, 154: 2649–2657.

Portenoy, R.K., Ugarte, C., Fuller, I. and Haas, G. (2004) Population-based survey of pain in the United States: differences among whites, African American and Hispanic subjects. *The Journal of Pain*, 5 (6): 317–328.

Raftery, M.N., Sarma, K., Murphy, A.W., de la Harpe, D., Normand, C. and McGuire, B.E. (2011) Chronic pain in the Republic of Ireland – community prevalence, psychosocial profile and predictors of pain-related disability: results from the Prevalence, Impact and Cost of Chronic Pain (PRIME) study, Part 1. *Pain*, 152: 1096–1103.

Raftery, M.N., Ryan, P., Normand, C., Murphy, A.W., de la Harpe, D. and McGuire, B.E. (2012) The economic costs of chronic noncancer pain in Ireland: results from the Prevalence, Impact and Cost of Chronic Pain (PRIME) study, Part 2. *The Journal of Pain*, 13: 139–145.

Rolland, Y., Abellan van kan, G., Benetos, A., Blain, H., Bonnefoy, M., Chassagne, P., Jeandel, C., Laroche, M., Nourhashemi, F., Orcel, P., Piette, F., Ribot, C., Ritz, P., Roux, C., Taillandier, J., Tremollieres, F., Weryha, G. and Vellas, B. (2008) Frailty, osteoporosis and hip fracture: causes, consequences and therapeutic perspectives. *The Journal of Nutrition, Health and Aging*, 12 (5): 319–330.

Smith, D.R., Mihashi, M., Adachi, Y., Shouyama, Y., Mouri, F., Ishibashi, N. and Ishitake, T. (2009) Menstrual disorders and their influence on low back pain among Japanese nurses. *Industrial Health*, 47: 301–312.

Sofaer, B., Moore, A.P., Holloway, I., Lamberty, J.M., Thorp, T.A.S. and O'Dwyer, J. (2005) Chronic pain as perceived by older people: a qualitative study. *Age and Ageing*, 34: 462–466.

Spink, M.J., Menz, H.B., Fotoohabadi, M.R., Wee, E., Landorf, K.B., Hill, K.D. and Lord, S.R. (2011) Effectiveness of a multifaceted podiatry intervention to prevent falls in community dwelling older people with disabling foot pain: randomised controlled trial. *British Medical Journal*, 342: d3411 (doi:10.1136/bmj.d3411).

Tracey, I. and Mantyh, P.W. (2007) The cerebral signature for pain perception and modulation. *Neuron*, 55: 377–391.

Treede, R.D., Jensen, T.S., Campbell, J.N., Cruccu, G., Dostrovsky, J.O., Griffin, J.W., Hansson, P., Hughes, R., Nurmikko, T. and Serra, J. (2008) Neuropathic pain: redefinition and a grading system for clinical research purposes. *Neurology*, 70: 1630–1635.

Turk, C. and Okifuji, A. (2010) Pain terms and taxonomies of pain. In S.M. Fishman, J.C. Ballantyne and J.P. Rathmell (eds), *Bonica's Management of Pain* (4th edn). Riverwoods, IL: Wolters Kluwer/Lippincott Williams and Wilkins.

United Nations Department of Economic and Social Affairs/Population Division (2012) *World Population Prospects: The 2012 Revisions: Highlights and Advance Tables*. New York: United Nations.

US Census Bureau (2012), www.census.gov (accessed 5 February 2014).

Waddell, G. (1992) Biopsychosocial analysis of low back pain. *Baillieres Clinical Rheumatology*, 6: 523–557.

Woolf, C.J. (2011) Central sensitization: implications for the diagnosis and treatment of pain. *Pain*, 152: S2–S15.

Woolf, C.J. and Salter, M.W. (2000) Neuronal plasticity: increasing the gain in pain. *Science*, 288: 1765–1768.

Wu, F., Guo, Y., Kowal, P., Jiang, Y., Yu, M., Li, X., Zheng, Y. and Xu, J. (2013) Prevalence of major chronic conditions among older Chinese adults: the Study on Global AGEing and Adult Health (SAGE) Wave 1. *PLOS One*, 8 (9).

# 5

# The assessment and measurement of pain

## Learning objectives

The learning objectives of this chapter are to:

- recognize the rationale for pain assessment and measurement
- understand the various components of comprehensive pain assessment
- identify the frequently utilized pain assessment and measurement tools
- select an appropriate tool for a particular patient population

## Introduction

This chapter discusses the principles of pain assessment and management and identifies several straightforward, recommended tools appropriate to the clinical and community setting for different populations across the life span.

## Rationale for pain assessment, measurement and documentation

Assessment of pain refers to evaluation of the overall characteristics of the patient's pain experience which include pain onset, location, intensity, chronology, pattern of pain duration, exacerbating and relieving factors, the patient's way of expressing their pain and the patient's stated impact of their pain on their quality of life. Pain measurement is asking the patient to give a numerical value to their subjective experience of pain intensity and associated distress.

Because pain is always subjective, the only way to really understand a person's pain experience is to ask him or her about that experience. 'Pain is whatever the experiencing person says it is, existing whenever the experiencing person says it does' (McCaffery, 1968: 95). This definition means that when the patient indicates he/she has pain, the healthcare team responds positively (McCaffery and Beebe, 1994: 15). There is an international effort to emulate the USA where the patient's pain experience in the clinical setting is documented according to VHA directives, which mandate pain as the fifth vital sign (Veterans' Health Administration, 2003, 2009) and according to recommendations by the Joint Commission on Accreditation of Healthcare Organizations (JCAHO) (2009; see also Berry and Dahl, 2000; Fink, 2000).

## Benefits of biopsychosocial pain assessment, measurement and documentation

There are three main benefits of the biopsychosocial assessment, measurement and documentation of pain:

1. The effectiveness of pain interventions can be monitored easily, over time.
2. Pain-related improvements or disimprovements in the patient's health status and quality of life can quickly be identified.
3. The patient is viewed as a person. Assessment and treatment have a biopsychosocial ethos in that there is a focus on rehabilitation and a maximal improvement in the health and quality of life of the patient (Gallagher, 2007; Gatchel et al., 2007; Helfand and Freeman, 2009; Williams, 1996).

## Individual differences in pain responses and pain experiences

Individual differences in pain responses and pain experiences are recognized and accepted as valid in the clinical setting. The intensity of the noxious clinical stimulus is often poorly related to the experience of subjective pain and varies from person to person. In order to obtain the best possible patient outcome in the clinical control of pain, the patient's subjective experience of pain needs to be measured. However, because the person's experience of pain can only be measured indirectly, progress in finding optimal, valid and reliable tools has until recently proved problematic. With carefully designed research methods these difficulties have been resolved (Chapman et al., 1985; Tracey and Mantyh, 2007).

Four types of procedures have been utilized in pain measurement studies on humans in the laboratory. These are:

- psycho-physical methods, which aimed to define the threshold for the pain experience;
- pain-rating methods, in which study participants rate their pain experience on structured scales with defined limits;
- procedures which estimate the magnitude or quality of stimulus intensity;
- measures of discrimination detection.

## Basic pain measurement terms

**Pain (perception) threshold:** this is the level at which the person perceives a noxious stimulus as painful and is therefore the minimal level at which the person reports that the sensation he or she feels is painful. Pain threshold measures have been useful for determining placebo effects and psychological variables relevant to pain management (Chapman et al., 1985). While it is considered that there isn't major variation between the pain perception threshold from person to person, studies show that cultural and gender differences play a role in what people consider acceptable in disclosing about their pain experience, so there may be discrepancies in how much pain a person feels compared to how much pain he or she reports feeling (Clark and Clark, 1980; Defrin et al., 2009; Nayak et al., 2000).

**Pain tolerance:** this is the amount of pain a person can tolerate before considering the pain unbearable and withdrawing from it. Pain tolerance varies from person to person. Pain tolerance can change depending on familiarity with the stimulus and the context (Chapman et al., 1985). Studies show that, again, cultural views about the acceptability of pain expression, as well as subjective pain beliefs, play a role in determining how much pain people can tolerate (Defrini et al., 2009; Nayak et al., 2000; Zborowski, 1952).

The **pain sensitivity range (PSR)** is the difference between the pain tolerance level and the pain threshold; the **drug request point** asks participants to consider the level of pain at which they would require a mild analgesia. Neither the pain sensitivity range nor drug request point have been particularly useful or widely used.

In **adjustment methods** participants are asked to tell the difference between a constant standard stimulus while adjusting a variable stimulus to the point where the two are perceived to be different, producing a **just noticeable difference (JND)**. The JND is the smallest step that can be discriminated during stimulation. Hardy et al. (1952) devised the Dol scale of JNDs, identifying 20 discernible degrees of pain (in response to radiant heat) between the pain threshold and the most excruciating level. The Dol scale was never properly validated or used (Skevington, 1996).

## Pain assessment and measurement

Some tools are unidimensional measures of pain intensity; other tools combine pain measurement with an assessment of multidimensional aspects of the pain experience.

Pain tools have been developed over recent years to meet requirements in both clinical and research contexts. The clinical and research settings differ in their requirements for the types of psychometric instruments used. The basic principle in the clinical setting is to assess and measure the patient's pain experience and to use that information to treat and control the patient's pain. This can be thought of as a three-step process:

1. Comprehensively assess, measure and document the patient's biopsychosocial pain experience; usually the nurse and physician work together to reduce patient burden.
2. The multidisciplinary care team utilizes the information provided by the patient to formulate an interdisciplinary management plan with appropriate pharmacological and nonpharmacological interventions, as required. The plan is documented by the nurse.
3. After an appropriate time interval the nurse reassesses, re-measures and re-documents the patient's pain as the fifth vital sign (and the patient's associated distress as the sixth vital sign, as appropriate), reporting changes in the patient's health status to the care team. The nurse develops competencies to be able to advocate for improvements in the patient's pain treatment, as required.

Selecting an appropriate pain tool requires consideration of which assessment type and quality of life domains are immediately important and would best suit the patient's optimal care and health outcome. For example, after initial comprehensive biopsychosocial assessment, many patients with acute pain will most likely require a straightforward rating-scale-type measurement of pain, whereas patients with chronic pain of a malignant or non-malignant origin require ongoing assessment of pain and how it impacts on the domains of quality of life (Breivik et al., 2008; de Rond and de Wit, 1999; Gatchel et al., 2007; Jensen, 2010; LeBel, 2006; McCaffery and Pasero, 1999; Williams, 1996).

## Domains of pain assessment

Appropriate assessment requires a knowledge of the classification of pain types. In considering what type of assessment tool is required, both the type and the domains of pain which require assessment need to be considered. The patient may have both acute pain and chronic pain at any one time, so there may be more than one type of pain to assess. In pain assessment, the domains of pain experience of primary consideration are:

- pain location: ask the patient to point to his or her body location where his or her pain(s) is/are located;
- pain intensity: this is measured numerically on a scale from zero to ten and supported by adjectival descriptors from no pain to worst pain imaginable;
- pain affect: what type of feeling is associated with the pain experience and the impact on the patient's emotions (e.g. tiring, sickening, punishing, distressing); distress can be measured numerically on a scale from zero to ten;

- pain quality: what words can best describe the nature of pain (e.g. aching, throbbing, sharp, stabbing);
- the temporal (chronological) characteristics of pain: how long does the pain last? Does the pain have a pattern: is it ongoing, rhythmic or intermittent? What time of day is the pain worst?
- exacerbating or relieving factors: are there positions/actions/remedies that reduce the pain sensation?
- interference of the patient's pain experience on different domains of quality of life; how much the patient's pain experience interferes with the different domains of their quality of life.

When the patient with pain first attends the GP or hospital clinical setting, a full biopsychosocial assessment is mandatory for accurate diagnosis and formulating a care plan. Other tools to measure the psychological impact of pain, particularly assessment tools for measuring distress, anxiety and depression and the impact of pain on the patient's quality of life, are regularly utilized.

## Validity, reliability and utility of pain tools

Like all measures, a pain assessment tool for use in the clinical setting needs to meet certain criteria to be able to effectively measure the patient's pain experience. Pain measure needs to have validity, reliability and utility. Older patients are more likely to have comorbidities and, possibly, more than one different type of pain to assess. The patient's pain may impact on different domains of quality of life, for example, sleep and functionality. How often the pain is documented and assessed is also an important point, depending on the patient's current health status and required level of pain intervention.

**Validity**: the main point to consider is whether the pain assessment tool optimally measures what it is required to measure. For example, the user needs to consider whether the pain assessment tool effectively feeds back on the patient's pain experience for a given domain, such as pain intensity.

**Reliability**: this considers how far the measure is free from error. Many factors can influence a person's subjective pain experience disclosure at any one time. How the person is asked about their pain experience (i.e. the communication interaction style between the healthcare professional and the patient) has a major bearing on the patient's willingness to disclose their subjective personal information – are they going to be believed? Factors can range from age, the social context of the person and their family, how culturally free they feel to disclose their pain experience, how distressed they are, and if they have any communication deficits associated, for example, with learning disabilities, or cognitive dysfunction associated with older-age neurodegenerative conditions such as Alzheimer's and similar dementias. Pain is a highly complex experience for any person, regardless of age, and can impact on concentration and cognition. The location of the pain assessment interview, whether the patient is at home, at the GP's surgery or at the hospital setting, whether they feel distressed or relaxed are factors that contribute to potential variation in the patient's disclosed pain score. The higher the variability, the lower the reliability. Therefore:

- a comprehensive biopsychosocial assessment is required in the first instance regardless of the setting where the patient presents;
- all members of the multidisciplinary care team, including the nurse, need to be highly skilled communicators;
- the patient's pain needs to be assessed and documented over time.

**Utility**: subjective pain is experienced in the context of the person's life, potentially impacting on all domains of their quality of life. It isn't usually practicable to measure the ongoing interference imposed by pain on all activities in a person's life, or to take pain measures on a very frequent basis. Utility is about deciding on the types of measure and application that are both practical and valid, which will not give the patient too great a burden and will give useful information to allow optimal and effective treatment intervention. A validated pain measure is useful, valuable and applicable to nursing care (de Rond and de Wit, 1999; Jensen, 2010).

## Description of the pain experience

The two major types of pain are nociceptive (physiological) and neuropathic (pathological). Nociceptive pain can be somatic or visceral in original (see Table 5.1). Superficial somatic pain arises from activation of cutaneous (body surface) nociceptors and is usually sharp, stabbing, and sometimes burning in quality, whereas deep somatic pain arises from nociceptors in muscles, bones, joints or connective tissue, and is described as dull, crampy and aching. Both superficial and deep somatic pain are usually well localized. Visceral pain arises from nociceptors in visceral organs such as the gastro-intestinal tract or the pelvic region, giving rise to a different type of pain according to organ involvement. (Other characteristics that help to identify visceral pain are that it can be vague, poorly defined and accompanied by marked neurovegetative signs. For a detailed review, see Giamberardino and Cervero (2007: 177–192).) For example, in the abdomen, obstruction of a hollow viscus, such as the bowel, can cause intermittent cramping, squeezing type pain, which is poorly localized. Neuropathic pain can vary from tingling 'pins and needles' to severe to unbearable gnawing, shooting, burning or lancinating jolts, often associated with allodynia. The descriptive language patients use to communicate the quality of their pain can help guide the identification of different pain conditions and indicate potential treatments (Griffin et al., 2010; Haroutinian et al., 2013; Jarrell et al., 2011; Jensen, 2010; Thakur et al., 2010).

**Table 5.1** Comparison of somatic and visceral nociceptive pain

| Pain | Somatic nociceptive | Visceral nociceptive |
| --- | --- | --- |
| Localization | More focused | More diffuse and poorly localized; pain felt in distribution innovated by the same spinal segment as organ; referred to other locations |
| Quality | Sharp, aching, burning, stabbing (cramping, tensive if deep somatic …) | Vague discomfort Hyperesthesia; hyperalgesia, allodynia |
| Associated symptoms | Accompanied by motor reflexes | Accompanied by motor and autonomic reflexes: associated muscle contraction/spasm, nausea/vomiting, pain sensation, circulatory changes in the region, decreased pulse/blood pressure, cold sweat |
| Triggers | Tissue injury | Distension, contraction, ischaemia, inflammation; pain not evoked from all viscera |

Source: Griffin, R.S., Fink, E. and Brenner, G.J. (2010) Functional neuroanatomy of the nociceptive system. In S.M. Fishman, J.C Ballantyne and J.P. Rathmell (eds), *Bonica's Management of Pain* (4th edn). Riverwoods, IL: Wolters Kluwer/Lippincott Williams and Wilkins. Copyright (2010). Republished with permission of Lippincott Williams and Wilkins.

## The concept of referred pain

A dermatome is an area of skin supplied by a sensory nerve arising from a spinal nerve ganglion structure (see Figure 5.1). The spinal cord is segmentally organized during embryonic development to receive afferent information about a specific dermatome band. Visceral pain in the abdomen tends to follow the structure of endo-dermal embryonic development, with pain from foregut structures perceived in the epigastrium. Pain from midgut structures is perceived in the peri-umbilical region and pain from hindgut structures is perceived in the lower abdomen. Pain symptoms resulting from visceral afferents are often felt in a location different from the organ itself. This is known as referred pain, and is considered to be a convergence of information from somatic structures and viscera at multiple sites of the central nervous system, giving rise to the experience of referred pain. One possible explanation for referred pain is that peripheral nociceptors from both somatic and visceral origins converge onto single projection neurons in the dorsal horn. Visceral afferents convey sensory information from the internal organs to the central nervous system, following autonomic nerves as they travel centrally. Most visceral receptors are free nerve endings with large receptive fields. They are able to respond to varied stimuli. Their free nerve endings relay information regarding disruption to the internal environment, such as distension, ischaemia, inflammation or irritation. Visceral afferents are sensitive

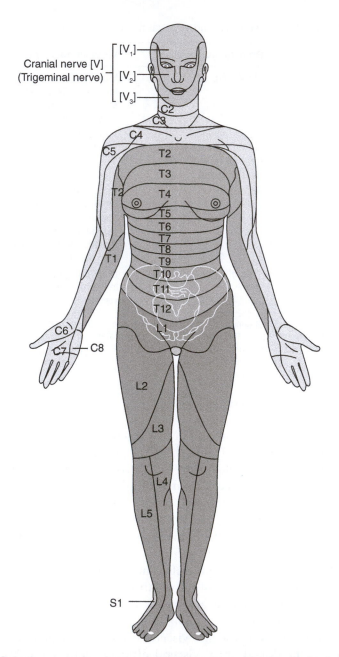

**Figure 5.1**    Spinal nerves give rise to peripheral nerves which innervate dermatomes

Source: *Gray's Anatomy for Students* (2nd edn), by Drake,R.L., Vogl, A.W. and Mitchell, A. W.M. (2010). Copyright Elsevier (2010). Republished with permission of Elsevier Mosby.

to distension and contraction, whereas somatic afferents are more sensitive to cutting and tearing. True visceral pain, irrespective of the affected organ, is usually perceived as being deep in the body in the midline of the thorax or abdomen (Giamberardino et al., 2010; Griffin et al., 2010; Jarrell et al., 2011; Joshi and Gehbart, 2000).

# The impact of chronic pain on quality of life

For the person with chronic pain an initial comprehensive biopsychosocial assessment (with regular follow-up) is required to determine the effect of their chronic pain on all domains of quality of life, work function and family/personal life (see Figure 5.2). Pasero and McCaffery, in *Pain Assessment and Pharmacologic Management* (2011), provide reproducible charts and nursing guidelines relevant to nursing pain management in the clinical setting (see Figure 5.3). Flor and Turk's *Chronic Pain: An Integrated Biobehavioural Approach* (2011) provides a CD with various useful patient care resources. PROQoLID is a quality of life instrument database which provides information about the conditions of use. Some measures are freely available, while other tools require a site licence and user agreement. The Hospital Anxiety and Depression Scale, which is used widely in the clinical setting, gives an indication of possible clinical anxiety or depression which can then be confirmed with a diagnostic

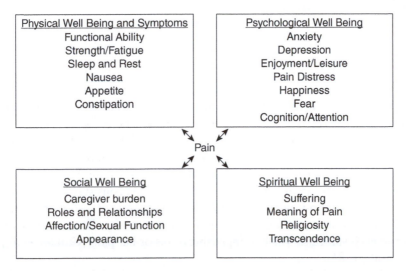

**Figure 5.2**  Pain impacts the dimensions of quality of life

Source: Copyright (1995). Republished with permission of Betty Ferrell and Marcia Grant, City of Hope Medical Center.

interview (Zigmund and Snaith, 1983). The Institute for Clinical Systems Improvement (ICSI) have created a comprehensive assessment and management algorithm for chronic pain based on the best-graded evidence available (Hooten et al., 2013).

An initial biopsychosocial nursing pain assessment tool (Pasero and McCaffery, 2011) with a number-rating scale, or age-appropriate scale, is utilized to assess both acute and chronic pain. For patients undergoing elective surgery, prior to surgery the nurse educates the patient about pain scale completion post-operatively, selecting an appropriate tool with the patient which the patient finds acceptable to measure their acute post-operative pain (usually using a Number Rating Scale alongside a Verbal (or Distress) Rating Scale or the Wong-Baker FACES® Pain Rating Scale or the Faces Pain Scale-Revised (Hicks et al., 2001); see section this chapter), to ascertain and record pain as the fifth vital sign, along with temperature, heart rate, respirations and blood pressure. Pain intensity and quality should be noted regularly in evaluating the effectiveness of analgesia. Immediate aspects of quality of life, particularly sleep, can be evaluated as well as over time. The nurse should ascertain the patient's pain score as soon as possible post-surgery and at appropriate, regular intervals after that, without overburdening the nurse or disturbing the patient if he or she is asleep and restful.

# Pain assessment tools for different population groups

## The McGill Pain Questionnaire as the basis for further developments of pain sssessment tools

The Gate Control Theory (Melzack and Wall, 1965) provided the basis for developing validated multidimensional pain measurement instruments. The first and best known multidimensional pain measurement instrument to be developed was the McGill Pain Questionnaire (MPQ) (Melzack, 1975; Melzack and Torgerson, 1971). Measures derived from the original MPQ are the Present Pain Intensity Index and the Pain Rating Index. The Present Pain Intensity Index is a numerical (1–5) scale and rates the current intensity of pain. The Pain Rating Index consists of a set of 78 verbal descriptors presented on one page in 20 lists (sub-classes) of 2–6 words each. Each list is arranged in a continuum from low to high intensity. The patient selects one word from each sub-class which is applicable to his or her pain (Graham et al., 1980; Kremer et al., 1981).

While the McGill Pain Questionnaire set the standard for understanding the importance of measuring the different domains of pain and identified verbal descriptors to accurately define and differentiate between the sensory, evaluative and affective components of pain, the MPQ can take anything from five to 20 minutes to complete, depending on whether the patient completes the form him or herself or receives assistance with completion. Recognizing the problems posed by the original

**Initial Pain Assessment Tool**

Date _____

Patients's Name _____    Age _____    Room _____

Diagnosis _____    Physician _____

Nurse _____

1. LOCATION: Patient or nurse mark drawing.

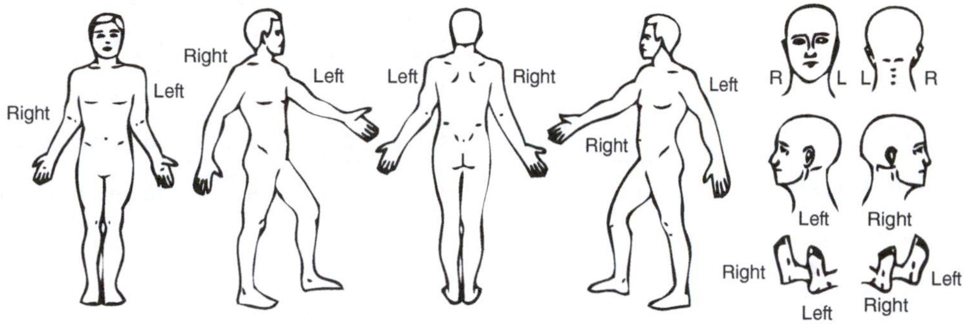

Right    Right    Left    Left    Left    Right    Right    Left    R  L  L  R    Left    Right    Right    Left    Right    Left

2. INTENSITY: Patient rates the pain. Scale used _____

Present pain: _____    Worst pain gets: _____    Best pain gets: _____    Comfort-Function goal: _____

3. IS THIS PAIN CONSTANT? _____    YES: _____    NO _____

IF NOT, HOW OFTEN DOES IT OCCUR? _____

4. QUALITY: (For example: ache, deep, sharp, hot, cold, like sensitive skin, sharp, itchy) _____

5. ONSET, DURATION, VARIATIONS, RHYTHMS: _____

6. MANNER OF EXPRESSING PAIN: _____

7. WHAT RELIEVES THE PAIN? _____

8. WHAT CAUSES OR INCREASES THE PAIN? _____

9. EFFECTS OF PAIN: (Note decreased function, decreased quality of life.)

Accompanying symptoms (e.g., nausea) _____

Sleep _____

Appetite _____

Physical activity _____

Relationship with others (e.g., irritability) _____

Emotions (e.g., anger, suicidal, crying) _____

Concentration _____

Other _____

10. OTHER COMMENTS: _____

11. PLAN: _____

**Figure 5.3**   Initial Pain Assessment Tool

Source: Pasero, C. and McCaffery, M. (2011) *Pain Assessment and Pharmacologic Management*. St Louis, MO: Elsevier Mosby. Copyright (2011). Republished with permission of Elsevier.

## Short-Form McGill Pain Questionnaire-2 (SF-MPQ-2)

This questionnaire provides you with a list of words that describe some of the different qualities of pain and related symptoms. Please put an X through the numbers that best describe the intensity of each of the pain and related symptoms you felt during the past week. Use 0 if the word does not describe your pain or related symptoms.

| | | | | | | | | | | | | | |
|---|---|---|---|---|---|---|---|---|---|---|---|---|---|
| 1. Throbbing pain | *none* | 0 | 1 | 2 | 3 | 4 | 5 | 6 | 7 | 8 | 9 | 10 | *worst possible* |
| 2. Shooting pain | *none* | 0 | 1 | 2 | 3 | 4 | 5 | 6 | 7 | 8 | 9 | 10 | *worst possible* |
| 3. Stabbing pain | *none* | 0 | 1 | 2 | 3 | 4 | 5 | 6 | 7 | 8 | 9 | 10 | *worst possible* |
| 4. Sharp pain | *none* | 0 | 1 | 2 | 3 | 4 | 5 | 6 | 7 | 8 | 9 | 10 | *worst possible* |
| 5. Cramping pain | *none* | 0 | 1 | 2 | 3 | 4 | 5 | 6 | 7 | 8 | 9 | 10 | *worst possible* |
| 6. Gnawing pain | *none* | 0 | 1 | 2 | 3 | 4 | 5 | 6 | 7 | 8 | 9 | 10 | *worst possible* |
| 7. Hot-burning pain | *none* | 0 | 1 | 2 | 3 | 4 | 5 | 6 | 7 | 8 | 9 | 10 | *worst possible* |
| 8. Aching pain | *none* | 0 | 1 | 2 | 3 | 4 | 5 | 6 | 7 | 8 | 9 | 10 | *worst possible* |
| 9. Heavy pain | *none* | 0 | 1 | 2 | 3 | 4 | 5 | 6 | 7 | 8 | 9 | 10 | *worst possible* |
| 10. Tender | *none* | 0 | 1 | 2 | 3 | 4 | 5 | 6 | 7 | 8 | 9 | 10 | *worst possible* |
| 11. Splitting pain | *none* | 0 | 1 | 2 | 3 | 4 | 5 | 6 | 7 | 8 | 9 | 10 | *worst possible* |
| 12. Tiring-exhausting | *none* | 0 | 1 | 2 | 3 | 4 | 5 | 6 | 7 | 8 | 9 | 10 | *worst possible* |
| 13. Sickening | *none* | 0 | 1 | 2 | 3 | 4 | 5 | 6 | 7 | 8 | 9 | 10 | *worst possible* |
| 14. Fearful | *none* | 0 | 1 | 2 | 3 | 4 | 5 | 6 | 7 | 8 | 9 | 10 | *worst possible* |
| 15. Punishing-cruel | *none* | 0 | 1 | 2 | 3 | 4 | 5 | 6 | 7 | 8 | 9 | 10 | *worst possible* |
| 16. Electric-shock pain | *none* | 0 | 1 | 2 | 3 | 4 | 5 | 6 | 7 | 8 | 9 | 10 | *worst possible* |
| 17. Cold-freezing pain | *none* | 0 | 1 | 2 | 3 | 4 | 5 | 6 | 7 | 8 | 9 | 10 | *worst possible* |
| 18. Piercing | *none* | 0 | 1 | 2 | 3 | 4 | 5 | 6 | 7 | 8 | 9 | 10 | *worst possible* |
| 19. Pain caused by light touch | *none* | 0 | 1 | 2 | 3 | 4 | 5 | 6 | 7 | 8 | 9 | 10 | *worst possible* |
| 20. Itching | *none* | 0 | 1 | 2 | 3 | 4 | 5 | 6 | 7 | 8 | 9 | 10 | *worst possible* |
| 21. Tingling or 'pins and needles' | *none* | 0 | 1 | 2 | 3 | 4 | 5 | 6 | 7 | 8 | 9 | 10 | *worst possible* |
| 22. Numbness | *none* | 0 | 1 | 2 | 3 | 4 | 5 | 6 | 7 | 8 | 9 | 10 | *worst possible* |

**Figure 5.4**   Short-Form McGill Pain Questionnaire-2 (SF-MPQ-2)

MPQ, a short-form McGill Pain Questionnaire (SF-MPQ-2) was developed and recently revised to measure both neuropathic and non-neuropathic pain in all settings (Figure 5.4). In a recent study the results suggest that the SF-MPQ-2 has excellent reliability and validity, with four readily interpretable subscales of continuous pain, intermittent pain, predominantly neuropathic pain, and affective descriptors, each measured on a 0–10 number rating scale. Adjectives 1–10 describe pain quality, adjectives 11–15 describe pain affect and adjectives 16–22 describe neuropathic symptoms. Measuring pain quality may help diagnose a pain problem as well as clarify the pain experience and determine pain treatment effectiveness. Recent research suggests that different pain qualities are associated with different causes and types of pain and that different pain mechanisms produce different pain sensations. While it is generally considered that the thinly myelinated A$\delta$ fibres may be substrates for sharp, stinging and shooting pain and unmyelinated C-fibres substrates for less localized dull, longer-lasting pain, these substrates need to be considered as part of the complexity of dermatomal developments, different spinal neuronal pathways and projections linked with the highly complex functioning of the central nervous system (Dworkin et al., 2009; Jensen, 2010).

## The Number Rating Scale to measure pain intensity

Apart from pain location, usually the most useful domains of pain measurement are pain intensity, affect and quality. As shown in the lower left box of Figure 5.5

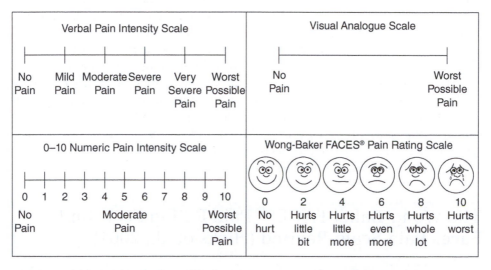

**Figure 5.5** Basic pain measurement tools: The Number Rating (Pain Intensity) Scale, Verbal Rating (Pain Intensity) Scale, Visual Analogue Scale and Wong-Baker FACES® Pain Rating Scale

Numeric Pain Intensity Scale (also called a Number Rating Scale, NRS) has an 11 point line. On the extreme left 0 represents no pain and 10 on the extreme right represents the worst possible pain. In pain assessment the rating chosen by the patient to describe their pain intensity also has a meaning in terms of the impact of pain on their functioning. Ratings on the NRS ranging from 1 to 4 represent mild pain, ratings of 5 and 6 indicate moderate pain, which has a greater impact on functioning. Ratings from 7 to 10 indicate severe pain which has the greatest impact on functioning (Jensen, 2010).

## The Verbal Rating Scale to measure pain intensity

In the top left box of Figure 5.5 is a Verbal Pain Intensity Scale, also known as the Verbal Rating Scale (VRS). No pain is represented on the far left of the line and the worst possible pain is represented on the far right of the line. The Number Rating Scale and the Verbal Rating Scale are recommended for use in the clinical setting. Patients often particularly like the Verbal Rating Scale to describe how their pain intensity feels.

## The Visual Analogue Scale to measure pain intensity

The top right box of Figure 5.5 shows a Visual Analogue Scale (VAS) that has anchor points for no pain or 0 on the far left of the line and the worst possible pain or 10 on the far right of the line. The patient is asked to grade their own pain level on this scale. The Visual Analogue Scale in theory has the psychometric properties of a ratio scale. However, it carries a greater psychological burden of comprehension as task completion is less clear than when using a Number Rating Scale. There are also implications regarding the scale's validity because the varied population of patients in the clinical setting (heterogeneous) differs to the more similar population (homogenous) of the clinical research context. Visual Analogue Scales show higher failure rates in the clinical setting and patients prefer the Number Rating Scale and Verbal Rating Scale to the Visual Analogue Scale.

## The Wong-Baker FACES® Pain Rating Scale and Faces Pain Scale-Revised (Hicks et al., 2001)

Some patients, regardless of age, may prefer the Wong-Baker FACES® Pain Rating Scale, see the lower right box of Figure 5.5 or the Faces Pain Scale-Revised (Hicks et al., 2001; see Figure 5.6). Both scales measure how the person 'feels inside', which is useful for young children and for mild to moderately cognitively impaired people.

Older and very mildly cognitively impaired patient can usually complete simple assessment tools after an initial demonstration, while patients with moderate to severe dementia may require tools validated for this population. For patients with any degree of cognitive impairment the question of whether their subjective pain sensation is being accessed by the assessment method is very important. The Verbal Rating Scale, Wong-Baker FACES® Pain Rating Scale and Faces Pain Scale-Revised are useful pain assessment measures for patients who have difficulty conceptualising bodily sensations, including pain, as a number. The Wong-Baker FACES® Pain Rating Scale is designed for people unable to or who prefer not to use numbers. Children may also respond well to a colour analogue scale, with a Number Rating Scale attached.

Patient education is vital in the clinical setting. Prior to surgical procedures it is important for the nurse to educate the cognitively competent patient, working with the patient to identify appropriate, preferred pain measurement scales. The nurse should explain to the patient how the patient's pain will be evaluated post-operatively by the nurse asking the patient, at regular intervals, to assign a number to their pain using the Number Rating Scale or the Wong-Baker FACES® Pain Rating Scale and supporting this value with an adjective from the Verbal Rating Scale, or by using the Faces Pain Scale-Revised (Hicks et al., 2001), as the patient prefers. The nurse should explain to the patient how the patient's pain will be evaluated post-operatively. The Number Rating (Pain Intensity) Scale is optimal for patients who comprehend and who are comfortable with numbers. The nurse explains how the patient will be asked, at regular intervals, to assign a number to their pain using the Number Rating Scale and supporting this value with an adjective from the Verbal Rating (Pain Intensity) Scale. The nurse should explain to the patient that 'zero is no pain and ten is the worst pain imaginable' and the patient is asked to assign a number to their pain experience now, with an explanation that the same procedure will be followed after the patient's surgery. The Number Rating Scale, alone, or with the Verbal Rating Scale can then be used more effectively post-operatively and post-procedure, as the patient understands that the purpose is to check the effectiveness of pain management interventions for their personal experience of pain. For patients unable, or

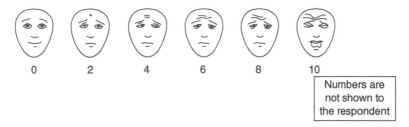

0  2  4  6  8  10

Numbers are not shown to the respondent

**Figure 5.6** Faces Pain Scale-Revised

Source: Hicks, C.L., von Baeyer, C.L., Spafford, P.A. van Korlaar, I. and Goodenough, B.L. (2001) The Faces Pain Scale-Revised: toward a common metric in pediatric pain measurement. *Pain*, 93: 173–183. Copyright (2001). Republished with permission of Elsevier.

who prefer not to use numbers, the Wong-Baker FACES® Pain Rating Scale and/or the Faces Pain Scale-Revised (Hicks et al., 2001) provide a method for the nurse to quantify the patient's pain. Patient education for the Wong-Baker FACES® Pain Rating Scale and/or the Faces Pain Scale-Revised (Hicks et al., 2001) focuses on ascertaining the patient's verbal description of his or her pain experience. The nurse demonstrates how, going from left to right, each face indicates an increased amount of pain compared to the one before. The nurse asks the patient to select the face which most accurately describes his or her current personal pain experience. The numbers on the Faces Pain Scale-Revised (Hicks et al., 2001) are not shown to respondents; the nurse instructs the patient: 'these faces show how much something can hurt. This face [point to left-most face] shows no pain. The faces show more and more pain [point to each from left to right] up to this one [point to right-most face] – it shows very much pain. Point to the face that shows how much you hurt (right now).' The nurse then quantifies the patient's pain with the corresponding number.

It should be made clear to the patient that they are not being 'tested' and that there is no 'right' or 'wrong' answer. Post-operative nursing pain assessment, especially in critical care, is acknowledged to be very challenging. It requires improvement in the standard of quality care, and should be addressed by hospital protocols and through the appropriate use of tools so that critical care nurses can properly assess post-operative pain. (Hicks et al., 2001; Gélinas et al., 2004; Jenson, 2010; Pasero and McCaffery, 2011; Paulson-Conger et al., 2011; Vickers et al., 2014)

## The assessment of pain and discomfort in infants and children

Determining adequate and accurate measures of infants' levels of pain and distress and differentiating infants' pain and distress experience has proved very challenging. The **CRIES Scale** is a 10-point scale based on the APGAR (1953) score and is an acronym for five physiological and behavioural measures shown to be associated with neonatal pain (Krechel and Bildner, 1995):

Crying

Requires oxygen (administration)

Increased vital signs

Expressions

Sleeplessness

Comfort is an absolute prerequisite for patient care, especially of infants and is a cardinal nursing responsibility (Wong and Baker, 1988). Pre- and full-term infants in intensive care units experience substantial numbers of invasive procedures on a

| Indicator | Finding | Points |
|---|---|---|
| Gestational age | ≥ 36 weeks | 0 |
| | 32 weeks to 35 weeks 6 days | 1 |
| | 28 weeks to 31 weeks 6 days | 2 |
| | < 28 weeks | 3 |
| Behavioural state | Active/awake, eyes open, facial movements | 0 |
| | Quiet/awake, eyes open, no facial movements | 1 |
| | Active/sleep, eyes closed, no facial movements | 2 |
| | Quiet/sleep, eyes closed, no facial movements | 3 |
| Heart rate maximum | 0–4 beats per minute increase | 0 |
| | 5–14 beats per minute increase | 1 |
| | 15–24 beats per minute increase | 2 |
| | ≥ 25 beats per minute increase | 3 |
| Oxygen saturation | 0 to 2.4% decrease | 0 |
| | 2.5 to 4.9% decrease | 1 |
| | 5.0 to 7.4% decrease | 2 |
| | 7.5 decrease or more | 3 |
| Brow bulge | None (≤ 9% of time) | 0 |
| | Minimum (10–39% of time) | 1 |
| | Moderate (40–69% of time) | 2 |
| | Maximum (≥ 70% of time) | 3 |
| Eye squeeze | None (≤ 9% of time) | 0 |
| | Minimum (10–39% of time) | 1 |
| | Moderate (40–69% of time) | 2 |
| | Maximum (≥ 70% of time) | 3 |
| Nasolabial furrow | None (≤ 9% of time) | 0 |
| | Minimum (10–39% of time) | 1 |
| | Moderate (40–69% of time) | 2 |
| | Maximum (≥ 70% of time) | 3 |

**Figure 5.7**  Premature Infant Pain Profile

Source: Stevens, B., Johnston, C., Pteryshen, P. et al. (1996) Premature Infant Pain Profile: development and initial validation. *Clinical Journal of Pain*,(1) 13–22. Republished with permission of Lippincott Williams and Wilkins. Copyright (1996). Republished with permission of Lippincott Williams and Wilkins.

daily basis. The **Neonatal Facial Coding System** is a widely accepted measure of pain-related distress in pain-specific contexts (Grunay and Craig, 1987). Studies with the Neonatal Facial Coding System show that infants undergoing painful procedures show behavioural indicators of arousal and distress. However, distinguishing between distress and pain in this population group is extremely challenging (Chimello et al., 2009; Kohut and Riddell, 2009).

The **Premature Infant Pain Scale (PIPP)** is a multidimensional measure which assesses acute pain in pre- and full-term infants by gestational age, behavioural state, heart rate, oxygen saturation and facial reactions of brow bulge, eye squeeze and naso labial furrow (Stevens et al., 1996; see Figure 5.7) The PIPP was utilized in a study by

Carbajal et al. (2003) with the French DAN Scale (Douleur Aiguë Nouveau-né), which evaluates acute pain in newborn infants with a behaviour scale comprised of ratings of facial expressions, limb movements and vocal expressions. The study explored the efficacy of breast feeding for pain relief during venepuncture procedures of full-term neonates. Nonpharmacological interventions are important for infants, who undoubtedly feel pain but usually do not receive analgesia for procedural pain because of concerns about effectiveness and side-effects. Importantly, this study found that breast feeding effectively reduced infants' responses to minor invasive procedural pain, probably through the provision of comfort, solace and close social contact, reflecting the biopsychosocial nature of human pain mechanisms.

The **FLACC Scale** (Merkel et al., 1997) is a behavioural scale for scoring postoperative pain in young children and is widely used in this population group. FLACC stands for:

Face

Legs

Activity

Cry

Consolability

Johansson and Kokinsky (2009) compared and evaluated the COMFORT B scale (Van Dijk et al., 2005) with the FLACC Scale for validity in pain assessment and sedation in intubated and ventilated infants and children. Children's self-reporting of pain is the gold standard. However, intubated children are sedated and receive analgesia and are therefore unable to self-report their pain experience and are at risk of physiological and psychological distress in the event of under-controlled pain or inadequate sedation. The study found the FLACC Scale showed construct validity for measuring pain, whereas the COMFORT B scale was a more reliable measure of sedation than of pain, giving substantially more information about sedation than the FLACC Scale. The FLACC Scale should not be used in older persons with dementia, who require assessment of different behavioural indicators for pain (Herr et al., 2006; Kovach et al., 2002).

## The assessment of pain and discomfort in older people

The Number and Verbal Rating scales and Faces Pain Scale-Revised (Hicks et al., 2001) are excellent generally for older people and for people with mild cognitive impairment who can comprehend the pain intensity rating task. Behavioural indicators, as recommended by the American Geriatric Society, are useful as measures of pain for older people who have Alzheimer's disease or similar dementia, or for an adult person who is severely cognitively impaired and unable to verbalize their experience of pain and associated distress.

The **Assessment of Discomfort in Dementia (ADD) Protocol** aims to make a differential assessment and treatment plan for both physical pain and affective discomfort (distress) experienced by people with dementia. The ADD is complex to utilize and nurses require extensive training in how to implement the five steps involved. Where it is feasible to implement it, particularly in residential settings for cognitively impaired adults, the ADD protocol is associated with a significant increase in the use of scheduled analgesics and nonpharmacological comfort interventions and a significant decrease in patient discomfort. It also has validity (Herr et al., 2006; Kovach, 2002).

The British Geriatrics Society (2013) has issued guidance on the management of pain in older people, stating that pain in cognitively impaired older people is often under-recognized and under-managed. Many older people in residential care have serious and very painful comorbidities and require regular assessment and treatment with 'at the clock' slow-dose non-opioid (paracetamol, acetaminophen) medications initially and then gradually titrated to their pain requirement. The administration of drugs should be monitored for effectiveness and side-effects (particularly for conditions associated with liver disease), changing to a slow release, stronger preparation if required to bring the person's pain under control. When using a scale to assess pain and discomfort, the question to ask is 'Does this scale work for its purpose?' If the scale identifies the patient's pain, then that is the scale to use.

However, care is required that the scale measures what it claims to measure. Behaviour indices do not substitute for pain intensity measures. The Abbey Scale (Abbey et al., 2004) purported to assess acute and chronic pain and acute on chronic pain, and is a quick scale for assessing behaviour indices in people with dementia who cannot verbalize, but lacks validity and reliability. The Abbey Scale includes four of the six pain behaviour indicators recommended by the American Geriatric Society's (AGS) Guidelines, but also includes a physiological pain measure which is not supported by the literature to assess chronic pain (American Geriatric Society Panel on Persistent Pain in Older Persons, 2002).

The PACSLAC (Pain Assessment Checklist for Seniors with Limited Ability to Communicate) has supporting evidence of scale validity for an older population and is comprehensive, addressing the six pain behaviour indicators recommended by the AGS Guidelines (facial expressions, verbalizations, body movements, changes in interpersonal interactions, changes in activity patterns or routines, and mental status changes) the PACSLAC should be completed on observing mobility and transfer in the older person and their behaviour over time in any one day (American Geriatric Society, 2002; Fuchs-Lacelle and Hadjistavropoulos, 2004; Herr et al., 2006).

The British Pain Society website (www.britishpainsociety.org) has downloadable Number Rating Scales for pain and distress in many different languages, making communication of their present pain intensity and distress easier for non-English-speaking patients.

Two further factors impact on nurses' decisions to utilize pain measurement tools. First is nurse education. Many nurses have resistant attitudes to using pain measures, which, studies show, can be changed by education. This is really important for the second factor, which is patients' expectations of and satisfaction with their care. Patients expect high-quality care. Ideally, pain assessment is aligned with a consideration of the patient's satisfaction with their pain treatment, care and management (Layman et al., 2006; Mason et al., 2011).

## Chapter summary

- Best practice and, increasingly, legislation require that the patient's pain experience is measured and documented as the fifth vital sign and that the information is believed and acted upon.
- Biopsychosocial nursing pain assessment requires measurement of pain intensity and evaluation of pain cause, onset, location, quality, affect, chronology, relieving and aggravating factors, associated symptoms and impact on quality of life.
- Appropriate validated and reliable pain assessment tools should be utilized. They need to take into consideration the patient's age, cognitive and health status, mental ability and clinical diagnosis. The patient's self-report is gold standard.
- Patients generally prefer the Number Rating Scale (NRS) used in conjunction with the Verbal Rating Scale (VRS). The Wong-Baker FACES® Pain Rating Scale and the Faces Pain Scale-Revised (Hicks et al., 2011) are helpful for measuring pain in children aged from 3–4 years and for people with mild cognitive impairment.
- A combination of physiological and behavioural measures are utilized to assess pain in neonates and very young children. Well-validated scales are CRIES, PIPP FLACC. Severely cognitively impaired people require tools validated for this population (PACSLAC and ADD).
- The revised McGill Pain Questionnaire SF-MPQ-2 has excellent reliability and validity, and may help to diagnose a pain problem, as recent research shows that different pain qualities are associated with different causes and pain types.
- The biopsychosocial assessment contributes essential information to the patient's care plan, together with regular unidimensional pain measurement to optimize pain treatment and management.
- Competency in the knowledge of anatomy and physiology involved in different types of pain (e.g. a patient's experience of 'electric shock' pain associated with a compressed sciatic nerve) improves the nurse's pain management skills.

## Reflective exercise

Consider how pain measurement and assessment can make a positive difference to a patient's health outcome.

## Recommended reading

Flor, H. and Turk, D.C. (2011) *Chronic Pain: An Integrated Biobehavioural Approach*. Seattle, WA: International Association for the Study of Pain.

Pasero, C. and McCaffery, M. (2011) *Pain Assessment and Pharmacologic Management*. St Louis, MO: Elsevier Mosby.

Turk, D.C. and Melzack, R. (2011) *Handbook of Pain Assessment* (3rd edn). New York: Guilford Press.

## Websites relevant to this chapter

Topics in pain management (a slide compendium; pain assessment): www.stoppain.org/for_professionals/compendium/

The British Pain Society (Pain Scales in Multiple Languages): www.britishpainsociety.org/pub_pain_scales.htm

Chronic pain Ireland online pain measurement tool: www.paintracker.ie/

PROQoLID: www.proqolid.org

# References

Abbey, J.A., Piller, N., DeBellis, A. Estermann, A., Parker, D., Giles, L. and Lowcay, B. (2004) The Abbey Pain Scale: a 1-minute numerical indicator for people with late stage dementia. *International Journal of Palliative Nursing*, 10 (1): 6–13.

American Geriatric Society Panel on Persistent Pain in Older Persons (2002) The management of persistent pain in older persons. *Journal of the American Geriatric Society*, 50: S205–S224.

Berry, P.H. and Dahl, J.L. (2000) The new JCAHO pain standards: implications for pain management nurses. *Pain Management Nursing*, 1 (1): 3–12.

Breivik, H., Borchgrevink, P.C., Allen, S.M., Rosseland, L.A., Romundstad, L., Breivik, E.K., Kvarstein, G. and Stubhaug, A. (2008) Assessment of pain. *British Journal of Anaesthesia*, 101 (1): 17–24.

British Geriatrics Society (2013) Guidance on the management of pain in older people. *Age and Ageing*, 42 (Suppl 1): i1–i57.

Carbajal, R., Veerapen, S., Couderc, S., Jugie, M. and Ville, Y. (2003) Analgesic effect of breast feeding in term neonates: randomised controlled trial. *British Medical Journal*, 326: 13.

Chapman, C.R., Casey, K.L., Dubner, R., Foley, K.M., Gracely, R.H. and Reading, A.E. (1985) Pain measurement. *Pain*, 22: 1–31.

Chimello, J.T., Gaspardo, C.M., Cugler, T.S., Martinez, F.E. and Linhares, M.B.M. (2009) Pain reactivity and recovery in preterm neonates: latency, magnitude and duration of behavioural responses. *Early Human Development*, 85: 313–318.

Clark, W.C. and Clark, S.B. (1980) Pain responses in Nepalese porters. *Science*, 209: 410–412.

de Rond, M. and de Wit, R. (1999) Daily pain assessment: value for nurses. *Journal of Advanced Nursing*, 29: 436–444.

Defrin, R., Shramm, L. and Eli, E. (2009) Gender role expectations of pain is associated with pain tolerance limit but not with pain threshold. *Pain*, 145: 230–236.

Department of Veterans Affairs (2013) *Pain as the 5th Vital Sign Toolkit*. Available at: www. va.gov/PAINMANAGEMENT/docs/TOOLKIT.pdf (accessed 5 June 2013).

Dworkin, R.H., Turk, D.C., Revicki, D.A., Harding, G., Coyne, K.S., Peirce-Sandner, S., Bhagwat, D., Everton, D., Burke, L.B., Cowan, P., Farrar, J.T., Hertz, S., Max, M.B., Rappaport, R.A. and Melzack, R. (2009) Development and initial validation of an wxpanded and revised version of the Short-form McGill Pain Questionnaire (SF-MPQ-2). *Pain*, 144: 35–42.

Ferrell, B.R. (1995) The impact of pain on quality of life: a decade of research. *Nursing Clinics of North America*, 30 (4): 609–624.

Fink, R. (2000) Pain assessment: the cornerstone to optimal pain management. *BUMC Proceedings*, 13 (3): 236–239. Retrieved from: www.ncbi.nlm.nih.gov/pmc/articles/PMC1317046/?tool=pubmed#B2 (accessed 23 June 2014).

Flor, H. and Turk, D.C. (2011) *Chronic Pain: An Integrated Biobehavioural Approach*. Seattle, WA: International Association for the Study of Pain (IASP).

Fuchs-Lacelle, S. and Hadjistavropoulos, T. (2004) Development and preliminary validation of the pain assessment checklist for seniors with limited ability to communicate. *Pain Management Nursing*, 5 (1): 37–49.

Gallagher, R.M. (2007) Selective, tailored, biopsychosocial pain treatment: our past is our future (Editorials). *Pain Medicine*, 8 (6): 471–474.

Gatchel, R., Peng, Y.B., Peters, M.L., Fuchs, P.N. and Turk, D.C. (2007) The biopsychosocial approach to chronic pain: scientific advances and future directions. *Psychological Bulletin*, 133: 581–624.

Gélinas, C., Fortier, M., Viens, C., Fillion, L. and Puntillon, K. (2004) Pain assessment and management in critically ill intubated patients: a respective study. *American Journal of Critical Care*, 13 (2): 126–135.

Giamberardino, M.A. and Cervero, F. (2007) The neural basis of referred visceral pain. In P.J. Parischa, W.D. Willis and G.F. Gebhart (eds), *Chronic Abdominal and Visceral Pain: Theory and Practice*. New York and London: Informa Healthcare. pp. 177–192.

Giamberardino, M.A., Costantini, R., Affaitati, G., Fabrizio, A., Lapenna, D., Tafuri, E. and Mezzetti, A. (2010) Viscero-visceral hyperalgesia: characterisation in different clinical models. *Pain*, 151: 307–322.

Graham, C., Bond, S., Gerkovich, M. and Cook, M. (1980) Use of the McGill Pain Questionnaire in the assessment of cancer pain: replicability and consistency. *Pain*, 8: 377–387.

Griffin, R.S., Fink, E. and Brenner, G.J. (2010) Functional neuroanatomy of the nociceptive system. In S.M. Fishman, J.C. Ballantyne and J.P. Rathmell (eds), *Bonica's Management of Pain* (4th edn). Riverwoods, IL: Wolters Kluwer/Lippincott Williams and Wilkins.

Grunay, R.V. and Craig, K.D. (1987) Pain expression in neonates: facial action and cry. *Pain*, 28: 395–410.

Hardy, J.D., Wolff, H.G. and Goodell, H.A. (1952) *Pain Sensations and Reactions*. Baltimore, MD: Lippincott Williams and Wilkins.

Haroutinian, S., Nikolajsen, L., Finnerup, N.B. and Jensen, T.S. (2013) The neuropathic component in persistent postsurgical pain: a systematic literature review. *Pain*, 154: 95–102.

Helfand, M. and Freeman, M. (2009) Assessment and management of acute pain in adult medical in patients: systematic review. *Pain Medicine*, 10 (7): 1183–1199.

Herr, K., Bjoro, K. and Decker, S. (2006) Tools for assessment of pain in nonverbal older adults with dementia: a state of the science review. *Journal of Pain and Symptom Management*, 31: 170–192.

Hicks, C.L., von Baeyer, C.L., Spafford, P.A. van Korlaar, I. and Goodenough, B.L. (2001) The Faces Pain Scale-Revised: toward a common metric in pediatric pain measurement. *Pain*, 93: 173–183.

Hooten, W.M., Timming, R., Belgrade, M., Gaul, J., Goertz, M., Haake, B., Myers, C., Noonan, M.P., Owens, J., Saeger, L., Schweim, K., Shteyman, G. and Walker, N. (2013) *Assessment and Management of Chronic Pain*. Minnesota: Institute for Clinical Systems Improvement.

Jarrell, J., Giamberardino, M.A., Robert, M. and Esfahahni, M.N. (2011) Bedside testing for chronic pelvic pain: discriminating visceral from somatic pain. *Pain Research and Treatment*, doi:10.1155/2011/692102.

Jensen, M.P. (2010) Measurement of pain. In S.M. Fishman, J.C. Ballantyne and J.P. Rathmell (eds), *Bonica's Management of Pain* (4th edn). Riverwoods, IL: Wolters Kluwer/Lippincott Williams and Wilkins.

Jensen, M.P. and Karoly, P. (2001) Self-report scales and procedures for assessing pain in adults. In D.C. Turk and R. Melzack (eds), *Handbook of Pain Assessment* (2nd edn). New York: Guilford Press.

Johansson, M. and Kokinsky, E. (2009) The COMFORT behavioural scale and the modified FLACC scale in paediatric intensive care. *Nursing in Critical Care*, 14 (3): 122–130.

Joint Commission on Accreditation of Healthcare Organizations (2009, October). *JCAHO Standards for Pain Management: Comprehensive Accreditation Manual for Hospitals (CAMH): The Official Handbook*. Joint Commission Resources. PC-7–PC-8. Update 2. Washington, DC: JCAHO.

Joint Commission on Accreditation of Healthcare Organizations (2012) *Pain Management: A Systems Approach to Improving Quality and Safety*. Joint Commission Resources. Washington, DC: JCAHO.

Joshi, S.K. and Gebhart, G.F. (2000) Visceral pain. *Current Review of Pain*, 4: 499–506.

Kohut, S.A. and Riddell, R.P. (2009) Does the Neonatal Facial Coding System differentiate between infants experiencing pain-related and non-pain related distress? *The Journal of Pain*, 10 (2): 214–220.

Kovach, C.R., Noonan, P.E. Griffie, J., Muchka, S. and Weisssman, D.E. (2002) The assessment of discomfort in dementia protocol. *Pain Management Nursing*, 3 (1): 16–27.

Krechel, S. and Bildner, J. (1995) A new neonatal postoperative pain measure score: initial testing of validity and reliability. *Pediatric Anesthesia*, 5 (1): 53–61.

Kremer, E., Hampton Atkinson, J. and Ignelszi, R.J. (1981) Measurement of pain: patient preference does not confound pain measurement. *Pain*, 10: 241–248.

Krueger, A.B. and Stone, A.A. (2008) Assessment of pain: a community-based diary survey in the USA. *Lancet*, 371: 1519–1525.

Layman, J.L., Horton, F.M. and Davidhizar, R. (2006) Nursing attitudes and beliefs in pain assessment and management. *Journal of Advanced Nursing*, 53 (4): 412–421.

LeBel, A.A. (2006) Assessment of pain. In J.C. Ballantyne (ed.), *The Massachusetts General Hospital Handbook of Pain Management* (3rd edn). Philadelphia, PA: Lippincott Williams and Wilkins.

Mason, S.T., Fauerbach, J.A. and Haythornthwaite, J.A. (2011) Assessment of acute pain, pain relief and patient satisfaction. In D.C. Turk and R. Melzack (eds), *Handbook of Pain Assessment* (3rd edn). New York: Guilford Press.

McCaffery, M. (1968) cited in McCaffery, M., Beebe, A., Latham, J. and Ball, D. (eds) (1994) *Pain: Clinical Manual for Nursing Practice*. London and St Louis, MO: Mosby.

McCaffrey, M. and Beebe, A. (1994) *Pain: Clinical Manual*. UK Edition. London: Mosby.

McCaffery, M. and Pasero, C. (1999) *Pain: Clinical Manual* (2nd edn). St Louis, MO: Mosby.

McGuire, D.B. (1992) Comprehensive and multidimensional assessment and measurement of pain. *Journal of Pain and Symptom Management*, 7: 312–319.

Melzack, R. (1975) The McGill Pain Questionnaire: major properties and scoring methods. *Pain*, 1: 277–299.

Melzack, R. and Torgerson, W.S. (1971) On the language of pain. *Anaesthesiology*, 34: 50–59.

Melzack, R. and Wall, P.D. (1965) Pain mechanisms: a new theory. *Science*, 150: 971–979.

Melzack, R. and Wall, P.D. (1982/1988) *The Challenge of Pain*. London: Penguin.

Merkel, S.I., Voepel-Lewis, T., Shayevitiz, J.R. et al. (1997) The FLACC: a behavioural scale for scoring postoperative pain in young children. *Pediatric Nursing*, 23 (3): 293–297.

Nayak, S., Shiflett, S., Eshun, S. and Levine, F.M. (2000) Culture and gender effects in pain beliefs and the prediction of pain tolerance. *Cross-Cultural Research*, 34: 135–151.

Ngamkham, S., Vincent, C., Finnegan, L., Holden, J.E., Wang, Z.J. and Wilkie, D. (2012) The McGill Pain Questionnaire as a multidimensional measure in people with cancer: an integrative review. *Pain Management Nursing*, 13 (1): 27–51.

Nworah, U. (2012) From documentation to the problem: controlling post operative pain. *Nursing Forum*, 47 (2): 91–99.

Pasero, C. and McCaffery, M. (2011) *Pain Assessment and Pharmacologic Management*. St Louis, MO: Elsevier Mosby.

Paulson-Conger, M., Leske, J., Maidl, C., Hanson, A. and Dziadulewicz, L. (2011) Comparison of two pain assessment tools in nonverbal critical care patients. *Pain Management Nursing*, 12 (4): 218–224.

Richardson, C. (2012) An introduction to the biopsychosocial complexities of managing wound pain. *Journal of Wound Care*, 2 (6): 267–273.

Skevington, S. (1996) *Psychology of Pain*. Chichester: Wiley.

Stevens, B., Johnston, C., Petryshen, P. and Taddio, A. (1996) Premature Infant Pain Profile: development and initial validation. *Clinical Journal of Pain*, 12 (1): 13–22.

Thakur, R., Kent, J.L. and Dworkin, R.H. (2010) Herpes zoster and postherpetic neuralgia. In S.M. Fishman, J.C. Ballantyne and J.P. Rathmell (eds), *Bonica's Management of Pain* (4th edn). Riverwoods, IL: Wolters Kluwer/Lippincott Williams and Wilkins.

Tracey, I. and Mantyh, P.W. (2007) The cerebral signature for pain perception and modulation. *Neuron*, 55: 377–391.

Van Dijk, M., Peters, J.W.B., van Deventer, P. and Tibboel, D. (2005) The COMFORT Behaviour Scale: a tool for assessing pain and sedation in infants. *American Journal of Nursing*, 105: 33–36.

Veterans' Health Administration (2003) *VHA Pain Outcomes Toolkit*. Available at: www1.va.gov/PAINMANAGEMENT/Clinical_Resources.asp (accessed 23 June 2014).

Veterans' Health Administration (2009) *VHA Directive 2009–053 (Pain Management)*. Available at: www1.va.gov/PAINMANAGEMENT/docs/VHA09PainDirective.pdf (accessed 23 June 2014).

Vickers, N., Wright, S. and Staines, A. (2014) Surgical nurses in teaching hospitals in Ireland: understanding pain. *British Journal of Nursing*, 23 (17): 924–929.

Williams, D.A. (1996) Acute pain management. In R.J. Gatchel and D.C. Turk (eds), *Psychological Approaches to Pain Management: A Practitioner's Handbook*. New York: Guilford Press.

Wong, D.L. and Baker, C.M. (1988) Pain in children: comparison of assessment scales. *Pediatric Nursing*, 14 (1): 9–17.

Zborowski, M. (1952) Cultural components in responses to pain. *Journal of Social Issues*, 8: 16–30.

Zigmond, A.S. and Snaith, R.P. (1983) The Hospital Anxiety and Depression Scale. *Acta Psychiatrica Scandinavica*, 67: 361–370.

# 6

# Communication in pain management

## Learning objectives

The learning objectives of this chapter are to:

- understand the components of the biopsychsocial model and patient-centred care
- be familiar with the conditions and skills for optimal nurse–patient communication
- recognize effective communication strategies in pain management
- recognize the need to listen to the patient's narrative of their pain experience

## Introduction

A humanistic approach to nursing care (i.e. an approach concerned with the welfare and dignity of humans) complements other nursing patient care approaches. The meaning of nursing derives from synonyms of the word 'nurse' which infer healing, fostering and sustaining. They signify that the aim of nursing is to promote an outcome of patient well-being through developmental, progressive and sustaining participatory processes. Nursing processes, through valuing the individual's or groups' capacity for innovative and creative change, transcend the boundary between nurse and patient. This chapter links the biopsychosocial model to principles of patient-centred care and explores the basic principles of nurse–patient communication relevant to pain management.

## Nursing and holistic patient care

Nursing is concerned with the human experiences of suffering, guilt, fear, anger and hopelessness, which often accompany the illness experience of the patient and his or her family. Nursing theory is influenced by a range of different theories from, for example, psychology, neurobiology, sociology, anthropology, ethics and counselling. Humanistic nursing offers a method for describing human phenomena from the patient's lived experiences, facilitating a truly patient-centred approach to nursing care. Modern nursing has moved away from the conceptualization of nursing as a 'doing for' process to one that regards the patient as a partner in his or her own healthcare (Arnold, 2003; Monti and Tingen, 2006; Reed, 2011).

## The modern-day return to an holistic approach to patient care

Later twentieth-century medicine became more accurate through the identification of diseases by the classification of sets of signs and symptoms, the use of clinical guidelines based on laboratory testing, technological advances such as biomarkers and imaging, and the implementation of decision systems based on an empirical paradigm. This mechanistic approach on its own does not address the patient's personal needs, views and concerns, and is less than satisfactory in fostering an optimal doctor/healthcare professional–patient relationship. Despite a lack of accurate knowledge of human anatomy and physiology, ancient holistic medicine systems focused on the whole patient, with the practitioner monitoring both the patient's bodily state and his or her illness experience and adjusting treatment accordingly. The modern-day return to an holistic approach to patient care is consistent with the first two principles of the World Health Organization's constitution:

1. Health is a complete state of physical, emotional and social well-being and not merely the absence of disease or infirmity.
2. The enjoyment of the highest attainable standard of health is one of the fundamental rights of every human being without distinction of race, religion, political belief, economic or social condition (WHO, 2006/1946).

## The evolution and definition of patient-centred care (PCC)

(In this section, the terms 'patient' and 'person' are used interchangeably.)

Patient-centred care (PCC), some concepts for which date back to Florence Nightingale, facilitates the development of a healthcare professional–patient relationship which focuses on the care recipient rather than the disease. The term *patient-centred medicine* was first used in the 1960s by Balint (1968), who emphasized that patient care should be provided on the basis of understanding each patient within the context of his or her personal circumstances. The concept of the patient-centred care (PCC) has been strongly promoted by the Institute of Medicine in its publication *Crossing the Quality Chasm* (Institute of Medicine, 2001; see also Morgan and Yoder, 2012). More recently, as shown in Table 6.1, more definitions of PCC have evolved.

**Table 6.1**  Definitions of patient-centred care, 2001–2012

| Author | Date | Definition of patient-centred care |
|---|---|---|
| Institute of Medicine | 2001 | Care that is respectful and responsive to individual patient preferences, needs, and values, and ensuring that patient values guide all clinical decisions. (p. 49) |
| Suhonen, Välimäki and Leino-Kilpi | 2002 | Comprehensive care that meets each patient's physical, psychological and social needs. |
| McCormack | 2003 | The formation of a therapeutic narrative between professional and patient that is built on mutual trust, understanding and sharing of collective knowledge. |
| Morgan and Yoder | 2012 | An holistic (bio-psychosocial-spiritual) approach to delivering care that is respectful and individualized, allowing negotiation of care and offering choice through a therapeutic relationship where persons are empowered to be involved in healthcare decisions at whatever level is desired by the individual who is receiving the care. |

# The biopsychosocial model and patient-centred care

It is now recognized that it is the interaction of the biopsychosocial model (which also assumes the inclusion of a 'spiritual' dimension within the 'psycho' element and a 'cultural' dimension within the 'social' element) with the patient-centred care (PCC) model (sometimes referred to as patient-centred medicine) that is fundamental to best practice. The World Health Organization has endorsed placing the person at the centre of (a) his or her own healthcare and (b) public health (WHO, 2006/1946). Landmark events in building person-centred medicine took place in the Geneva Conferences of 2008 and 2009, through the collaboration of 16 major global medical and health organizations and committed individuals to form the International College of Person-Centered Medicine (ICPCM, 2009/2011). The International Council of Nurses (ICN) is among the collaborators of this major development in improved patient care. The ICPCM (2009, 2011) stated that: 'The basic thrust of person-centered clinical care is to place the person in context at the centre of health care, shifting the focus of the field from disease to patient to person.'

The conceptual bases of person-centred care include:

- a broad bio-psycho-socio-cultural-spiritual theoretical framework;
- attention to positive-health and ill-health as components of a broad concept of health;

- enhancement of person-centered communication, diagnosis, treatment, prevention and health promotion;
- respect for the autonomy, responsibility and dignity of every person involved;
- promotion of person-centered relationships and partnerships at all levels;
- articulation of person-centered clinical medicine and people-centred public health (taken from the byelaws of the ICPCM (2011)).

Figure 6.1 shows the common and distinct components of patient-centred and biopsychosocial models of care. The patient is at the centre of both models, and the juncture of overlap locates understanding of the patient's subjective experience of illness.

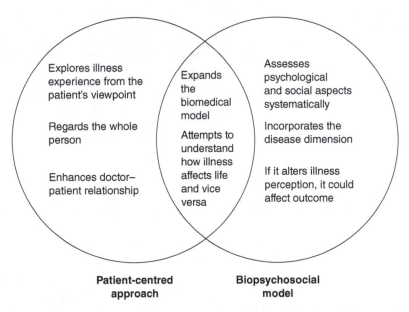

**Figure 6.1** The common and distinct components of the patient-centred approach and biopsychosocial model

Source: Creed, F. (2005) Are the patient-centered the biopsychosocial approaches compatible? In P. White (ed.) *Biopsychosocial Medicine: An Integrated Approach to Understanding Illness*. Oxford: Oxford University Press. Copyright (2005). Republished with permission of Oxford University Press.

## Patient-centred care in nursing

At the inaugural Geneva Conference on patient-centred medicine in 2008, Claudia Bartz (2010) of the International Council of Nurses (ICN), Geneva, Switzerland stated:

> Person-centered care is of utmost importance to the nursing profession. Nurses focus on the person across multiple settings, such as ambulatory,

hospital, and home care, and also in community and public health settings. At any level of care, nurses use the nursing process to structure care delivery as they assess (clients) patients, develop nursing diagnoses, plan and carry out interventions, and evaluate patient outcomes. The nurse's interventions are based on the nursing diagnosis and in support of the medical plan of care for the patient. The patient's outcomes would be in response to the nurse's interventions and the medical plan of care. The International Council of Nurses' (ICN) Code of Ethics notes that 'Inherent in nursing is respect for human rights, including cultural rights, the right to life and choice, to dignity and to be treated with respect. Nursing care is respectful of and unrestricted by considerations of age, colour, creed, culture, disability or illness, gender, sexual orientation, nationality, politics, race or social status' (ICN, 2006).

The International Council of Nurses gives the following definition of nursing:

- Nursing encompasses autonomous and collaborative care of individuals of all ages, families, groups and communities, sick or well and in all settings.
- Nursing includes the promotion of health, prevention of illness, and the care of ill, disabled and dying people.
- Advocacy, promotion of a safe environment, research, participation in shaping health policy and in patient and health systems management, and education are also key nursing roles (ICN, 2009).

Studies show that nurses play a vital role in the provision of PCC. In professional nursing practice, the concept of holism as a fundamental orientation of the nurse to the care of the patient as a person is recognized as a prerequisite to best quality practice. A study by McCormack and McCance (2006) identified four constructs in the person-centred nursing framework:

1. Prerequisites: focusing on the attributes of the nurse.
2. The care environment: focusing on the context in which care is delivered.
3. Person-centred processes: focusing on delivering care through a range of activities.
4. Expected outcomes: the results of effective person-centred nursing.

A narrative review by Kitson et al. (2013) identified three main themes in PCC:

1. Patient participation and involvement.
2. Relationship between the patient and the healthcare professional.
3. The context where the care is delivered.

# Prerequisite conditions and skills for person-centred nurse–patient communication

This section describes the nursing attributes and skills required for optimal nurse–patient communication with relevant, well-recognized theories and guidelines.

## The provision of core conditions by the nurse to the patient: empathy, congruence, unconditional positive regard and spiritual way of being

The humanistic concepts developed by the American psychologist **Carl Rogers** for person-centred counselling are highly relevant to nursing practice and patient-centred care (Rogers, 1961). Rogers introduced the term 'person-centred' to reflect the human values and mutuality between the person and the therapist. The central hypothesis of the person-centred approach is that the vast resources for self-understanding and for change can be activated within any person, if facilitated by the helper's provision of the three core conditions of empathy, congruence and unconditional positive regard. These three attitudes on the part of the helper emphasize the primacy of the person being helped, who, through the type of helping relationship provided, finds the capacity for personal development and change within him- or herself. The practice of person-centred counselling emphasizes the quality of the interpersonal relationship. Rogers later added a spiritual way of being as another helper core condition. Rogers encouraged other people and colleagues to develop his theory further (Arnold, 2011; Nelson-Jones, 1995; Rogers, 1961).

## The provision of attitudes of caring, love and compassion between nurse and patient

**Jean Watson** is an internationally renowned nurse, philosopher, theorist and teacher, Distinguished Professor of Nursing and Founder Director of the Watson Institute of Caring Science, Colorado, USA, who founded the theory of human caring. Watson's theory of human caring has given a substantial philosophical, scientific, ethical and spiritual foundation to nursing internationally (Foster, 2007). According to Watson, caring transcends models and theories and is central to the professional discipline of nursing (Watson and Smith, 2002). Watson's theory of human caring emphazises caring as a moral and scientific commitment to humanity, the enactment of which, in nursing practice, preserves both human dignity and humanity in systems and society. Watson's theory of human caring has helped to distinguish nursing from medicine and has influenced teaching and nursing practice and research internationally. It is considered a benchmark for the quality of care in the US Magnet hospitals' initiatives (Clarke et al., 2009).

Watson's theory of human caring drew on a wide range of philosophical and psychological theories. In particular, the humanistic concepts developed by carl Rogers have influenced Watson's work (Arnold, 2011). A caritas (love of human-kind) process is the core element to Watson's theory of human caring to guide nurses to practice human caring in an authentic, transpersonal, healing relationship (Lukose, 2011). Watson has described Caritas nursing as 'making new connections between caring and love as the energetic basis for sustaining humanity. Increasingly, hospitals, educational programmes' representatives and people committed to expanding and implementing caring implement theory/caritas nursing models' (Clarke et al., 2009). In 1995 The American Nurses' Association revised its definition and policy statement of nursing to include caring (Watson and Smith, 2002). Caring, as a framework for nursing, fits with generalist nurse practices. Holistic nursing care, which emphasizes the caring–healing relationship between the nurse and the patient, thus ensuring that the patient's quality of life and inner healing experiences are at the centre of the relationship, impacts positively on patient outcomes and the success of the system delivering care. In an article about caring science, presented through an interview and dialogue format, Watson stated that:

> Humanitarian healing and caring science is becoming trans-disciplinary, whereby the nursing focus on caring is relevant to all healthcare professionals and scholars. ... The central task of all health professionals' education in nursing, medicine, dentistry, public health, psychology, social work, and the allied health professionals must be to help students, faculty and practitioners learn how to form caring healing relationships with patients, their communities, with each other and themselves. (Clarke et al., 2009)

In patient-centred care, quality of care also depends on the healthcare professional's state of mind, body and spirit. Caring begins with the nurse acknowledging the patient's suffering, with the patient describing his or her experience of suffering in terms of subjective meaning (Ellis, 1999). Caring is the heart of nursing, and is therefore an obligation to patients, families, communities and the universe. Figure 6.2 shows the practice model comprising the four elements of Watson's theory of human caring, which are:

- caritas process;
- transpersonal caring relationship;
- caring moment;
- caring healing modalities.

The nurse treats the patient as a whole person and the nurse–patient relationship is authentic, transpersonal and caring (Lukose, 2011).

As well as the core conditions for personal change and development put forward by Rogers, practical skills derived from Rogers' counselling and psychotherapy work are helpful in improving healthcare professional–patient communication

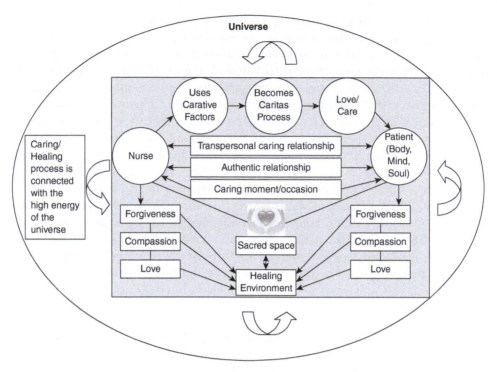

**Figure 6.2**    Watson's theory of human caring – a practical model

Source: After Lukose, A. (2011) Developing a practice model for Watson's Theory of Caring. *Nursing Science Quarterly*, 24: 27–30.

(Arnold, 2003, 2011; Nelson-Jones, 1995). While the terms 'client' and 'service-user' are used throughout the counselling, nursing and healthcare literature, for the purposes of this text the term 'patient' will be used to denote the person who is the primary care recipient.

Psychologist Gerard Egan developed the SOLER acronym to accompany his book, *The Skilled Helper* (1975, 2009), which is a renowned counselling textbook based on Rogers' work. Egan's SOLER (1975) acronym continues to be used extensively by all interdisciplinary team healthcare professionals, including nurses, to optimize a physical way of being when communicating with patients and families.

## SOLER: Guidelines for visibly 'tuning-in' to the patient

S stands for: Sit facing the patient Squarely. Adopting this posture non-verbally indicates interest, involvement and availability to listen to the patient. Body orientation should be congruent with what the nurse is trying to do in terms of making contact that is empathic and non-threatening with the patient.

O represents adopting an **O**pen position and posture which, in many countries, is indicated by sitting facing the patient with arms and legs uncrossed, in order to increase the non-verbal communication of openness and availability. In order to convey non-verbally his or her attitudes of empathy and open-mindedness to the patient, the nurse's posture should mirror what is in his or her heart.

L stands for **L**eaning towards the patient and indicates the nurse's involvement and interest. Postural position and flexibility is important so that the nurse's upper body can easily move towards and away from the patient, as appropriate.

E stands for maintaining good **E**ye contact without staring, which conveys interest, involvement and a desire to listen to the person. Looking away too frequently may give the idea to the person that the nurse is reluctant to be with them. Eye contact is a highly culturally sensitive behaviour, so it is important to know the patient's cultural background and their probable interpretation of eye contact for both the nurse and the patient to be comfortable.

R is for being **R**elaxed and natural in these behaviours, which helps the patient to be more at ease with the nurse.

Voice direction is very important for blind or visually impaired patients. Egan (2009) has suggested that, rather than using the letter 'E' in SOLER, for people who are visually impaired or blind, the letter 'E' becomes 'A' (SOLAR) for **A**im. Aiming the head and body in the direction of the person with the sight impediment, so that he or she can hear the speaker's voice, indicates that the speaker is addressing him or her directly. What is particularly important is that blind and visually impaired people are very sensitive to the orientation of the speaker. For both sighted and blind or visually impaired patients, anything that distracts from the nurse's non-verbally 'being there' can harm the interaction and quality of the dialogue. In order to be respectful, empathic, genuine and caring, internal attitudes have to be reflected in the nurse's external behaviours (Egan, 2009).

# Culture and competency

An adaptation of the acronym SOLER is the acronym SURETY, which stands for 'Sit at an angle', 'Uncross legs and arms', 'Relax', 'Eye contact', 'Touch', and 'Your intuition'. The SURETY model advances the SOLER model to include the use of touch and the importance of individual intuition and thinking about therapeutic space. It is necessary to be aware that touch, personal space and direct eye contact are highly culturally determined patient preferences, and the nurse needs to be sensitive to these aspects of communication in each patient interview and dialogue and to adjust non-verbal behaviour accordingly (Buscemi, 2011; DeVito, 2009; Stickley, 2011).

While cognizant of his or her own cultural background and identity, the culturally competent nurse respects the values, beliefs and attitudes of diverse populations. (The reader is referred to the work of Campinha-Bacote (2002) regarding becoming culturally competent in healthcare delivery.) Awareness of the patient's cultural and social context helps the nurse to understand the meaning of the impact of the patient's pain experience on their quality of life and their family. Globally, people of different racial and ethnic backgrounds relocate to other countries, retaining elements of their former culture and acquiring elements of their new culture. Competency in understanding cultural mores is vital for the nurse who has regular contact with patients and their families from different ethnic and racial backgrounds. Time taken to ascertain the ethnicity of the patient and their expectations with regard to communication and social interaction can be very beneficial for optimal nurse–patient interactions (Arnold, 2011; DeVito, 2009; Hadjistavropoulos et al., 2011).

## Active listening to facilitate optimal nurse–patient communication

While the holistic (biopsychosocial) care model incorporates all aspects of the patient as individual, that is, mind, body and spirit, the patient-centred care model (PCC) empowers the patient by allowing him or her to identify and determine his or her own needs. This approach to care requires that the healthcare professional is also a skilled listener and that the patient is able to communicate his or her needs, or be able to rely on close family to assist if required. PCC also encourages the healthcare professional to reflect on his or her practice and to strive for personal and professional growth (Ellis, 1999).

PCC promotes an egalitarian healthcare professional–patient relationship so that the patient's voice is heard and the patient is empowered to convey the personal meaning of illness (Mead and Bower, 2000). Having regard to the person means listening to their story to understand the impact of pain on their lives. This is relevant both in acute and chronic pain because understanding the person empowers him or her to adopt a partnership approach to care and therefore helps to maximize his or her health outcomes. The relief of pain and suffering is a primary nursing goal linked to patient empowerment. In pain management, both the measurement of the patient's subjective pain experience and the patient's narrative of their pain experience provide the means to effectively intervene, treat and prevent pain (Lovell and Boyle, 2010). Listening is the major skill requirement for all healthcare professionals in optimal patient–healthcare communication regardless of their role in the interdisciplinary team and in the care setting. Research has shown that good communication skills can be taught. Brief educational interventions in communication skills for both patients and healthcare professionals have been shown to benefit both groups (Cegala and Lenzmeier, 2003).

Active listening requires an attentive focus on the content of what the person is trying to say in order to understand both the meaning and feelings behind the words. This means being attentive both to the verbal and non-verbal language. Active listening is especially important and is a core communication skill (Moss, 2008). The nurse's personal actions, attributes and skills interact within the contextual requirements to effect communication which include people as message sources–receivers; their processes of message encoding–decoding interact with communication channels, which can be face to face, via telephone or mobile or other technology as in texting, email, conference calls and Skyping.

## Communication as transaction/interaction

Each person involved in communication gives and receives messages, that is, each person is both a source (or speaker) and a receiver (or listener). Each person who is speaking, writing/texting, gesturing or smiling is sending a message and each person listening, reading, watching, observing non-verbal behaviour is receiving a message. Therefore, people who are communicating are both sending and receiving messages within a context, via a channel. The channel can be verbal, that is, oral or written, in person or via technology, and non-verbal, such as how a person dresses, their body gestures and body language.

The act of putting thoughts and ideas into words is called **encoding**, while the act of receiving and understanding messages is called **decoding**. Because the person is often listening, or observing the non-verbal behaviour of the receiver, and speaking at the same time, encoding and decoding are usually performed simultaneously (DeVito, 2009).

Communication is an active and dynamic transactional event. The transactional nature of communication means that all the elements are in a constant state of change. Each element of communication is linked to the other elements, for example, each message received requires a message source. While each person participating in the communication in person interacts in the present time, or if communicating using modern technology in the present or the past time, their message content and quality and tone of interaction is influenced by many factors, some of which are: how they feel, how past experience is relevant to the communication, their attitudes, self-image, and cultural beliefs.

Frequently, there is no clear-cut beginning or ending in conversations between two people. Usually communication as dialogue in the present time is a circular, dynamic, transactional process, segmented into smaller sections: one person speaks and the other responds in a cause-and-effect manner. Often people punctuate the continuity of the communication to allow for a two-way conversation.

Effective communication requires that each person understands the point of view of the other person, which requires both listening and speaking at appropriate intervals. One of the essential skills of communication is to check on the meaning of the message imparted, as two people listening to the same message may derive very different meanings, depending on the cultural background and experience of each.

The meaning of the message may be distorted by physical (e.g. external sounds), social-psychological (e.g. distractions to attention), and semantic (i.e. cultural and linguistic misinterpretations) 'noise', and the nurse needs to be sensitive to this possibility. Paraphrasing what the patient has said to check back that she or he has really understood the content and meaning of each patient's communication is a vital aid to effective communication (DeVito, 2009). For example, patient education is an important care element in medication management. The nurse needs to check with the patient that he or she fully understands instructions provided about taking medications and especially instructions regarding pain medications.

## Communication skills requirements for nurses

Reflection is the nurse's ability to know him or herself, to reflect on their own skills, to identify where knowledge deficits exist, and to endeavour to enhance learning through new information acquisition and application to nursing practice. Building on the humanistic theory of interpersonal communication developed by Martin Buber (1958), in which individuals respond to each other as unique persons in a mutually respectful 'I–Thou' manner, Duldt's (1991) interpersonal communication in nursing theory recognized the human need to communicate and that the way in which a person communicates determines what the person becomes. Interpersonal communication is a humanizing factor in the nursing process which involves patient assessment, treatment and care planning, and interventions and evaluation (Duldt, 1991). As shown in Table 6.2, Duldt (1991) identified humanizing and dehumanizing communication attitudes, with humanizing communications by the nurse being more likely to result in humanizing communication from patients and colleagues.

**Table 6.2**  Humanizing and dehumanizing communication attitudes

| Humanizing | Dehumanizing | Humanizing | Dehumanizing |
|---|---|---|---|
| Dialogue | Monologue | Empathy | Tolerance |
| Individual | Categories | Authenticity | Role-playing |
| Holistic | Parts | Caring | Careless |
| Choice | Directives | Irreplaceable | Expendability |
| Equality | Degradation | Intimacy | Isolation |
| Positive regard | Disregard | Coping | Helpless |
| Acceptance | Judgement | Power | Powerless |

Source: Duldt, B.W. (1991). 'I–Thou': research supporting humanistic nursing communication theory. *Perspectives of Psychiatric Care*, 27 (3): 5–12. Copyright (1991). Republished with permission of John Wiley and Sons.

In patient-centred care (PCC) the nurse tries to 'get inside the skin' of the patient through empathic listening, establishing a dialogue to create a therapeutic relationship with the patient. Rogers described empathy as an ability to communicate a sensing of the patient's feelings as though they are the listener's own, but without losing the 'as if' quality (Rogers, 1961). Therefore, the nurse is aware of the distinction of self and other (Williams and Stickley, 2010). A trained empathy state can be defined as transient behaviours enacted to convey understanding of another person (Alligood, 2005). A detailed clarification of the derivation of the word 'empathy' and the relevance of empathy in the nurse–patient relationship is given by Määttä (2006).

The basic skills of active listening are:

- being as open, intuitive, empathic and as self-aware as possible;
- maintaining good eye contact;
- having an open and attentive body orientation of posture;
- paying attention to non-verbal forms of communication and meaning;
- allowing for appropriate silence as a form of communication;
- taking up an appropriate physical distance;
- picking up and following cues;
- being aware of your own distracting mannerisms and behaviour;
- avoiding vague, unclear and ambiguous comments;
- being aware of the importance of people finding their own words in their own time;
- remembering the importance of the setting and the general physical environment;
- minimizing the possibility of interruptions and distractions;
- being sensitive to the overall mood of the interview, including what is not being communicated;
- listening for the emotional content of the interview and adapting questions as appropriate;
- checking out and seeking feedback whenever possible and appropriate;
- being aware of the importance of timing, particularly where strong feelings are concerned;
- remembering the importance of tone, particularly in relation to sensitive and painful issues;
- avoiding the dangers of pre-conceptions, stereotyping or labelling, or making premature judgements or evaluations;
- being as natural, spontaneous and relaxed as possible (Trevithick, 2005).

## Nurse communication attributes and the work environment

A study by Wilkinson (1991) investigated the facilitating and blocking factors that influence how nurses communicate with patients with cancer. Table 6.3 outlines categories of facilitative and blocking behaviours used by nurses in Wilkinson's (1991) study. The study found that predictors for facilitating verbal behaviours, in descending order, were:

- the ward the nurse worked on;
- nurses feeling stressed from giving poor care;
- the amount of support given by nurse managers;
- completion of an oncology course;
- nurses' feelings about communicating with patients;
- the number of hobbies (substantially more hobbies equated with fewer facilitating verbal behaviours).

Blocking behaviours (i.e. behaviours which indicate to the patient that the nurse is not interested in listening or which discourage the patient from communicating) were associated with, in descending order:

- the ward the nurse worked on;
- their stated religion or none;
- their own self-awareness of their own verbal behaviours;
- fear of dying;
- level of anxiety;
- the number of hobbies (substantially more hobbies equated with more blocking verbal behaviours);
- conflicts with staff members.

The study highlighted that while nurses have the skills to facilitate patients' open communications, the work environment was particularly important in facilitating effective communication between nurse and patient (Wilkinson, 1991).

**Table 6.3** Facilitative and blocking behaviours used by nurses when communicating with patients with cancer

| Nurses' facilitating verbal behaviours | Nurses' blocking verbal behaviours |
| --- | --- |
| Introduction of self | Normalizing/stereotyped comments |
| Purpose of interview | Premature/false reassurance |
| Acknowledging patient | Inappropriate advice |
| Open questions | Closed/leading multiple questions |
| Encouragement | 'Passing the buck' |
| Pick-up of cue | Requesting an explanation |
| Reflection | Disapproving/disagreeing |
| Clarification | Approving/agreeing |
| Empathy | Defending |
| Confrontation challenge | Change topic/ignoring/selective attention to cue |
| Information giving | Change of focus to relative |
| Summarising problems | Jollying along |
| Patient questions | Personal chit-chat |
| Consultation of plan of action | |

Source: Wilkinson, S. (1991) Factors which influence how nurses communicate with cancer patients. *Journal of Advanced Nursing*, 16, 677–688. Copyright (1991). Republished with permission of John Wiley and Sons.

Effective communication strategies in pain management require an interdisciplinary team approach which requires collaborative working based on:

**Common goals:** the patient care starting point and comfort – care functions as agreed by the team – for pain management, which also includes a pain assessment tool relevant for the patient's age and cognitive status.

**Common language:** the team works with a common language that is understood by the team, and pain assessment tools are included in this approach. The adequate management of the person's pain requires assessment and treatment skills that address potential individual psychological and social differences. Empathic listening is essential. It is also essential to address the pain-related behaviours and cues of neonate patients, patients with speech and language deficits, and patients with varying levels of cognitive impairment.

**Common knowledge base:** the team works with a set of agreed clinical practice guidelines to achieve end goals in patient pain and health outcome and education.

**Regular communication:** the team meets and communicates regularly. Patient care plans, pain assessment tools, and nursing outcomes and reports are correctly completed and documented. Guidelines and fact sheets can be distributed to the patient and interdisciplinary care team members as required. Pain is a relatively new discipline, even for physicians, and many team members appreciate having a brief guideline to follow when questions arise about pain assessment and treatment.

**Patient education:** facts sheets also help patients to understand medication regimens and potential medication side-effects (Craig, 2009; Hadjistavropoulos et al., 2011; Pasero and McCaffery, 2011).

## Patient barriers to reporting pain

Anxiety can increase the pain experience and patients can be admitted to hospital with high levels of pain and anxiety and low expectations of pain relief. Poor nurse–patient communication, lack of use of pain assessment tools and poor nursing documentation can result in the patient's pain experience being disregarded by the nurse and the care team. The patient can be depersonalized by the processes of becoming a patient; for example, changing from personal clothes to a hospital gown, lying for long periods on a hospital trolley, being examined by a number of clinicians and possibly having personal privacy less than fully regarded. The patient can be made to feel fearful of the authority of the medical and nursing team and that the pain they feel is of less interest than their medical condition. Particularly, patients often feel they should not make a fuss or become a 'nuisance patient'.

## The role of cultural influences, empathic listening and patient narrative in accessing the patient's subjective pain experience

A person's culture has a major influence on the development of their neural systems, cognitions and behaviours, which can influence pain sensation and the person's expression of their pain experience (Giordano et al., 2009). Culture may mean the family, the immediate social or work environment or the wider community, and the ethnic and racial aspects of the person's country of residence. Pain is an intermittent feature of the lived experience of each individual in the context of their social world and historical experience. A study by Fabrega and Tyma (1976) showed how sensory neuronal information conveyed to the central nervous system was modified by hormonal, affective and perceptual processes. These processes were influenced by cultural and social factors, demonstrating the complex, multilayered nature of the pain experience and endorsing the individuality of the pain experience.

Considerable suffering can be avoided by addressing the person's individual psychological and social differences. While often pain arises from a mechanical injury to afferent neurons or diseases which destruct the nervous system, a percentage of people suffering pain do not have identified viable tissue pathology or evidence of a pathophysiological process. Narrative competence is the ability to absorb, interpret, understand and respond to the meaning and significance of the patient's story, the healthcare professional responding with empathy, reflection, listening, action and trustworthiness. The narrative approach requires active listening for the especially hidden concerns of the patient. Expression of suffering does not have to be verbal. Art therapies are an important therapy of expression for those suffering from pain and for raising public awareness of the problem of pain (Benedetti, 2011; Braš et al., 2013; Charon, 2001; Đorđević et al., 2012; Egan, 2009; Finset, 2010).

## Conclusion

It is now accepted that mind and body have a circular influence on each other and that the patient's psychological state and social circumstances influence disease pathophysiology and treatment outcomes. The acceptance that the patient's psychological state is influenced by biological factors means that the 'whole' patient, along with his or her emotional, cognitive and motivational experiences, must be at the centre of care. The biopsychosocial model when linked with the patient-centred care model allows for the targeting of psychosocial factors which may influence the patient's therapeutic outcome. Studies show that psychosocial factors, including culture, are linked to brain functions, affirming body and mind interaction, and thus the potential for influencing therapeutic outcome.

# Chapter summary

- Patient-centred care (PCC) places the patient at the centre of his or her care and aims to understand the impact of the patient's illness on his or her quality of life. PCC complements and overlaps with the biopsychosocial model and is endorsed by the World Health Organization.
- PCC reflects a humanistic orientation to nursing care and complements other modern nursing theories and patient care approaches. The patient is regarded as an experiencing individual rather than the object of some disease entity.
- A key role in nursing is preserving the patient's basic integrity, supporting the patient as a person through his or her illness experience, preventing further injury, and providing interventions and educational and emotional support to the patient and his or her family.
- Effective communication skills are prerequisites for appropriate attitudes of caring, love and compassion between the nurse and the patient. They should be exercised to form caring, healing relationships with patients. Reflective practice is important in improving nurse–patient communication.
- Verbal and non-verbal body language comprises essential aspects of communication skills. The useful skills and attitudes developed by renowned counselling and nurse theorists are commonly integrated into nursing care. Active listening is the major skill requirement.
- Communication is active, dynamic and transactional. It is a two-way process in which both people are simultaneously 'sender' and 'receiver' and 'encoder' and 'decoder'. Physical, social, psychological and semantic 'noise' can interfere with the message meaning.
- Empathy, caring and compassion are vital for effective listening and for ascertaining the patient's pain experience. The ethos of the work environment, the nurse's attributes, the patient's participation and the nurse–patient interaction all influence the patient's health outcomes.
- Studies show how the nurse's ability to implement PCC and to communicate effectively are impacted by the culture of the care organization and environment, particularly the nursing unit. Effective staff relationships and supportive organizational systems are essential.

# Reflective exercise

Practice the SOLER and SURETY acronyms in the clinical setting; observe for improvements in your communications with patients and caregivers.

## Recommended reading

Benedetti, F. (2011) *The Patient's Brain: The Neuroscience behind the Doctor–Patient Relationship*. Oxford: Oxford University Press.
Carr, B., Loeser, J.D. and Morris, D.B. (eds) (2005) *Narrative, Pain and Suffering*. Seattle, WA: International Association for the Study of Pain.
Coakley, S. and Kaufman Shelemay, K. (2007) *Pain and its Transformations: The Interface of Biology and Culture*. Cambridge, MA: Harvard University Press.
White, P. (ed). (2005) *Biopsychosocial Medicine: An Integrated Approach to Understanding Illness*. Oxford: Oxford University Press.

## Websites relevant to this chapter

International College of Person-Centered Medicine (ICPCM):
    http://personcentredmedicine.org/mission.php
Watson Caring Science Institute and International Caritas Consortium:
    http://watsoncaringscience.org/
International Council of Nurses, Geneva, Switzerland (definition of nursing):
    www.icn.ch/definition.htm
The Process of Cultural Competence in the Delivery of Healthcare Services Model:
    www.transculturalcare.net/Cultural_Competence_Model.htm

## References

Alligood, M.R. (2005) Rethinking empathy in nursing education: shifting to a developmental view. *Annual Review of Nursing Education*, 3: 299–309.
Arnold, E.C. (2003) Theoretical perspectives and contemporary issues. In E.C. Arnold and K. Underman Boggs, *Interpersonal Relationships: Professional Communication Skills for Nurses*. Philadelphia, PA: Elsevier Saunders.
Arnold, E.C. (2011) Theoretical perspectives and contemporary dynamics. In E.C. Arnold and K. Underman Boggs, *Interpersonal Relationships: Professional Communication Skills for Nurses*. Philadelphia, PA: Elsevier Saunders.
Balint, E. (1968) The possibilities of patient-centred medicine. Paper presented at the symposium conducted at the American Psychiatric Association, New Orleans, LA.
Bartz, C.C. (2010) International Council of Nurses and person-centered care. *International Journal of Integrated Care*, 10: 24–26.
Benedetti, F. (2011) *The Patient's Brain: The Neuroscience behind the Doctor–Patient Relationship*. Oxford: Oxford University Press.

Braš, M., Đorđević, V. and Janjanin, M. (2013) Person-centered pain management: science and art. *Croatian Medical Journal*, 54: 296–300.

Buber, M. (1958) *I and Thou* (2nd edn). Translated and edited by R. Smith. New York: Scribner. Cited in Arnold, E.C. (2003) Theoretical perspectives and contemporary issues. In E.C. Arnold and K. Underman Boggs, *Interpersonal Relationships: Professional Communication Skills for Nurses*. Philadelphia, PA: Elsevier Saunders.

Buscemi, C.P. (2011) Acculturation: state of the science in nursing. *Journal of Cultural Diversity*, 18 (2): 39–42.

Campinha-Bacote, J. (2002) The process of cultural competence in the delivery of healthcare services: a model of care. *Journal of Transcultural Nursing*, 13 (3): 181–129.

Cegala, D.J. and Lenzmeier, S. (2003) Provider and patient communication skills training. In T.L. Thompson, A.M. Dorsey, K.I. Miller and R. Parrott (eds), *Handbook of Health Communication*. Englewood Cliffs, NJ: Lawrence Erlbaum.

Charon, R. (2001) Narrative medicine: a model for empathy, reflection, profession and trust. Journal of the American Medical Association, 286: 1897–1902.

Clarke, P.N., Watson, J. and Brewer, B.B. (2009) From theory to practice: caring science according to Watson and Brewer. *Nursing Science Quarterly*, 22: 339–345.

Craig, K.D. (2009) The social communication model of pain. *Canadian Psychology*, 50: 22–32.

Creed, F. (2005) Are the patient-centred and biopsychosocial approaches compatible? In P. White (ed.), *Biopsychosocial Medicine: An Integrated Approach to Understanding Illness*. Oxford: Oxford University Press.

DeVito, J.A. (2009) *Human Communication: The Basic Course* (11th edn). London Pearson/Allyn Bacon.

Đorđević, V., Braš, M. and Brajković, L. (2012) Person-centered medical interview. *Croatian Medical Journal*, 53: 310–313.

Duldt, B.W. (1991) 'I–Thou': research supporting humanistic nursing communication theory. *Perspectives of Psychiatric Care*, 27 (3): 5–12.

Egan, G. (1975) *The Skilled Helper: A Systematic Approach to Effective Helping*. Pacific Grove, CA: Brooks/Cole.

Egan, G. (2009) *The Skilled Helper: A Problem Management and Opportunity Development to Helping* (9th edn). Belmont, CA: Brooks Cole.

Ellis, S. (1999) The patient-centred care model: holistic/multi professional/reflective. *British Journal of Nursing*, 8 (5): 296–301.

Fabrega, H. and Tyma, S. (1976) Culture language and the shaping of illness: an illustration based on pain. *Journal of Psychosomatic Research*, 20: 323–337. Cited in M. Delvecchio Good, P.E. Brodwin, B.J. Good and A. Kleinman (eds) (1992) *Pain as Human Experience: An Anthropological Perspective*. Berkeley, CA: University of California Press.

Finset, A. (2010) Emotions, narratives and empathy in clinical communication. *International Journal of Integrated Care*, 10: 53–56.

Foster, R.L. (2007) Tribute to the theorists: Jean Watson over the years. *Nursing Science Quarterly*, 20 (7).

Giordano, J., Engebretson, C. and Benedikter, R. (2009) Culture, subjectivity and the ethics of patient-centred pain care. *Cambridge Quarterly of Healthcare Ethics*, 18: 47–56.

Hadjistavropoulos, T., Craig, K.D., Duck S. et al. (2011) A biopsychosocial formulation of pain communication. *Psychological Bulletin*, 137 (6): 910–939.

Institute of Medicine (2001) *Crossing the Quality Chasm*. Washington, DC: National Academies Press. Available at: http://iom.edu/Reports/2001/Crossing-the-Quality-Chasm-A-New-Health-System-for-the-21st-Century.aspx (accessed 23 June 2014).

International College of Person-Centered Medicine (ICPCM) (2009/2011) *By-Laws of the International College of Person-Centred Medicine*. Available at: http://personcentred-medicine.org/docs/participants.pdf (accessed 11 July 2013).

International Council of Nurses (2006) *ICN Code of Ethics*. Geneva: International Council of Nurses.

International Council of Nurses (2009) Definition of nursing. Geneva: International Council of Nurses. Available at: www.icn.ch/definition.htm (accessed 23 June 2014).

Jesse, D.E. (2010) 'Watson's Philosophy and Theory of Transpersonal Caring'. In Alligood, M.R. and Tomey, A.M. *Nursing Theorists and Their Work* (7th edn). St Louis, MO: Elsevier, Mosby.

Kitson, A., Marshall, A., Bassett, K. and Zeitz, K. (2013) What are the core elements of patient-centred care? A narrative review and synthesis of the literature from health policy, medicine and nursing. *Journal of Advanced Nursing*, 69: 4–15.

Lovell, M. and Boyle, F. (2010) Communication strategies and skills for optimal pain control. In D.W. Kissane, B.D. Bultz, P.M. Butow and I.G. Finlay (eds), *Handbook of Communication in Oncology and Palliative Care*. New York: Oxford University Press.

Lukose, A. (2011) Developing a practice model for Watson's Theory of Caring. *Nursing Science Quarterly*, 24: 27–30.

Määttä, S.M. (2006) Closeness and distance in the nurse–patient relation; the relevance of Edith Stein's concept of empathy. *Nursing Philosophy*, 7: 3–10.

McCormack, B. (2003) A conceptual framework for person-centered practice with older people. *International Journal of Nursing Practice*, 9: 202–209.

McCormack, B. and McCance, T.V. (2006) Development of a framework for person-centered nursing. *Journal of Advanced Nursing*, 56: 472–479.

Mead, N. and Bower, P. (2000) Patient-centredness: a conceptual framework and review of the empirical literature. *Social Science and Medicine*, 51: 1087–1110.

Monti, E.J. and Tingen, M.S. (2006) Multiple paradigms of nursing science. In W.K. Cody (ed.), *Philosophical and Theoretical Perspectives for Advanced Nursing Practice* (4th edn). Burlington, MA: Jones and Bartlett Learning.

Morgan, S. and Yoder, L.H. (2012) Concept analysis of person-centered care. *Journal of Holistic Nursing*, 30 (1): 6–15.

Moss, B. (2008) *Communication Skills for Health and Social Care*. London: Sage.

Nelson-Jones, R. (1995) *The Theory and Practice of Counselling* (2nd edn). London: Cassell.

Pasero, C. and McCaffery, M. (2011) *Pain Assessment and Pharmacological Management*. St Louis, MO: Mosby.

Reed, P.G. (2011) Nursing: the ontology of the discipline. In W.K. Cody (ed.), *Philosophical and Theoretical Perspectives for Advanced Nursing Practice* (5th edn). Burlington, MA; Jones and Bartlett Learning (4th edn, 2006).

Rogers, C.R. (1961) *On Becoming a Person*. Boston, MA: Houghton Mifflin.

Stickley, T. (2011) From SOLER to SURETY for effective non-verbal communication. *Nurse Education in Practice*, 11 (6): 395–398.

Suhonen, R., Välimäki, M. and Leino-Kilpi, H. (2002) Individualised care from patients', nurses' and relatives' perspective: a review of the literature. *International Journal of Nursing Studies*, 39: 645–654.

Trevithick, P. (2005) *Social Work Skills: A Practice Handbook* (2nd edn). Maidenhead: Open University Press. Cited in B. Moss (2008) *Communication Skills for Health and Social Care*. London: Sage.

Watson, J. and Smith, M.C. (2002) Caring science and the science of unitary human beings: a trans-theoretical discourse for nursing knowledge development. *Journal of Advanced Nursing*, 37 (5): 45–461.

Wilkinson, S. (1991) Factors which influence how nurses communicate with cancer patients. *Journal of Advanced Nursing*, 16: 677–688.

Williams, J. and Stickley, T. (2010) Empathy and nurse education. *Nurse Education Today*, 30: 752–755.

World Health Organization (2006/1946) Constitution of the WHO. In *Basic Documents* (45th edn). Supplement, October 2006. Amendment WHA 51.23. Geneva: World Health Organization.

# 7

# Pharmacological and interventional pain management

## Learning objectives

The learning objectives of this chapter are to:

- know the definition of and systems associated with the analgesic response
- be cognizant of the endogenous opioid system and implication for therapeutics
- know the basic concepts of pharmacology for pain management in nursing practice
- be aware of the mechanisms of a range of pharmacological and nonpharmacological pain interventions

## Introduction

This chapter outlines the major therapeutic intrinsic and extrinsic drug systems utilized in pain treatment and management, as well as the pharmacological and nonpharmacological interventions that are particularly useful for chronic non-malignant and cancer pain.

## Definitions of pharmacology and analgesia

Pharmacology can be defined as 'the study of the effects of drugs on the function of living systems' (Rang et al., 2012: 1). A drug for therapeutic purposes can be defined as 'a chemical substance of known structure, other than a nutrient or an essential dietary ingredient, which, when administered to a living organism, produces a biological effect' (Rang et al., 2012:1). A medicine usually contains one or more drugs and is administered with the intention of producing a therapeutic effect. Medicines also contain other substances to make them more convenient to use, such as stabilizers and solvents (Rang et al., 2012).

Analgesia can be defined as the 'absence of the spontaneous report of pain or pain behaviours in response to stimulation that would normally be expected to be painful. The term 'analgesia' implies a defined stimulus and defined response and both can be tested in animals and humans (Turk and Okifuji, 2010: 15). The analgesic response in humans can be brought about through:

- an intrinsic analgesia system;
- an endogenous opioid system;
- exogenously, through the administration of analgesic drugs.

## The intrinsic analgesia system

As previously described, responses to pain stimulation vary from person to person and are partly the result of an **intrinsic pain analgesia system,** which has three major components (see Figure 7.1):

- neurons from the midbrain periaqueductal gray (PAG) and periventricular areas of the mesencephalon and upper pons, surrounding the aqueduct of Sylvius and parts of the third and fourth ventricles send signals to:
- the nucleus raphe magnus in the lower pons and upper medulla and the gigantocellular reticular nucleus located laterally in the medulla; second-order signals are transmitted from these nuclei down the dorsolateral columns in the spinal cord to:
- a pain inhibitory complex located in the dorsal horn of the spinal cord where the analgesia signals can block pain signals prior to their being relayed to the brain. (Hall, 2011: 587; see also Haines, 2012)

## The endogenous opioid system

In 1975 the discovery of **endogenous opioids,** enkephalins, followed the identification of the opioid receptor in 1973. Both of these discoveries were predated by research by Reynolds (1969) which showed that abdominal surgery could be performed on awake rats during focal electrical stimulation applied near the midbrain PAG, while the rats continued to respond to tactile stimulation, demonstrating that the midbrain PAG stimulation produced analgesia rather than anaesthesia. These major advances provided important directions for the clinical use of opioid analgesics (Moulin, 2005).

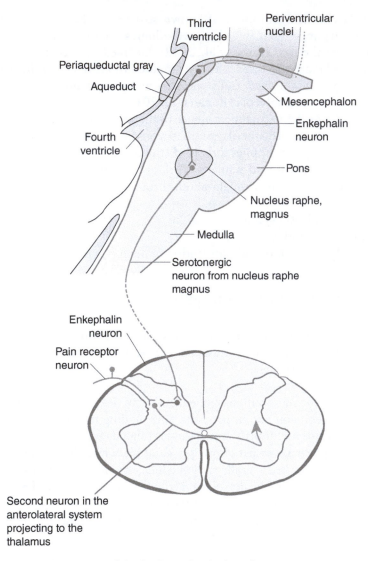

**Figure 7.1** Analgesia system of the brain and spinal cord

Most drugs that alter neuronal excitability act on synaptic receptors. After Reynolds' 1969 publication, further studies sought natural opiates in the brain, leading to the discovery of about a dozen opiate-like substances to date, found at different places in the nervous system. The most important of these are three families of opioid peptides: (a) β-endorphin (located in the hypothalamus and pituitary gland), (b) met-enkephalin and leu-enkephalin (both located in the brain stem and spinal cord), and (c) dynorphin (in smaller quantities also in the brain stem and spinal cord). These three opioid peptides, together with three families of receptors, μ (MOR), δ (λ, DOR) and κ (KOR) comprise the **endogenous opioid system**. Preferentially, enkephalins interact with the δ receptor, dynorphins interact with the κ receptor, and β-endorphins bind to both μ and δ receptors (Benarroch, 2012; Hall, 2011).

- The μ receptor is the most abundant receptor in the amygdala, thalamus and brainstem. The μ receptor is also highly expressed at all levels of the central pain control network, including the anterior cingulate cortex, amygdala, hypothalamus, midbrain PAG, rostral ventromedial medulla (RVM), and superficial dorsal horn, and contributes to multiple aspects of pain modulation.
- The δ receptor is mostly expressed in the cerebral cortex, olfactory system, striatum and limbic cortex. The δ receptor is also expressed in pain modulatory areas of the forebrain and dorsal horn and, to a lower extent, in the brain stem, suggesting that the δ receptor is involved in the primary processing, cognitive and emotional aspects of pain.
- The κ receptor is mostly distributed in the claustrum, striatum and hypothalamus (Benarroch, 2012; Hall, 2011).

## Mechanisms and consequences of opioid receptor activation

- In the dorsal horn and the periphery, μ and δ receptors inhibit the release of glutamate, substance P and calcitonin gene-related peptide from primary dorsal root ganglion (DRG) afferents.
- In the cerebral cortex all opioid receptors inhibit presynaptic glutamate release.
- In many brain regions activation of μ or δ receptors facilitates neuronal output by inhibiting gamma-aminobutyric acid (GABA) release from local inhibitory neurons (Benarroch, 2012).

Enkephalin and serotonin are the two neurotransmitter substances that are especially involved in the analgesia system, along with several others. Suppression of pain signals from the periphery takes place by activation of the analgesic system or by inactivation of pain pathways by the endogenous opioids. Many detailed mechanisms of the body's intrinsic opiate system have yet to be fully explained.

## Endogenous opioids, placebo and nocebo

A **placebo** is a substance (dummy medicine) or procedure (dummy therapeutic intervention) without therapeutic effect that is provided as a treatment, and is frequently used to control patients' expectations for the efficacy in testing a treatment intervention (Turk and Okifuji, 2010). The patient believes the placebo is (and in the context of a controlled trial the patient believes the placebo could be) the real thing. The placebo response is the beneficial effect that follows the administration of a placebo, that is, an inert treatment (Benedetti, 2011). The use of placebo interventions, particularly for pain medicine, poses ethical and moral risks to patients and must only be undertaken in the context of approved clinical trials (Rang et al., 2012). The discovery of endogenous opioids led to research to identify the physiological mechanisms underpinning the placebo response. Studies have shown that the placebo response is certainly, in part, mediated by endogenous opioid mechanisms (Lenz et al., 2010).

The phenomenon of placebo analgesia demonstrates how psychological factors, that is, the patient's belief in the analgesic effectiveness of the treatment, can influence pain perception. A recent fMRI study demonstrated that psychological factors (i.e. expectation and anticipation) can influence nociceptive processing at the dorsal horn of the spinal cord and that one possible mechanism of placebo analgesia is the inhibition of spinal cord nociceptive processing, mediated by the descending pain control system in a gate control manner (Eippert et al., 2009). This important study showed that it is possible to measure modulatory influences on spinal cord activity, indicating the potential for further research and new developments in pain treatment. While currently the exact mechanism is not yet fully understood, it is likely that, in placebo analgesia, endogenous opioids play a major role in the descending pain control system. Research into the placebo effect has crucially helped to clarify how the psychosocial context of the patient impacts on the patient's brain to lead to positive therapeutic outcomes. In the experimental context (when a patient has consented to participate), when the placebo (inert treatment) is given with verbal suggestions of clinical improvement, sometimes the outcome is positive for the patient. The placebo is therefore a psychobiological phenomenon which happens in the patient's brain. There are many mechanisms that underpin placebo effect, particularly expectation and anticipation of clinical benefit (Benedetti, 2011).

A **nocebo** refers to negative treatment effects induced by a substance or procedure containing no toxic or detrimental substance (Turk and Okifuji, 2010). Thus, a nocebo can be considered as a negative outcome; it is given in a negative context (Benedetti, 2011; Tracey, 2010). Studies on placebo analgesia and nocebo hyperalgesia have increased the understanding of neurobiological mechanisms underpinning placebo and nocebo. Descending modulatory mechanisms from supraspinal regions to the dorsal horn of the spinal cord involve the rostral anterior cingulate cortex (rACC), hypothalamus, amygdala and midbrain PAG which are combined in the brain stem rostral ventromedial medulla (RVM), where output impacts on nociceptive inputs to the spinal cord, which are then processed prior to transmission to the brain. The descending modulatory system involving the endogenous opioid system is both facilitatory (i.e. pronociceptive) and inhibitory (i.e. antinociceptive), so that cognitive, emotional and contextual reappraisal can potentially change subjective pain experience, as demonstrated by fMRI studies. Frontal and limbic regions are also involved in the cognitive control of pain and contribute to the descending modulatory process. Studies to date show that cognitive and emotional mechanisms mediate pain experience via prefrontal-limbic-brainstem interactions (Tracey, 2010).

# The exogenous administration of analgesic drugs

The study of medical pharmacology addresses drug interactions with the human body according to two categories:

- pharmacodynamics: effects of the drug on the body;
- pharmacokinetics: the way the body affects the drug with time, in terms of absorption, distribution, metabolism and excretion.

## Pharmacodynamics

Most drugs act on specific protein molecules, called receptors, that are located in the cell membrane. Receptors respond to endogenous chemicals such as transmitter substances or hormones. Chemicals or drugs which activate receptors are called agonists. Drugs known as antagonists reduce or block the action of the transmitter substance or another agonist. Many drugs reduce or enhance synaptic transmission, some block transmitter inactivation, others inhibit enzymes or transport processes. While drug prescription is intended to produce a therapeutic effect, many drugs potentially have side-effects, varying in impact from minor to serious to fatal (Neal, 2012).

## Pharmacokinetics: metabolism, absorption, distribution and excretion

### Drug metabolism and absorption

While the main organ of metabolism is the liver for most drugs, other organs play a major role in drug absorption. Drugs given orally are usually absorbed in the small intestine, entering the portal system to the liver to be extensively metabolized. This is known as first-pass metabolism, which includes both the intestinal and liver mechanisms.

The two important effects of drug metabolism are:

- The drug is made more hydrophilic, enabling rapid renal excretion.
- Metabolites are usually made less active, but not always, so each drug needs to be checked for the activity of the metabolites.

The two types of reaction in liver metabolism are:

- Phase 1: in which the drug is biotransformed, either through oxidation, reduction or hydrolysis.
- Phase 2: drugs and phase 1 metabolites undergo conjugation (of different types) with endogenous substances, becoming less active and more readily excreted by the kidneys.

Hepatic metabolism and renal function are both reduced at birth and in pre-term infants, and in the older population, so these populations require the calculation of smaller drug doses.

**Drug toxicity**: acetaminophen (a generic name, with many proprietary names: Paracetamol, Tylenol, etc.) is a very widely used analgesic, which, when administered above recommended doses, can result in fatal liver necrosis. This happens through a conjugation process. When the phase 2 liver conjugation of high doses of acetaminophen results in glucuronidation and sulphation saturation, an additional conjugation with glutathione takes place. A potentially lethal hepatotoxic metabolite then accumulates when the glutathione supply is depleted: intravenous or oral acetylcysteine and oral methionine act as antidotes to paracetamol poisoning as both increase synthesis of liver glutathione. Four hours or more following ingestion a blood plasma drug concentration should be determined before administering. Intravenous acetylcysteine, given within 8 hours of paracetamol ingestion, is the most effective antidote. Activated charcoal should be given as an immediate antidote (< 1 hour since ingestion) (Neal, 2012: 12).

## Distribution and excretion

When a drug reaches the circulation it is distributed around the body and must penetrate tissues to act. **Plasma half-life** is the time taken for the drug (blood) plasma concentration to reduce to one half of its value.

**Steady state**: to be therapeutically effective, a drug requires steady plasma levels of concentration. This is the reason for giving drugs at dosages scheduled 'at the clock' (ATC), that is, for example, at four or six hourly intervals, or at other time dosage intervals as prescribed. This is so that the **drug blood plasma level can maintain therapeutic levels at target tissues and cell sites of action**. An analgesic drug (as with any therapeutic drug), if given at dosages which result in a drug plasma concentration which is too low, is not therapeutic, and is therefore ineffective; a drug plasma concentration level which is too high can result in serious adverse reactions and events for the patient, with potentially significant organ damage or fatal consequences, such as acetaminophen overdose causing liver damage or too high a dose of morphine causing respiratory depression.

Knowing the plasma half-life ($t_{1/2}$) of a drug allows an approximate calculation of the time for the drug to reach a steady state. For most drugs, a steady state is reached at approximately five times the half-life of the drug. Drugs with a longer half-life require a longer time to arrive at the drug plasma concentration steady state, so may require an initial loading dose followed by a smaller maintenance dose. Drugs with shorter half-lives need more frequent administration (Greenstein, 2009).

**It is important to remember that:**

- the therapeutic steady state of a drug cannot be maintained by giving a single dose. Drugs given PRN ('pro re nata', or as needed) require patients to request analgesia. PRN drugs are important when the dosage for an ATC drug is either insufficient or ineffective (e.g. in cancer 'breakthrough pain') or given prior to painful procedures, sometimes in addition to the ATC regimen.
- there are many disadvantages to PRN dosing because of the potential for inadequate and ineffective drug treatment, so each situation where PRN dosing is potentially required should be carefully evaluated. Some therapeutic situations require the use of both ATC and PRN dosing for effectiveness (Pasero and McCaffery, 2011).

In effective treatment a steady state plasma concentration is established by an appropriate therapeutic dosage over time. **A steady state is achieved when the rate of drug entering the systemic circulation equals the rate of elimination** (Neal, 2012: 13).

**Clearance** is the volume of blood or plasma cleared of drug in unit time (Neal, 2012: 13). It gives an idea of the efficiency of the liver and kidneys to metabolize and eliminate a particular drug, which in pain treatment, may be one of several drugs at any one time undergoing metabolism and elimination by the liver and kidneys and may be competing for enzyme resources.

**Drug bioavailability** describes the proportion of administered drug which reaches the systemic circulation (Neal, 2012: 13). **Drug bioavailability varies according to the route of drug administration.** Drugs given orally go through **first-pass metabolism**, usually by the liver, and consequently have a variable amount of bioavailability. Drugs given sublingually and intravenously have 100% bioavailability in the circulation as they bypass absorption barriers. Taking patient safety and drug suitability into consideration, a rapid therapeutic effect can be obtained by giving a patient a smaller dose of a drug intravenously rather than a larger dose orally.

**Renal excretion** is aided by a drug becoming less lipid-soluble through metabolism. The renal tubules reabsorb lipid-soluble drugs in the renal glomerular filtrate by passive diffusion, giving a longer-lasting effect in the body (Neal, 2012: 13).

Drugs concentrated in the bile and subject to **biliary excretion** may be reabsorbed by the intestine, also giving a longer-lasting effect in the body (Greenstein, 2009; Neal, 2012).

## Attention to safety issues [*]

The nurse needs to be aware of factors in each patient's situation which might increase the risks of drug treatment side-effects, for instance, younger age, debilitation, chronic hypertension, gastric ulceration, older age and frailty; respiratory, cardiac, hepatic or renal impairments; current medications that might give unwanted side-effects or interact negatively with pain medication; a history of drug allergies; a history of addiction with prescription drugs (American Pain Society, 2008).

**For each patient, care is required in selecting and/or checking the following:**

(a) an appropriate, effective analgesic medication, dosage (according to patient age, body weight and health status), administration mode, timing and frequency intervals;
(b) potential drug treatment side-effects;
(c) potential interactions of selected medication with other medications;

For these details, nurses should be competent in checking the most up-to-date Formulary utilized by their country and *Mosby's Drug Guide for Nursing Students* (Skidmore, 2013). The nurse must be cognizant of medication regulations, management, storage and record-keeping procedures, in keeping with national nursing board requirements and legislation relevant to the country of their practice.

## Routes of drug administration (Neal, 2012; Greenstein, 2009; NMC)

The **oral** route of drug administration is the most widely used and frequently the most convenient. Orally administered drugs pass through the gut wall into the bloodstream. The drug absorption process, usually proportional to the lipid solubility of the drug, is influenced by several factors, among which are drug formulation, gut motility, food content of stomach and stability to acid and enzymes of the drug. The large surface area of the small intestine facilitates drug absorption. Absorbed drugs enter the portal circulation and first-pass metabolism of most drugs takes place as they pass through the liver. Liquid or soluble preparations, if stable in solution, may be helpful for young and older patients. Modified-release preparations aim to delay, prolong or target drug delivery and maintain plasma drug concentration for extended periods and must not be crushed or broken, otherwise the full

---

[*]Please note: a nurse must have an appropriate postgraduate qualification to prescribe drugs.

dose may be released at once, with potential for toxicity. The oral route is the preferred route for morphine, which is given either as an immediate release (liquid) or as a modified-release (tablet) preparation.

The **sublingual** route provides rapid absorption into the systemic circulation. Veins from the **buccal** cavity avoid portal liver circulation, which is useful for drugs subject to a high degree of first-pass metabolism, which can render drugs inactive. Preparations of Fentanyl, a very strong synthetic opioid, are available for sublingual, buccal and nasal spray routes for severe chronic pain and cancer breakthrough pain.

**Inhalation** is the route of administration for volatile anaesthetics and some drugs used in asthma treatment.

**Topical** skin application makes the drug more available near the intended target site, such as topical NSAID for relieving musculoskeletal pain or a capsaicin cream for the relief of osteoarthritis or neuropathic pain. Topical drug application is directly to the surface where drug action is required, so also includes giving eye-drops and eye ointments, giving drugs by means of inhalations as well as medicines delivered by vaginal or rectal routes.

**Transdermal drug delivery system (TDDS)** is the mode of administration, in a controlled, programmed rate, of a predetermined drug (molecules) amount through systems which deliver active ingredients to reach the systemic circulation. This route is extremely helpful for patients with chronic pain to be able to maintain a blood plasma steady state (TDDS is not suitable for acute pain, which requires rapid and varying titration). A 72-hour Fentanyl '12' patch is approximately equivalent to a 30 mg daily dose of morphine, while a Buprenorphine BuTrans '10' – 7-day patch – is approximately equivalent to a 24 mg daily dose of morphine. When converting from transdermal Fentanyl to oral morphine the ratio is 1:100 (see BNF (2014a, 2014b) for equivalent dosages).

The **intranasal** route is a developing technology for some drugs. Now in Phase 3 trials, it allows rapid, patient-controlled analgesic onset.

The **rectal** route avoids portal circulation and gives quite rapid absorption. Rectal administration, where acceptable, can be an effective route for urgently required breakthrough pain relief in palliative care; for administration of acetaminophen suppositories for patients who cannot swallow; when the oral route is no longer appropriate, especially for frail, cachectic patients, or for the treatment of nausea and vomiting; for additional post-operative analgesia required urgently, and for the administration of steroids by enema for treatment of inflammatory bowel disease.

Drugs which are destroyed by acid or enzymes in the gut must be given by a non-oral and non-gastro-intestinal route. Drug administration routes, other than oral or gastrointestinal routes, are called parenteral, which usually refers to injection directly into the body, bypassing the skin and mucous membranes.

The **parenteral** route includes drugs administered in the following ways:

- **Intravenous** injection, in which the drug enters circulation directly, bypassing absorption barriers. An intravenous injection allows for continuous administration by infusion, where rapid effect and/or large volumes may be required and where local tissue damage may be caused by giving drugs via other routes. Patient-controlled anaesthesia (PCA) of intravenous opioids is frequently utilized in the post-operative setting.

- **Intramuscular and subcutaneous** injections, which allow for fairly rapid absorption of drugs in aqueous solutions.
- **Spinal route: intrathecal (subarachnoid) infusion** into the space between the pia mater and the arachnoid mater membrane surrounding and bathing the spinal cord with cerebrospinal fluid. The intrathecal route is used for implantable morphine pump devices for types of chronic pain.
- **Epidural infusion** into the epidural space, between the dura (comprised of arachnoid mater membrane lying against the dura mater membrane) and surrounding bone, is a potential space containing a venous plexus, connective tissue and fat, and is utilized for analgesia infusion and patient-controlled epidural infusion (PCEA).
- **NB neuroaxial**: spaces into which analgesic drugs can be administered. It usually refers to epidural and subarachnoid spaces.
- **Regional nerve block**: injection of local anaesthetic or corticosteroid into the perineural space.

Increasingly, regional anaesthesia is used for invasive procedures on large body areas or limbs. Nerve blocks can provide continued analgesia, reducing nociceptive inputs to sensitized neuronal systems for patients with chronic pain. Joint and muscular injections are also a valuable component of chronic pain management.

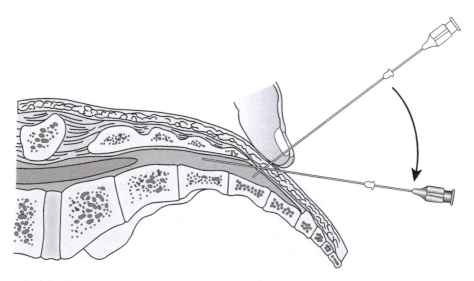

**Figure 7.2** Caudal epidural block

Combined steroid and local anaesthetic injections into inflamed joints can reduce inflammation and pain. Myofascial pain syndrome, characterized by tight muscle bands with tender trigger points and referred pain, requires physiotherapy to regain the function of affected muscle. Local anaesthetic injections into the trigger points can reduce sensitivity and facilitate exercise to regain muscle elasticity, resulting in considerable pain relief (O'Connor and Abram, 2014).

**Epidural injections** and **nerve blocks** are often comprised of a combination of steroid for reducing inflammation and a local anaesthetic which reduce nociceptive inputs to the spinal cord or brain. The cause and type of pain (e.g. nerve inflammation, joint irritation, muscle contraction) and location of the pain determine both the spinal level site of the injection or nerve block and the strength of the local anaesthetic and the type of steroid. For example, there is evidence for the effectiveness of caudal epidural steroid injections for short-term and long-term relief of chronic low back pain. For the caudal epidural block (see Figure 7.2), local anaesthetic Lidocaine 1% 5-15ml is combined with a corticosteroid (e.g. triamcinolone diacetate 50mg). Lidocaine has a rapid onset. Epidural lidocaine appears to block small unmyelinated C-fibres and may work with further, as yet unclarified, mechanisms. Procedural equipment and drugs are prepared. Resuscitation drugs are immediately accessible. The patient is assisted to a specific position, depending on the procedure. For the caudal epidural block, the patient lies prone with a pillow under the abdomen, on the operating table to allow flexion of the lumbo-sacral spine. A set procedure is followed with a high emphasis on patient safety and aseptic technique. A successful block is confirmed by relief of pain with anaesthesia or diminished sensation in the region of the blocked nerves. Potentially serious immediate side-effects include: intravascular or intrathecal injection, hypotension, exacerbated pain, headache, allergic reaction. Longer-term side-effects include: infections, cushingoid symptoms from repeated injections, epidural hematoma (O'Connor and Abram, 2014).

**Spinal Cord Stimulation (SCS)** is a method of electro-analgesia delivered through electrodes implanted in the epidural space which is thought to work on the same Gate Control Theory principles as TENS: activation of Aβ non-nociceptive fibres by SCS decreases the nociceptive input from small C-fibre afferents at the dorsal horn. Recent research suggests there are multiple additional neurological mechanisms underpinning the efficacy of spinal cord stimulation, possibly through various neuronal pathways. For example, descending inhibition controls on spinal neuronal output, with suppression of neuronal hyperexcitability, including reducing dorsal horn WDR neuronal hyperactivity as one of these. SCS may have relevant neurological application for sensory, autonomic and motor disturbances. Studies show that SCS is effective for neuropathic, visceral and ischaemic pain. The device consists of a power source (see Figure 7.3) implanted under the skin. An extension lead runs under the skin to the implanted electrodes which deliver electrical pulses in the epidural space, to nerves in the dorsal aspect of the spinal cord, at different points on the neuroaxis depending on the clinical condition to be treated. The procedure aims to obtain pain relief in the area of pain/paresthesia (abnormal sensations of

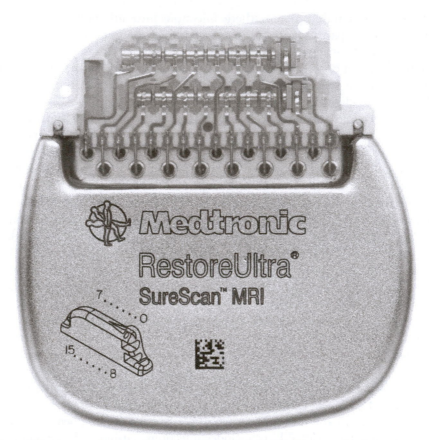

**Caution: diathermy must not be used for patients implanted with neurostimulators because energy from diathermy can be transferred through the implanted system, causing tissue damage at the locations of the implanted electrodes, resulting in severe injury or death. See Medtronic Safety Guidelines.**

**Figure 7.3**　Power device for spinal cord stimulation, the Restore Utra® SureScan® Neurastimulator

tingling) overlap. Appropriate patient selection is vital, with an emphasis on pain location, intensity, duration and characteristics as well as psychological screening for the patient, who may benefit from psychological therapy. Patients with a major psychiatric diagnosis must have treatment before undergoing an SCS screening trial.

Skilled clinical expertise and optimal training with the correct equipment contribute to a successful outcome, which is the reduction of pain. SCS requires a screening trial to be able to predict success. NICE recommends SCS for the treatment of chronic neuropathic pain of at least six months' duration which is not controlled by conventional pharmacotherapy. SCS, an underused therapy, is increasingly used for patients with chronic pain as trials confirm the efficacy for different clinical applications. SCS is increasingly seen as a cost-effective treatment for certain severe chronic pain conditions. Medtronic have recently developed an MRI-compatible SCS system which eliminates the need to perform an inconvenient and costly explanation (Ciampi de Andrade et al., 2010; NICE, 2008; North and Linderoth, 2010).

# The World Health Organization's Analgesic Ladder for pain relief

The World Health Organization (1986, 1996) Analgesic Ladder is a set of principles to guide the prescription of appropriate analgesia, on the basis of the patient's pain type and intensity. The principles and application of the ladder to cancer pain is detailed in Chapter 10. This chapter outlines the relevancy of the WHO Analgesic Ladder for acute pain. For each type of analgesia the side-effects profile and dosage risks for each population need to be carefully assessed, with very particular care to dosage calculations in neonates, pre-term and young infants and frail, older people. The potential hazards of each analgesic and adjuvant drug for pregnant and breast-feeding women must be considered in terms of the risk to the mother and the foetus.

## The principles and five phrases of the WHO Analgesic Ladder

The principles of the WHO Analgesic Ladder are to administer analgesia: 'by mouth'; 'at the clock' (ATC); 'by the ladder'; with the additional phrases 'for the individual' and 'with attention to detail', to treat and control the patient's pain and associated symptoms. The WHO Analgesic Ladder addresses pain intensity treatment in a stepwise progression. It uses the term 'adjuvant' in the context of additional non-analgesic medications prescribed to reduce the symptoms that the patient may also experience concurrent with pain (Pasero and McCaffery, 2011).

Step 1 of the WHO Analgesic Ladder addresses mild pain (rated on a Number Rating Scale as 3 or below and described by the patient as mild) by advising a non-opioid analgesia, either acetaminophen or a non-steroidal anti-inflammatory drug (NSAID). The NSAIDs comprise acetylsalicylic acid (aspirin) and non-selective COX (cyclo-oxygenase) inhibitor and selective COX (cyclo-oxygenase) 2 inhibitor NSAIDs.

## Choosing between acetaminophen, aspirin and other non-steroidal anti-inflammatory analgesics

(The following medication information is based on information from the most recent British National Formulary (2014a, 2014b) and similar formularies and Sinatra et al. (2011); please consult the relevant National Formulary for your country.)

On the first step of the Analgesic Ladder for mild pain, considerations are required in regard to potential side-effects in a particular patient population and for each individual patient when choosing between acetaminophen or aspirin and other non-steroidal anti-inflammatory drugs (NSAIDs), all of which are particularly suitable for mild nociceptive pain of musculoskeletal origin or sickle-cell disease. Acetaminophen, while a nonsalicylate, has a similar analgesic and antipyretic (temperature lowering) potency as aspirin and the other NSAIDs, but no antiplatelet or anti-inflammatory effects. It does not damage the gastric mucosa and so is often preferred over aspirin, especially in children and older people. Aspirin (acetylsalicylic acid) is contra-indicated in children under the age of 16 due to the risk of Reye's syndrome, a potentially fatal disease impacting on all organs, especially the brain and liver.

Acetaminophen is often the preferred drug of choice for children requiring analgesia for pain, pyrexia and discomfort. Analgesic effect is mediated by central nervous system action which is not yet understood. Acetaminophen can be given via a number of routes. Given orally, acetaminophen is well absorbed, reaching peak plasma concentrations within 60 minutes. In a child with a body weight under 50 kg, the maximum daily dose of acetaminophen, in divided doses of 15 mg/kg every 4–6 hours, is 60 mg/kg daily. The maximum therapeutic dose, in divided doses, of acetaminophen for a child with a body weight over 50 kg and an adult is up to 4 grams per day.

The potential risks associated with acetaminophen can be severe. The most common of these are:

(a) an underlying risk of hepatotoxicity compared to non-use in patients without underlying liver disease;

(b) a risk of over anticoagulation for patients taking warfarin anticoagulation therapy, so this patient group requires particular vigilance to prevent over-anticoagulation when taking acetaminophen;

(c) a risk of fatal hepatic necrosis following an acute overdose (particularly attempted suicide), while an overdose in a child, equally potentially fatal, may cause hepatic damage that may not be detected for some days.

Non-steroidal anti-inflammatory drugs interrupt the arachidonic acid cascade that produces pain-associated local inflammation, vasodilation and increased vascular permeability by inhibiting the production of cyclo-oxygenase (COX) and synthesis of prostaglandins and other pro-inflammatory substances (see Vane, 1971; Vane and Botting, 2003). Aspirin (acetylsalicylic acid) is the oldest known NSAID, with a duration of action of about four hours. It is well absorbed orally through the stomach and large surface of the upper small intestine. Aspirin is a prodrug which is metabolized in the body to the active drug salicylate and to acetic acid. Salicylates are converted in the liver to water-soluble conjugates which are excreted by the kidneys. Aspirin is rapidly metabolized and excreted, so an oral dosage of 300–900 mg every 4–6 hours is required to maintain the adult patient's pain-free status.

Aspirin works at the periphery (Lim et al., 1964), is effective for relieving mild-to-moderate nociceptive dental pain, transient musculoskeletal pain, dysmenorrhoea, headache and sore throat. Aspirin has an antipyretic action in a raised body temperature by inhibiting endogenous pyrogen-associated prostaglandin production in the heat regulating mechanism in the hypothalamus. Aspirin is particularly effective for relieving continuous chronic inflammatory conditions with low-level pain intensity (e.g. rheumatoid arthritis), through a combined effect of analgesic and anti-inflammatory action.

Antibiotic therapy, especially Penicillin (or erythromycin if the patient is allergic to penicillin), is the treatment of choice in primary prevention and treatment of group A streptococcal pharyngitis. Antibiotic therapy is given in order to reduce the risk of complications, particularly acute rheumatic fever, for which children in less developed countries are more at risk. The treatment of joint pain and inflammation is addressed by anti-inflammatory medicines, especially NSAIDS, or by acetaminophen (Cilliers, 2006; Low, 2011: 1827; Wessels, 2011). Although aspirin is not generally recommended for children under 16 years of age (because of the risk of Reye's syndrome), an exception is made in acute rheumatic fever as aspirin is highly effective in reducing inflammation and pyrexia.

The most common potential risks and adverse side-effects associated with aspirin medication are the possibility of bleeding in patients taking anticoagulant drugs, or in patients with a history of liver disease or peptic ulcer, haemophilia and other bleeding disorders. Aspirin is contraindicated in all these patient groups.

Aspirin can prompt allergic reactions and has the potential for poisoning in larger doses. When treating adult patients with high doses of aspirin (orally 300–900 mg every 4–6 hours, max 4 grams daily; rectal administration 450–900 mg every 4 hours, max 3.6 grams daily) (e.g. patients with acute rheumatic fever), it is essential to have a urine alkalinization protocol in place. Urine alkalinization should be considered as a first-line treatment for patients with moderately severe salicylate poisoning who do not meet the criteria for hemodialysis. Urine alkalinization is achieved through intravenous administration of sodium bicarbonate which produces increased urine output (diuresis) with a pH of about 7.5, increasing poison elimination. (See position paper on urine alkalinization by Proudfoot et al. (2004).)

- Aspirin is strictly contraindicated for children under 16 years of age due to the risk of Reye's Syndrome.
- Aspirin is contraindicated for treatment of/in patients with gout.

While pain relief is rapid with NSAIDs, full analgesic effect may take some days and for anti-inflammatory effect up to three weeks. There is wide individual variation in response to different NSAIDs. Patients had different preferences for different types of NSAIDs. Only one NSAID should be prescribed at a time, and given for a maximum of two weeks, after which time, if the treatment effect is not achieved, the patient's treatment should be switched to another NSAID. The lowest dose that is effective should be prescribed. NSAIDs are indicated for pain and stiffness associated with rheumatic disease, gout, osteoarthritis and soft tissue disorders, often experienced by older patients. Particular care should be taken with regard to side-effects in this patient group, as well as in patients with tendencies for gastrointestinal bleeding. On rare occasional, NSAIDS can bring about irreversible kidney damage in patients with cardiac, hepatic and renal impairments, so renal function should always be checked regularly in patients with these disorders. Ibuprofen and Naproxen are good NSAIDs with which to begin analgesic treatment as they have lower side-effect profiles. NSAIDs matched to the type of pain and monitored carefully can give very effective pain relief. Ibuprofen and Diclofenac relieve mild-to-moderate dental pain (but always as a temporary measure as the cause of dental pain must be addressed directly), pain due to inflammation, other musculoskeletal disorders, migraine and post-immunisation pyrexia in children.

Selective COX (cyclo-oxygenase) 2 inhibitor NSAIDs selectively inhibit COX (cyclo-oxygenase) 2, the enzyme isoform which synthesizes inflammatory prostaglandins while sparing COX (cyclo-oxygenase) 1, the latter protecting the stomach from damaging effects of acid which might otherwise be caused by inhibition of prostaglandins synthesis in the gastric mucosa.

Selective COX (cyclo-oxygenase) 2 inhibitor NSAIDs Celecoxib, Etoricoxib and Parecoxib, which are indicated for patients with a particularly high risk of gastrointestinal bleeding, are contraindicated for patients with ischaemic and vascular heart diseases. All NSAIDs are associated with a risk of myocardial infarction and stroke, especially selective COX (cyclo-oxygenase) 2 inhibitor NSAIDs. Early side-effects can be severe, particularly for those with cardiac impairment or any kind of heart disease. NSAIDs are contraindicated in patients with a history of hypersensitivity to aspirin or any other NSAIDs. All NSAIDs are potentially associated with serious gastrointestinal toxicity. It is advised that the NSAID with the lowest risk is used to start with, at the lowest required dose, and monitored carefully for effectiveness and side-effects. Many NSAIDs are not suitable for children. Diclofenac is suitable for children with chronic inflammatory pain and acute post-operative pain and can, as with adults, be administered via different routes according to patient need.

As with all analgesics, nurses and prescribers should always check the most up-to-date Formulary of their country for appropriate drug dosage, route and frequency of administration and potential side-effects. Nurses are advised to have immediate access also to *Mosby's Drug Guide for Nursing Students* (Skidmore, 2013), which outlines nursing assessment, diagnoses and patient education points as well as dosage and side-effects for each drug.

**Step 2** of the WHO Analgesic Ladder, mostly for nociceptive pain that is rated as mild to moderate on the Verbal Rating Scale and about 4–6 on the Number Rating Scale, is to introduce opioid medication, which works in the central nervous system at spinal and supra spinal level. The optimal Step 2 treatment regime is the weak opioid agonist tramadol in combination with non-opioid acetaminophen. Tramadol is less constipating and has fewer toxic side-effects than morphine, particularly less respiratory depression and less nausea and vomiting. Both codeine, which is very constipating, and tramadol have an affinity for the μ receptor.

At Step 3 (transitioning to Step 4 for interventional techniques), opioid medication to treat or prevent severe acute pain may be given neuraxially for prevention of post-operative pain for post-ceasarian section, and epidurally and intravenously for post-operative pain, both methods allowing the patient to control the analgesic dosage. The importance of properly controlled use and monitoring of opioid medication to effectively alleviate pain in these and other contexts cannot be over-emphasized. Opioid use requires comprehensive knowledge and skilled management. Each type of opioid has particular drug-related adverse effects and shares common effects with morphine. The most common effects are circulatory and respiratory depression, nausea and vomiting, constipation and itch. Each side-effect needs medical and nursing prevention and management.

## Side-effects of morphine and other opioids

Cardiovascular and respiratory effects include bradyarrhythmia – cardiac or respiratory depression leading to possible cardiac arrest:

- **Reversal of respiratory depression:** the administration of Naloxone is required to reverse opioid-induced respiratory depression.

Gastro-intestinal effects most commonly include nausea and vomiting, which can have a high incidence rate which **can be treated with an antiemetic** appropriate to the cause of vomiting (opioid), for example phenothiazines or metoclopramide. Constipation requires careful prevention and management with laxatives and/or stool softeners.

Histamine release (which is more likely with morphine compared with other opioids) can lead to pruritus (itch; especially after neuraxial injection), orthostatic hypotension, circulatory depression, palpitations, central nervous system excitation, and shock.

- Pruritis is treated with antihistamines.

Neurological side-effects include dizziness, confusion, insomnia, headache, seizures and coma.

May cause psychological (delirium, depression and psychotic) symptoms, urinary retention and nephrotoxic effects.

**Step 3** opioid medications, which are essential in the prevention and treatment of severe acute pain, produce an immediate analgesic effect. However, after a while normal tolerance and dependence can occur. **Tolerance,** which is a normal consequence of medication use, is a physiological state in which a person requires an increased dosage of a psychoactive substance to sustain a desired effect (Turk and

Okifuji, 2010). **Physical dependence** is a pharmacological property of a drug (e.g. an opioid) that is characterized by the occurrence of an abstinence syndrome following the abrupt discontinuation of the substance or administration of an antagonist. It does not imply an aberrant psychological state or behaviour or addiction (Turk and Okifuji, 2010).

Chronic non-maligant pain and acute pain have directional differences to the approach of treatment interventions. For moderate to severe acute pain, analgesia is titrated to the level of the patient's pain intensity, aiming to reduce the pain score, bring the pain under control and reduce the analgesia requirement to zero, as appropriate. For chronic pain, treatment interventions may begin at Step 1 with non-opioids, depending on the level of the patient's pain intensity and functionality.

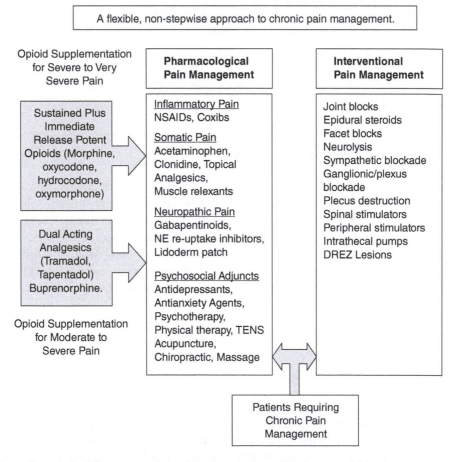

**Figure 7.4**   A flexible, non-stepwise approach to chronic pain management

Source: *The Essence of Analgesia and Analgesics*. Sinatra, R.S., Jahr, J.S. and Watkins-Pitchford, J.M. (eds), p.70, Copyright (2011). Republished with permission of Cambridge University Press.

Adjuvant medications, which are often opioid sparing, are recommended for all types of pain, and are prescribed according to each person's individual requirement for pain and symptom control. Sometimes a trial is required to obtain the maximally efficient pain treatment regimen. This may require opioid switching, that is, changing from an immediate release preparation to an extended release preparation, which may be in a transdermal delivery system. A low-dose buprenorphine patch for an older person with chronic pain of osteoarthritis can help prevent fluctuations in blood plasma levels with potential for fewer opioid-induced side-effects. The resultant improvement in pain management positively impacts the patient's sleep, quality of life and functioning. Careful patient selection is required. Vigilant observation and management of opioid side-effects is essential in this patient group, particularly to prevent constipation and falls and fall-related injuries (Breivik et al., 2010; James et al., 2010).

There is increasing evidence that opioids prescribed for chronic pain can cause hyperalgesia in some patients, although the causative mechanism are not yet clear. It is recognized that chronic pain is associated with deficits in some aspects of cognitive function which may be worsened by the long-term use of opioid therapies (Schiltenwolf et al., 2014). Figure 7.4 shows a flexible, non-stepwise approach to chronic pain management, with either dual-acting opioid analgesic tramadol (a weak opioid agonist that inhibits norepinephrine (noradrenaline) re-uptake), Tapentadol (a strong opioid agonist that inhibits noradrenaline re-uptake), or Buprenorphine (a partial agonist with a much longer duration of action than morphine and with less severe side-effects) as a treatment option, in addition to non-opioid analgesia and appropriate interventional pain management. The non-stepwise approach allows an individualized and flexible chronic pain care plan to be developed from a broad range of treatment options.

The goal of flexible pain management is to maximize the patient's quality of life and functionality in a way that is patient-centred and facilitates the patient's participation in a care plan. Flexible pain management aims to give optimal pain relief and restore the patient's maximum functioning across all domains of their quality of life.

## Chapter summary

- Analgesia can be defined as 'absence of the spontaneous report of pain or pain behaviours in response to stimulation that would normally be expected to be painful'. The term 'analgesia' implies a defined stimulus and response and both can be tested in animals and humans.
- The analgesic response in humans can be brought about through an intrinsic analgesia system, as well as through an endogenous opioid system and exogenously through the administration of analgesic drugs.

*(Continued)*

*(Continued)*

- Three opioid peptides, together with their receptors, μ (MOR), δ (λ, DOR) and κ (KOR) comprise the endogenous opioid system. Enkephalins interact with the δ receptor, dynorphins with the κ receptor and β-endorphins bind to both μ and δ receptors.
- A placebo is a substance (dummy medicine) or procedure (dummy therapeutic intervention) without therapeutic effect that is provided as a treatment and is frequently used to control patients' expectations for the efficacy in testing a treatment intervention.
- Pharmacology addresses drug interactions with the human body according to two categories: pharmacodynamics is the effects of the drug on the body, whereas pharmacokinetics is the way the body affects the drug with time, in terms of absorption, distribution, metabolism and excretion.
- Epidural injections and nerve blocks usually comprise a steroid for reducing inflammation and a local anaesthetic to reduce nociceptive inputs to the spinal cord or brain. The cause, type and location of the pain determine the spinal site of the injection or nerve block.
- Spinal Cord Stimulation (SCS) is delivered through electrodes implanted in the epidural space and is thought to work on the same Gate Control Theory principles as TENS. Recent research suggests there are multiple mechanisms underpinning the efficacy of spinal cord stimulation.
- The WHO Analgesic Ladder for pain relief was proposed for the management of persistent cancer pain in 1986 (2nd edn, 1996). Acute and chronic pain have opposite directions for pain relief. Opioid sparing analgesia and adjuvants should always be used.

## Reflective exercise

How would you as the nurse on the multidisciplinary team contribute to the discussion about developing a care plan for an older, female patient living in the community who is suffering severe pain as a result of osteoarthritis?

## Recommended reading

Downie, G., Mackenzie, J. and Williams, A. (2010) *Calculating Drug Doses Safely: A Handbook for Nurses and Midwives* (2nd edn). Edinburgh: Churchill Livingstone.

Greenstein, B. (2009) *Trounce's Clinical Pharmacology for Nurses* (18th edn). Edinburgh: Elsevier Churchill Livingstone.

McPherson, M.L. (2010) *Demystifying Opioid Conversion Calculations: A Guide for Effective Dosing*. Bethesda, MD: American Society of Health Systems Pharmacists.

Niblett, V. (2005) *A Nurses' Guide to Dosage Calculations.* Philadelphia, PA: Lippincott, Williams and Wilkins.

Skidmore, L. (2013) *Mosby's Drug Guide for Nursing Students* (10th edn). St Louis, MO: Elsevier Mosby.

## Websites relevant to this chapter

UK Medicines Information: www.ukmi.nhs.uk

British National Formulary: www.bnf.org

Buprenorphine: A Guide for Nurses: http://buprenorphine.samhsa.gov/bwns/TAP_30_Certified.pdf

Medtronic neurostimulators: www.medtronic.com/patients/chronic-pain/device/neurostimulators/our-neurostimulators-for-pain/restore-sensor/index.htm

Nursing and Midwifery Council *Standards for Medicines Management*: www.nmc-uk.org/Documents/NMC-Publications/NMC-Standards-for-medicines-management.pdf

# References

American Pain Society (2008) *Principles of Analgesic Use in the Treatment of Acute Pain and Cancer Pain: Research, Education, Treatment, Advocacy* (6th edn). Chicago, IL: APS.

Benarroch, E.E. (2012) Endogenous opioid systems: current concepts and clinical correlations. *Neurology*, 79: 807–814.

Benedetti, F. (2011) *The Patient's Brain: The Neuroscience behind the Doctor–Patient Relationship.* Oxford: Oxford University Press.

Boswell, M.V., Trescot, A.M., Datta, S., Schlutz, D.M., et al. (2007) Interventional techniques: evidence-based practice guidelines in the management of chronic spinal pain. *Pain Physician*, 10: 7–111.

Breivik, H., Ljosaa, T.M., Stengaard-Pedersen, K., Persson, J., Aro, H., Villumsen, J. and Tvinnemose, D. (2010) A 6-months, randomised, placebo-controlled evaluation of efficacy and tolerability of a low-dose 7-day buprenorphine transdermal patch in osteoarthritis patients naïve to potent opioids. *Scandinavian Journal of Pain*, 1: 122–141.

British National Formulary (2014) BNF 66 for Adults September 2013–March 2014. London: Pharmaceutical Press.

British National Formulary (2014) BNF for Children July 2013–July 2014. London: Pharmaceutical Press.

Ciampi de Andrade, D., Bendib, B., Hattou, M., Keravel, Y., Nguyen, J.P. and Lefaucher, J.P. (2010) Neurophysiological assessment of spinal cord stimulation in failed back syndrome. *Pain*, 150: 485–491.

Cilliers, A.M. (2006) Rheumatic fever and its management. *British Medical Journal*, 333: 1153–1156.

Downie, G., Mackenzie, J. and Williams, A. (2010) *Calculating Drug Doses Safely: A Handbook for Nurses and Midwives* (2nd edn). Edinburgh: Churchill Livingstone.

Eippert, F., Finsterbusch, J., Bingel, U. and Buchet, C. (2009) Direct evidence for spinal cord involvement in placebo analgesia. *Science*, 326: 404.

Greenstein, B. (2009) *Trounce's Clinical Pharmacology for Nurses* (18th edn). Edinburgh: Elsevier Churchill Livingstone.

Haines, D. (2012) *Neuroanatomy: An Atlas of Structures, Sections and Systems* (8th edn). Riverwoods, IL: Wolters Kluwer/Lippincott Williams and Wilkins.

Hall, J.E. (2011) *Guyton and Hall Textbook of Medical Physiology* (12th edn). Philadelphia, PA: Saunders Elsevier.

James, I.G.V., O'Brien, C.M. and McDonald, C.J. (2010) A randomised , double-blind double-dummy comparison of the efficacy and tolerability of low-dose transdermal buprenorphine (Butrans seven-day patches) with buprenorphine sublingual tablets (Temgesic) in patients with osteoarthritis pain. *Journal of Pain and Symptom Management*, 40 (2): 266–278.

Lenz, F.A., Casey, K.L., Jones, E.G. and Willis, W.D. (2010) *The Human Pain System: Experimental and Clinical Perspectives*. New York: Cambridge University Press.

Lim, RKS., Guzman, F., Rodgers, D.W., Goto, K., Braun, C., Dickerson, G.D. et al. (1964) Site of action of narcotic and non-narcotic analgesics determined by blocking bradykinin-evoked visceral pain. *Archives internationales de pharmacodynamie et de thérapie*, 152: 25–58.

Low, D.E. (2011) Nonpneumococcal streptococcal infections, rheumatic fever. In: Goldman, L. and Schafer, A.I. (eds), *Cecil Medicine* (24th edn). Philadelphia, PA: Saunders Elsevier. p. 1827.

Moulin, D. (2005) Opioid treatment for cancer pain and chronic noncancer pain. In H. Merskey, J.D. Loeser and R. Dubner (eds), *The Paths of Pain, 1975–2005*. Seattle, WA: International Association for the Study of Pain.

Neal, M.J. (2012) *Medical Pharmacology at a Glance* (7th edn). Chichester: Wiley-Blackwell.

Niblett, V. (2005) *A Nurses' Guide to Dosage Calculations*. Philadelphia, PA: Lippincott, Williams and Wilkins.

NICE (2008) Spinal Cord Stimulation for Chronic Pain of Neuropathic or Ischaemic Origin. London: National Institute for Health and Clinical Excellence.

North, R.B. and Linderoth, B. (2010) Spinal Cord Stimulation. In S.M. Fishman, J.C. Ballantyne and J.P. Rathmell (eds), *Bonica's Management of Pain* (4th edn). Riverwoods, IL: Wolters Kluwer/Lippincott Williams and Wilkins.

Nursing and Midwifery Council (2006) *Standards for Medicines Management*. Available at: www.nmc-uk.org/Documents/NMC-Publications/NMC-Standards-for-medicines-management.pdf (accessed 4 November 2014).

O'Connor, T. and Abram, S. (2014) *Atlas of Pain Injection Techniques* (2nd edn). Edinburgh: Elsevier Churchill Livingstone.

Pasero, C. and McCaffery, M. (2011) *Pain Assessment and Pharmacologic Management*. St Louis, MO: Elsevier Mosby.

Pita, G. (1998) Disturbances in recent memory and behavioural changes caused by the treatment with intraventricular morphine administration in severe cancer pain. *Human Psychopharmacology: Clinical and Experimental*, 13: 315–323.

Proudfoot, A.T., Krenzelok, E.P and Vale, J.A. (2004) Position paper on urine alkalinization. *Journal of Toxicology: Clinical Toxicology*, 42 (1): 1–26.

Rang, H.P., Dale, M.M., Ritter, J.M., Flower, R.J. and Henderson, G. (2012) *Rang and Dale's Pharmacology* (7th edn). Edinburgh: Elsevier Churchill Livingstone.

Rastogi, V. and Yadav, P. (2012) Transdermal drug delivery system: an overview. *Asian Journal of Pharmaceutics*, 6: 161–170.

Reynolds, D.V. (1969) Surgery in the rat during electrical analgesia induced by focal brain stimulation. *Science*, 164: 444–445. Cited in F.A. Lenz, K.L. Casey, E.G. Jones and W.D. Willis (2010), *The Human Pain System: Experimental and Clinical Perspectives*. New York: Cambridge University Press.

Rosa, J. and Patel, S. (2011) Morphine-oral and parenteral. In R.S. Sinatra, J.S. Jahr and J.M. Watkins-Pitchford (eds), *The Essence of Analgesia and Analgesics*. New York: Cambridge University Press.

Salway, J.G. (2012) *Medical Biochemistry at a Glance* (3rd edn). Chichester: Wiley-Blackwell.

Schiltenwolf, M., Akbar, M., Hug, A., Pfuller, U., Gantz, S., Neubauer, E., Flor, H. and Wang, H. (2014) Evidence of specific cognitive deficits in patients with chronic low back pain under long-term substitution treatment of opioids. *Pain Physician*, 17: 9–19.

Sinatra, R.S. (2011) A stepwise approach to pain management. In R.S. Sinatra, J.S. Jahr and J.M. Watkins-Pitchford (eds), *The Essence of Analgesia and Analgesics*. New York: Cambridge University Press.

Skidmore, L. (2013) *Mosby's Drug Guide for Nursing Students* (10th edn). St Louis, MO: Elsevier Mosby.

Tracey, I. (2010) Getting the pain you expect: mechanisms of placebo, nocebo and reappraisal effects in humans. *Nature Medicine*, 16 (11): 1277–1285.

Turk, D.C. and Okifuji, A. (2010) Pain terms and taxonomies of pain. In S.M. Fishman, J.C. Ballantyne and J.P. Rathmell (eds), *Bonica's Management of Pain* (4th edn). Riverwoods, IL: Wolters Kluwer/Lippincott Williams and Wilkins.

Vale, A. (2012) Salicylates. *Medicine*, 40 (3): 156–157.

Vane, J.R. (1971) Inhibition of prostaglandin synthesis as a mechanism of action for Aspirin-like drugs. *Nature: New Biology*, 231: 232–235.

Vane, J.R. and Botting, R.M. (2003) The mechanism of action of aspirin. *Thrombosis Research*, 110: 255–258.

Wessels, M.R. (2011) Streptococcal pharyngitis. *The New England Journal of Medicine*, 364 (7): 648–655.

World Health Organization (1986) *Cancer Pain Relief*. Geneva: World Health Organization.

World Health Organization (1996) *Cancer Pain Relief (with a Guide to Opioid Availability)* (2nd edn). Geneva: World Health Organization.

Williams, B.S. and Buvanendran, A. (2011) Multimodal analgesia (sites of analgesic activity). In R.S. Sinatra, J.S. Jahr and J.M. Watkins-Pitchford (eds), *The Essence of Analgesia and Analgesics*. New York: Cambridge University Press.

# 8

# Acute pain

## Learning objectives

The learning objectives of this chapter are to:

- understand that biopsychosocial pain assessment is vital in the context of acute pain
- appreciate the severity of post-operative tonsillectomy pain and the need for pre-operative parent and child education
- understand the different components of shock-associated acute pain
- recognize the need for early examination and pain relief for patients with acute pain

## Introduction

This chapter gives an overview of the etiology and management of acute pain. Because causes of acute pain are extensive and diverse, some examples of the most commonly occurring acute pain types are outlined. For some human body regions, distinguishing between acute and chronic pain can be diagnostically challenging. This is particularly the case for abdominal pain and chest pain, which, when acute, carry potentially life-threatening consequences if not diagnosed and treated accurately.

## Acute pain in neonates, infants and children

The diagnosis and pharmacological treatment of acute pain in infants and neonates requires careful consideration of the immature body systems; the potential for drug-induced toxicity is increased because rates of hepatic metabolism and renal excretion are reduced. Aspirin is contraindicated in children under 16 years of age. Many drugs have not been formally assessed in clinical trials in paediatric pollutions and often preparations trialled for adults are used for children (Kumar and Clark, 2012).

Consideration of respiratory depression and sedation effects makes non-opioid medication the first-line choice for infants and children for mild to moderate pain. Acetaminophen, while viewed as the safest medication for children, can be particularly dangerous if an overdose is taken as there is a high likelihood of liver failure. See the National Formulary of your country for specific dosing regimens. Non-steroidal anti-inflammatory drugs (NSAIDs) are widely used post-operatively for children from aged 6 months onwards, and have an opioid-sparing effect. They have a good safety record for short-term post-operative pain relief, particularly in healthy children in whom the risk of clinically significant bleeding is uncommon.

# Procedural pain

Infants, especially if pre-term or receiving investigations and/or treatment for complex conditions, often undergo frequent skin-piercing procedures. Most research regarding the safety of eutectic mixture of local anesthetics (EMLA) has been carried out with pediatric populations and studies strongly support the use of topical analgesics for painful skin-penetrating procedures, except for infants and children allergic to amide local anesthetics. EMLA is comprised of lidocaine 2.5% and prilocaine 2.5%, and has a melting point lower than either of the anesthetics alone, so that the drug can easily penetrate the skin, giving non-toxic serum blood levels. Blistering, skin blanching and eruptions are possible side-effects. EMLA should be given with caution in conjunction with other preparations as there is the potential for drug interaction. EMLA should be applied with caution to the skin of an infant (to minimize the risk of methemoglobinemia, a reduced ability of haemaglobin to transport oxygen, due to systemic absorption of prilocaine) and removed as soon as possible after the procedure. Sufficient time needs to be given prior to the painful procedure to allow the EMLA application to be effective. Precautions require that the maximum recommended dose is not exceeded and any residual substance is removed promptly following each procedure (Pasero and McCaffery, 2011).

Children often react to routine immunization with fever and irritability and minor adverse reactions, for which antipyretics are frequently recommended. Results of a study by Dhingra and Mishra (2011) of 'immediate' versus 'as-needed' doses of acetaminophen syrup (10–15 mg/kg single dose) for post-immunization pyrexia, pain and irritability supports the use of 'as needed' acetaminophen to reduce fever, pain and/or irritability in children following immunization. Adverse reactions can be distressing for both child and parent, and may be a deterrent to further immunization. The careful use of 'as needed' over-the-counter acetaminophen can allay fears and give comfort to child and parent.

# Post-operative tonsillectomy pain in children

Tonsillectomy in children is often accompanied by the possibility of high levels of nausea and vomiting and potentially life-threatening bleeding from the tonsil bed. Tonsillectomy and adeno-tonsillectomy carry different levels of risk for haemorrhage, depending on the surgical procedure utilized, with laser and certain types of electro-surgery associated with a higher risk of post-operative bleeding. Therefore, there is widespread concern among surgeons about post-tonsillectomy bleeding (haemorrhage) even though procedures to ensure optimal haemostasis, the first stage of wound healing, are followed. While NSAIDs are widely prescribed for children following tonsillectomy, some institutions do not prescribe NSAIDs because of the potential risk for bleeding from the tonsil bed.

Post-tonsillectomy pain can be very severe in children, adolescents and young adults. The oropharynx and tonsillar fossae, which are highly represented in the somatic cortex, are innervated by branches of the trigeminal and glossopharyngeal nerves and are extremely sensitive. The nerve innervations increase the risk of sensitization and hyperalgesia from the tonsil bed site, which also has nociceptive pain from inflamed connective tissue and muscle. Adequate and appropriate post-operative pain relief is therefore essential to prevent sensitization, reduce patient distress and aid recovery. Immediate post-operative relief is given by peritonsillar infiltration after surgery; for example, infiltrated tramadol has been shown to give effective analgesia in the immediate post-tonsillectomy period (Atef and Aly Fawaz, 2008). Where permitted, appropriate doses of NSAIDs, to reduce local inflammation, depending on age and weight, should be given with caution orally or rectally, the latter for a limited time period, usually 2–4 days, and the patient monitored very carefully. NSAID suppositories, while very effective analgesics for post-tonsillectomy pain, are problematic for storing for home use in hot countries, due to melting at high temperatures. Pediatric formats of acetaminophen alone are not sufficient for immediate post-tonsillectomy pain. A combination of acetaminophen and opioid is more effective for the combination for pain types in post-tonsillectomy pain and may be prescribed for use at home, in which case stimulant laxatives must also be prescribed. The US FDA advise that the use of opioid medications post-tonsillectomy (and/or adenoidectomy) at home should be on an 'as needed' (PRN) basis only. The US FDA have issued a black box warning (FDA, 2013) against the use of codeine as a post-operative medication for children following tonsillectomy, as children with a genetic variant encoding the enzyme P4502D6 convert codeine via the liver rapidly into high levels of morphine, with the increased potential for fatalities due to respiratory depression or sleep apnoea. See the National Formulary of your country for licence limitations regarding age and specific dosing regimens (Howard et al., 2014; Stanko et al., 2013).

# Key issues in the care of the child undergoing tonsillectomy

Early patient and parent education preparation is very important. In keeping with hospital protocol, prior to surgery the nurse plays a major role in educating the child and parent about what to expect regarding the procedure, how to prepare and how to manage after the surgery. Anxiety pre- and post-surgery may be experienced by both parent and child, potentially increasing the child's pain intensity. Education and information can substantially alleviate apprehension. Information leaflets, child-friendly educational material, books and videos can help with the preparation. Sutters et al. (2011) have developed the pediatric PRO-SELF programme, which is an educational programme by nurses supporting parents through their child's post-tonsillectomy period with home management instruction, demonstration and discussion of pain assessment and pharmacological and nonpharmacological pain management techniques (Sutters et al. 2011; see also Howard et al., 2014).

Severe post-operative pain associated with tonsillectomy should not be underestimated, and can easily last for longer than a week, causing distress for both child and parent. Frequently, the child is discharged home early and, while parents have been educated about possible post-operative complications, many parents are at a loss about how to cope with their child's pain and when to seek help. Parental education regarding pain management advice about the child's need for post-operative analgesia and appropriate prescribing of acetaminophen and an opioid suspension, the latter on an 'as needed' (PRN) basis, together with stimulant laxatives, should be included in the educational meeting with the child and the parent before surgery and reinforced immediately following surgery. Parents require education particularly about the need for regular 'at the clock' medication to maintain a steady state of blood plasma levels of the non-opioid analgesic drug, especially for the first 48 hours and very possibly longer, to avoid unnecessary patient suffering. The nurse advises the parent about promoting the child's optimal sleep hygiene, rest and relaxation, distraction and comfort, as well as the importance of drinking plenty of cold fluids to reduce inflammation and the risk of infection. The parent and patient should be reassured that, as the pain reduces, and sometimes this does not happen until the second week post-surgery, the 'as needed' (PRN) opioid preparation doses can be gradually stopped to minimize possible gastric side-effects of withdrawal and to continue with doses of acetaminophen on an 'as needed' (PRN) basis until no longer required.

The parent and child should be instructed in how to keep a pain dairy, and have access to a liaison hospital nurse in the two-week post-operative period to discuss any pain control and symptom-related problems the parent and child are experiencing about high pain levels, nausea and vomiting, or poor fluid intake and to carefully monitor the side-effects of opioid medication, particularly if the child has any breathing problems, chest infection or constipation. The pediatric tonsillectomy pain management should be according to a specific hospital protocol to cover the period to the child's full recovery.

Comfort and nonpharmacological measures are really important to reduce anxiety. A salient issue is the healing of the tonsil bed, associated inflammation, bleeding and the risk of infection. A recent randomized controlled trial found that the use of flavoured ice lollies significantly lowered the pain score of children aged between 2 and 12 years post-tonsillectomy, with or without adenoidectomy in the immediate post-operative period, compared with a control (no ice-lolly). The aim is to reduce tonsil-bed inflammation with cooling, which, studies suggest, may inhibit nociception, reduce muscle spasms and pain-related metabolic enzyme activity (Sylvester et al., 2011). Another study found that eating and drinking in the immediate pediatric tonsillectomy post-operative period reduced nausea, vomiting and pain.

In the first study of its type, Sertel et al. (2009) carried out a randomized controlled trial of the benefits of one session of acupuncture in addition to NSAIDs. The study (of 123 patients aged 16 years and above) evaluated the efficacy of acupuncture against swallowing pain between the first and fifth post-operative day following tonsillectomy. The acupuncture group experienced significant additional pain relief as well as longer lasting analgesic benefit from the NSAID analgesia. Music, imagery, video games and other distraction cognitive behavioural activities may all help to maintain the child's equilibrium, reduce distress, raise the pain threshold and facilitate recovery (Howard et al., 2014).

## Post-operative patient-controlled analgesia (PCA) for children

For the management of post-operative pain and acute pain associated with sickle cell occlusive crisis, which require opioid medication, **patient**-controlled analgesia (PCA) for children is feasible where the child is adequately cognitively developed to understand the relationship between pushing the button and obtaining pain relief. **Nurse**-controlled analgesia (NCA) is effective in younger children, for whom PCA can have a failure rate due to a lack of understanding the cause-and-effect relationship between button-pushing and obtaining pain relief. The benefit of opioid medication given by PCA is to avoid variations in blood plasma concentration levels, which impact negatively on analgesic effect and increase drug side-effects. **Parent**-controlled analgesia is strongly discouraged in the acute care setting unless linked with stringent protocols and frequent nurse assessment, as the risk of adverse events has been shown to be very high.

All opioid medication is potentially constipating, even if taken for a few doses, so a proactive approach should always be taken, with laxatives as part of the preventative regimen. Table 8.1 shows the typical starting doses for patient-controlled (first-line opioid analgesia) analgesia for children, with lock-out time. The nurse observes, measures, documents and monitors the patient's five vital signs and fluid intake and output from the time of the patient's admission to the pediatric acute care setting and post-operatively, documenting pain medication and monitoring effectiveness, checking for adverse opioid and other medication side-effects, especially respiratory depression, sedation, nausea and vomiting, and pruritus (itch), advocating for medication adjustment and communicating as required with the acute care team and with the infant's or child's parents (Greco and Berde, 2010; Kennedy, 2014).

**Table 8.1** Starting dose for patient-controlled analgesia

| Drug | Bolus dose (µg/kg) | Continuous rate (µg/kg/h) | 4-hour limit (µg/kg) |
|---|---|---|---|
| Morphine | 20 | 4–15 | 300 |
| Hydromorphone | 5 | 1–3 | 60 |
| Fentanyl | 0.25 | 0.15 | 4 |

Source: Greco, C. and Berde, C.B. (2010) Acute pain management in children. In S.M. Fishman, J.C. Ballantyne and J.P. Rathmell (eds), *Bonica's Management of Pain* (4th edn). Riverwoods, IL: Wolters Kluwer/Lippincott Williams and Wilkins.

## Acute abdominal pain in adolescents and adults

This section highlights the frequent signs and symptoms associated with acute abdominal pain, and the nurse's role in observing, documenting and monitoring vital signs and communicating with the patient and with the acute pain care team.

Acute abdominal pain signals a warning about possible tissue damage for injury to abdominal organs and is frequently visceral (associated with the visceral organs of the gastro-intestinal tract) in origin, whereas acute pain of somatic origin, arising from bone, joint, muscle, skin or connective tissues, depending on the cause of the pain, may allow the person to identify the cause and withdraw or remove the stimulus, or seek help to do so. Acute visceral pain, in contrast, prompts involuntary autonomic reflex responses; it is the body's mechanism to remove, expel or otherwise counteract the harmful stimulus. Virtually all acute abdominal pain has an acute inflammatory component, so the person with acute abdominal pain associated with an inflamed gastro-intestinal tract may have nausea, vomiting, and/or diarrhoea as well as other symptoms indicative of autonomic stress (Hall, 2011; Kumar and Clark, 2012; Maybin and Serpell, 2012; Mayer et al., 2013).

## Etiology of acute abdominal pain

Causes of acute abdominal pain are associated with:

> inflammation of organs within the region of the parietal peritoneum (thin serous covering the abdominal inner walls which gives rise to somatic pain from

the spinal nerves) and the visceral organs within the visceral peritoneum (thin serous covering the visceral peritoneum). Examples include (but are not limited to) acute appendicitis, acute diverticulitis or perforated viscus.

vascular causes: an example includes (but is not limited to) acute ischemic colitis, in which the blood supply to the colon is interrupted.

visceral obstruction: examples include (but are not limited to) cancer invading the intestine or kidney stones which have travelled to the ureter.

distention of the capsules covering the visceral organs. (Mayer et al., 2013)

Each of these types of acute pain has distinguishing typical features of pain location. The quality of visceral pain is usually aching or gnawing and poorly localized, in contrast to pain from the parietal peritoneum, which is sharp, more defined, somatic pain transmitted via the spinal nerves. The nature of onset is rapid, sudden or gradual, and the chronology is constant or colicky. Aggravating and associated factors often include a fever (a raised temperature) and leucocytosis (in inflammatory conditions, the bone marrow releases neutrophils which limit bacterial infection by phagocytosis), and, depending on the underlying cause, include nausea, vomiting, bloody stools and/or diarrhoea and other specific symptoms. For example, a perforated viscus (i.e. an internal body organ, which, in the context of appendicitis, is a ruptured appendix) may present with a paralytic ileus, a loss of bowel function due to an autonomic feature of motor inhibition of nerves and muscles, which is the body's method of trying to prevent the further drainage of toxins into the peritoneal cavity. Paralytic ileus is a type of acute colonic pseudo-obstruction in which the bowel is distended by gas and painful (and which is also a potential post-operative complication following bowel manipulation in intestinal surgery) (Flynn Makie, 2014; Kumar and Clark, 2012; Mayer et al., 2013).

## Acute pain and shock

As all acute pain is potentially associated with shock, nursing responsibilities include measurement and observation, documentation and ongoing monitoring of the five vital signs of temperature, pulse, respiration, blood pressure and pain as well as body fluid intake and output, including frequency and type and rate of vomiting, urinary and faecal excretion (bloody stools, diarrhoea). These observations are taken from the time of the patient's admission to the emergency department and at regular intervals thereafter.

Shock is a clinical syndrome affecting all body systems in which cells lack an adequate blood supply, depriving them of oxygen and nutrients. Hypoperfusion of tissues, hypermetabolism and activation of the inflammatory response are common to all types of shock as a consequence of the body's response in activating the autonomic sympathetic nervous system and the onset of 'fight or flight' arousal mechanisms. Blood is shunted away from the body periphery in order to supply vital organs to cope with the stressor. Table 8.2 shows the harmful effects of unrelieved pain from a biopsychosocial perspective (McCaffery and Pasero, 1999).

**Table 8.2**   Harmful effects of unrelieved pain

| Domains affected | Specific responses to pain |
|---|---|
| Endocrine | ↑ Adrenocorticotrophic hormone (ACTH), ↑ cortisal, ↑ antidiuretic hormone (ADH), ↑ epinephrine,↑ norepinephrine,↑ growth hormone (GH),↑ catecholamines, ↑ renin, ↑ angiotensin 11,↑ aldosterone,↑ glucagon,↑ interleukin-1; ↓ insulin, ↓ testosterone |
| Metabolic | Gluconeogenesis, hepatic glycogenolysis, hyperglycemia, glucose intolerance, insulin resistance, muscle protein catabolism, ↑ lipolysis |
| Cardiovascular | ↑ Heart rate, ↑ cardiac output, ↑ peripheral vascular resistance, ↑ systemic vascular resistance, hypertension, ↑ coronary vascular resistance, ↑ myocardial oxygen consumption, hypercoagulation, deep vein thrombosis |
| Respiratory | ↓ Flows and volumes, atelectasis, shunting, hypoxemia, ↓ cough, sputum rentention, infection |
| Genitourinary | ↓ Urinary output, urinary retention, fluid overload, hypokalemia |
| Gastrointestinal | ↓ Gastric and bowel motility |
| Musculoskeletal | Muscle spasm, impaired muscle function, fatigue, immobility |
| Cognitive | Reduction in cognitive function, mental confusion |
| Immune | Depression of immune response |
| Developmental | ↑ Behavioural and physiologic responses to pain, altered temperaments, higher somatization, infant distress behaviour; possible altered development of the pain system, ↑ vulnerability to stress disorders, addictive behaviour, and anxiety states |
| Future pain | Debilitating chronic pain syndromes: post-mastectomy pain, post-thoracotomy pain, phantom pain, postherpetic neuralgia |
| Quality of life | Sleeplessness, anxiety, fear, hopelessness, ↑ thoughts of sucide |

Source: McCaffery, M. and Pasero, C: Pain: *Clinical Manual*, p. 24. Copyright 1999. Republished with permission of Elsevier Mosby. Information from Cousins M: Acute postoperative pain. In Wall P.D., MelZack, R., (eds), *Textbook of Pain* (3rd edn), pp. 357–385, New York, 1994, Churchill Livingstone; Kehlet .H. Modification of responses to surgery by Neural blockade. In Cousins, M.J., Bridenbaugh, P.O., (eds), *Neural Blockade*, pp. 129–175, Philadelphia,1998, Lippincott-Raven; Mcintyre, P.E., Ready, L.B. *Acute Pain Management: A Practical Guide*, Philadelphia, 1996, WB Saunders.

# The three stages of shock

In stage 1 (compensatory), the blood pressure remains within normal limits. For the patient's survival, it is necessary to address shock at this stage. The patient in shock will look pale and have cool skin, increased respirations and a reduced urinary output, brought about by physiological mechanisms to try to keep the blood pressure stable. Cardiac output and vasoconstriction are increased.

In stage 2 (progressive), the blood pressure falls to hypotensive levels of less than 90 mm Hg or below 65 mm Hg mean arterial pressure. At stage 2 shock, all organs are hypoperfused and the patient is critically ill, requiring skilled, interdisciplinary care in the intensive care unit. The heart becomes dysfunctional through overwork and a highly complex feedback of failure in all organs and systems ensues.

At stage 3 shock, the severe organ damage precludes a response to treatment. Multiple organ failure precedes death (Flynn Makie, 2014).

## Essential nursing practice in acute pain and shock

Pain acts as a stressor, stimulating the sympathetic nervous system. The secretion of epinephrine (adrenaline) and norepinephrine (noradrenaline) in increased efforts maintains tissue perfusion and adequate blood supply to vital organs. The patient in severe pain with an infection is at high risk for shock and associated complications. The primary nursing practice responsibility is ongoing monitoring of the patient's five vital signs and body fluid intake and output to identify shock and facilitate intervention at the earliest possible opportunity by the acute care team. The lead physician prescribes treatments which are usually administered by the nurse.

- Pain should be measured as the fifth vital sign, documented, addressed and treated at the earliest opportunity to reduce shock and to prevent sensitization. Morphine is the drug of choice for acute severe pain and is especially beneficial for visceral pain. In acute abdominal pain in the older child or adult, the doctor may prescribe an initial reduced slow intravenous injection starting dose (morphine < 5mg) over at least five minutes. The dose is dependent on the age, weight and the health status of the patient, and is reduced for the older person. This acts to reduce the pain level, counter the ongoing development of the shock process, and help the patient feel more comfortable, while not impeding diagnosis. The patient will require an antiemetic, usually cyclizine or a similar drug, to prevent further nausea and vomiting associated with abdominal pain and autonomic stress as well as opioid-related nausea (Macaluso and McNamara, 2012).
- Blood pressure: the patient's blood pressure must be monitored regularly. If the patient's blood pressure is falling, the nurse alerts the acute care team before the systolic blood pressure reduces to below systolic < 90 mm Hg or mean arterial pressure of < 65 mm Hg, at which point serious, potentially irreversible cellular and tissue damage has taken place. Intravenous fluids are administered at stage 1 shock to increase blood volume and improve cardiac output. Careful nursing monitoring of intravenous fluids intake and urinary output (the latter compromised in shock) is required at all stages as possible side-effects include cardiovascular overload and pulmonary oedema.
- Pulse/heart rate (stage 1 > 100 beats per minute or 25 beats per 15 seconds): oxygen is administered at stage 1 shock, which, together with intravenous fluids, helps to increase tissue oxygen perfusion throughout the body and to reduce cardiac strain.
- Respirations: > than 20 breaths per minute; inadequate tissue perfusion results in metabolic acidosis which prompts an increase in respirations with the aim

of removing excess carbon dioxide from the blood. As a measure of tissue hypoperfusion, improved sublingual capnometry technologies allow blood carbon dioxide levels to be determined by the blood flow in the mucosal bed by a probe placed under the patient's tongue. Increased blood levels of carbon dioxide indicate poor tissue perfusion of oxygen.

- Tissue oxygen can also be measured by a near-infrared spectroscope by a probe placed to the thenar muscle on the palm of the hand. Infrared light absorption indicates the level of skeletal muscle oxygenation saturation.
- Temperature: a raised temperature contributes to the body's stress response and efforts to regain homeostasis by the autonomic nervous system.
- The nurse has close contact with the patient and his or her family, all of whom may be anxious and require empathic, supportive communications and explanations of procedures, what to expect and changes in the patient's health status. The patient may be confused or agitated (Flynn Makie, 2014).

## A case of acute pain

A 14-year-old white adolescent male, Jack, presented at the emergency department at 7 pm on a Tuesday evening, accompanied by his father. Checking his observations, the nurse found that Jack had a fever (T 38.5C; 101.3F). When the nurse asked Jack where his pain was, Jack indicated his right lower abdomen (right lower quadrant). Jack rated his pain as 9 (on a 0–10 Number Rating Scale) and described his pain as the worst pain possible (on a Verbal Rating Scale), and as aching and gnawing and sharp in quality. Jack had rapid breathing, very rapid pulse-tachycardia and lowered blood pressure. The nurse documented the five observations, with pain as the fifth vital sign. Jack's father indicated that Jack had vomited frequently all day, had had no food and only a little water to drink, vomiting back any fluids taken. Jack lay on his left side on the hospital trolley with his hips and knees flexed to try to reduce the severe pain sensation and did not feel like talking. The nurse gently asked Jack: (a) when the pain started – Jack replied that the pain started in the middle of his tummy over the past day; (b) when Jack had last eaten – Jack replied he had eaten the previous day; and (c) when Jack had last passed urine and had a bowel movement – Jack replied that he had passed urine and had a bowel movement the previous day (Monday morning) and the nurse documented this information. The nurse also asked Jack if he had taken any recreational drugs or alcohol recently and told Jack this information was very important to prevent any side-effects from his hospital treatments. Jack replied that he had not taken recreational drugs or alcohol and the nurse documented this information.

- Q1. How are Jack's immediate nursing intervention requirements addressed?
  A: The immediate nursing interventions are:
- Observation/measurement and documentation of Jack's temperature, pulse, respirations and blood pressure and pain (as the fifth vital sign).
- Ensuring that Jack is not left alone by asking Jack's father to stay with Jack at all times, while seeking immediate clinical medical attention for Jack.

*(Continued)*

CLINICAL EXAMPLE

*(Continued)*

Q2. How will Jack's immediate medical and nursing care interventions proceed?
A: Immediate medical and nursing care interventions are:

- From both a nursing and medical perspective, for safe and optimal care, a biopsychosocial medical history is absolutely essential and Jack's father may be able to assist the nurse and the doctor with all information, including drug allergies.
- Jack requires an immediate medical clinical examination by the doctor. Jack has an urgent requirement for rehydration with intravenous fluids, oxygen and for immediate pain relief. The nurse and doctor work with the care team to address these needs.

Q3. Are there competing issues in this instance? If so, how does current knowledge and patient-centred interdisciplinary care address them?
A: The patient needs an early examination and early pain relief, conducted in the light of an accurate biopsychosocial medical history. Although controversial traditionally, through reviews of relevent studies, the Agency for Healthcare Research and Quality (Brownfield, 2001) concluded that an appropriate and judicious use of immediate opioid analgesics in patients with acute abdominal pain:

(a) did not impair physicians' or surgeons' ability to accurately diagnose, evaluate or treat patients with acute abdominal pain or their treatment decision, facilitating more accurate diagnosis in some patients
(b) is more humane (Brownfield, 2001; Macaluso and McNamara, 2012).

........................................................................................................

# Evaluation of abdominal pain by physical examination

The cornerstone of accurate diagnosis of the underlying cause of acute pain is a comprehensive patient biopsychosocial medical history. Social and behavioural issues inform the diagnosis. For example, social drug use (especially cocaine and alcohol) and domestic violence can cause gastric symptoms. The examination of the patient with acute abdominal pain by the nurse and the doctor is helped by using the PQRST mnemonic:

P3 – positions, and interventions (if any), which make the pain better and factors which make the pain worse
Q – pain quality
R3 – region where the pain is felt, and if and where the pain radiates to another location
S – pain severity
T3 – time and mode of onset of the pain, how the pain has progressed and whether there have been previous episodes. (Macaluso and McNamara, 2012: 789)

Acute appendicitis is frequently diagnosed through a combination of information provided by the patient's past and current medical history, together with laboratory tests (white cell (WBC) and absolute neutrophil counts (ANC) and C-reactive protein (CRP)), physical examination, ultrasound and CT Scan. Children often have difficulty talking about their symptoms and pain experience. Overlap with other diseases such as gastro-enteritis may complicate diagnosis (Allister et al., 2011; Snyder, et al. 2012).

Appendicitis is regularly misdiagnosed and is a major cause of litigation. The diagnostic indicators must be placed in the context of Jack's social history, which does not give any indication for gastric pain in Jack's case. Jack's father indicates that there is a family history of appendicitis. There are indicators that Jack's pain is visceral in origin as he has complained of 'aching and gnawing' pain and has nausea and vomiting. Jack's pain has also changed location from the middle of the abdomen, localizing to the right iliac fossa, within the past few hours.

The appendix is a long diverticulum situated at the end of the caecum at the start of the large bowel. In appendicitis, the initial distension of the appendix (most often with a faecolith, a hardened stool mass, sometimes with acute inflammation, tumour, foreign body or lymphoid hyperplasia) causes a periumbilical visceral pain which is poorly localized and generated by spinal afferents innervating visceral organs. The visceral and somatic afferent nerve fibres converge onto the same spinal neurons. When the inflammation is limited to the appendix, the visceral pain is felt as gnawing and aching. When the inflammation increases, and the inflamed appendix comes into contact with the parietal peritoneum, the pain becomes somatic and sharp in quality and more localized (Mayer et al., 2013).

There are two classic diagnostic tests for appendicitis:

(a) The psoas sign: with the patient lying on his or her side, the psoas sign, which is increased pain of the psoas muscle by an inflammatory process near the muscle, is elicited by the examiner passively extending the contralateral hip joint.

(b) The Rovsing sign is elicited by the examiner applying pressure in the left lower abdominal quadrant. The test is positive if the patient feels rebound pain in the right lower quadrant on pressure release. For a detailed description of the physical examination of the patient with abdominal pain, see Macaluso and McNamara (2012).

# Diagnosis, treatment and nursing care of the patient with myocardial infarction

**Acute coronary syndrome** (ACS) is an acute onset of myocardial ischemia which can result in myocardial death (myocardial infarction) and which requires prompt and specific high-level emergency interventions to prevent fatalities. In Europe, up to 200,000 people each year experience acute coronary syndrome. In the USA, more than a quarter of a million people each year experience an acute myocardial infarction, resulting in many deaths, which occur before the person has even arrived at hospital (Dressler and Weitmann, 2014; Edmondson et al., 2012).

## Pathophysiology of acute coronary syndrome

The term acute coronary syndrome (ACS) was derived from the similarity of the symptoms of unstable angina pectoris (in which the rupture of an atherosclerotic plaque results in further reduction in blood flow in a coronary artery) with myocardial infarction, so that the two conditions are indistinguishable by symptoms. In unstable angina, the coronary artery is not completely occluded (closed), whereas atherosclerotic plaque eruption and thrombus formation completely occlude the coronary artery in myocardial infarction. The common mechanism for acute coronary syndrome is the rupture or erosion of a coronary artery fibrous plaque, which leads to platelet aggregation and adhesion, localized thrombosis, distal thrombus embolization and vasoconstriction, resulting in myocardial ischaemia due to the reduction of coronary blood flow.

## Diagnosis of myocardial infarction

In acute coronary syndrome (ACS), the key factor in patient survival is rapid and accurate diagnosis of myocardial infarction. Patients may present with severe chest pain, along with a range and combination of symptoms, such as difficulty with breathing (dyspnoea), anxiety, nausea and vomiting, and gastric indigestion. Their vital signs may show autonomic, sympathetic nervous system arousal associated with early shock, with rapid pulse and respiration, lowered or raised blood pressure and cool, clammy, pale skin.

Pain cannot be used as an indicator to distinguish between myocardial ischemia and myocardial infarction. Sometimes myocardial ischemia does not present with pain and is 'silent'. This is considered to be due to reduced sensitivity because of 'neural stunning' by previous ischaemia or because of individual variations in cardio-pathophysiology or pain sensitivity.

The chest is highly innervated by nerve plexi to different visceral organs. Chest pain, while severe, is often poorly localized and referred because of dermatomal origin to another location (see Figure 8.1). The pain of myocardial infarction typically refers to the left arm, neck and jaw. Myocardial infarction (MI) occurs when cardiac myocytes die due to myocardial ischaemia. MI can be diagnosed on the basis of appropriate clinical history, 12-lead ECG and elevation of biomarkers cardiac troponin 1, which is a highly sensitive test of myocite necrosis, as well as elevation of biomarkers troponin T and C, creatine-kinase-MB (CK-MB) and myoglobin (Dressler and Weitmann, 2014; Edwards et al., 2013; Kumar and Clark, 2012).

**Visceral pain referral**

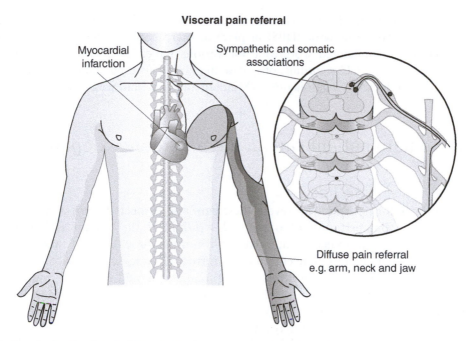

A. Syrimis, Cardiac Pain Referral Mechanism, www.clinicalexams.co.uk

**Definition:** The manifestation of cardiogenic pain at a somatic site adjacent or distal to the actual site of injury. Cardiac referred pain is the sensation of pain in the left side of the face, neck, chest, and left upper limb which can sometimes occur on the right in cases of dextrocardia.

**Causes:** The usual causes of cardiac referred pain include: myocardial infaction or heart attack, dissecting aortic aneurism. The precise mechanism behind the referred pain phenomenon remains poorly understood. Cardiac visceral afferent fibres run with the sympathetics back to the spinal cord, where their cell bodies are located in the dorsal root ganglia of T1 to T5. The central nervous system interprets cardiogenic pain as of somatic origin corresponding to the T1 to T5 segments. In addition to this, the dermatomes corresponding to this spinal level (T1 to T5) have their cell bodies located in the dorsal root ganglia, and synapse at the same spinal segment as the visceral afferents from the heart. It is suggested that there is some sort of confusion in the interpretation and differentiation of pain.

**Examination:** In a clinical setting, one must consider cardiac referred pain when assessing a patient complaining of pain in the sites corresponding to this referral pattern. The case history and the character of the pain are important determinants in the diagnosis or clinical exclusion of cardiac referred pain. It is uncommon for a visceral pathology to be aggravated by provocative stimulation of the soma. A full cardiovascular examination is indicated to rule out cardiac referred pain.

**Figure 8.1**   Pain of myocardial infarction is often poorly localized and referred because of dermatomal origin in another location

A 12-lead ECG is performed on admission to the emergency department. It detects electrocardiographic evolution of myocardial infarction. If the ST segment is elevated, together with positive biomarkers and a relevant patient/family clinical history, ST-elevation myocardial infarction (STEMI) is diagnosed (Kumar and Clark, 2012).

A recent warning publication has highlighted the need to check whether the patient has a deep brain stimulator (DBS) in place as increasing numbers of deep brain stimulators are implanted worldwide for various indications. The DBS must be turned off during ECG recording, otherwise the ECG recording and reading may be inaccurate and lead to a misdiagnosis (Mindermann and Maurer, 2013).

# Immediate patient care in the emergency department

## Time is muscle

The priority for patients with severe chest pain and suspected myocardial infarction is the administration of oxygen (2–4 L/min if the patient is hypoxic), intravenous opioid analgesia and glyceryl trinitrate for pain relief, and aspirin (162–325 mg) as an anti-platelet to prevent further clotting. Other anticoagulation medication can be given. An intravenous antiemetic should be given. Immediate pain relief helps to reduce the work burden on the heart, limit further damage to the heart muscle and restore supply and demand between the myocardial requirement for tissue perfusion by oxygenated blood and the coronary artery supply. Comprehensive treatment guidelines for acute myocardial infarction are available at www.guideline.gov/content.aspx?id=39320&search=chest+pain+and+acute+coronary+syndrome.

Speed of diagnosis is vital so the patient's close others may help with providing information about patient and family medical history, previous adverse cardiac events and risk factors for coronary heart disease that the patient may have (Dressler and Weitmann, 2014).

## CLINICAL EXAMPLE

## A case of acute coronary syndrome

Mrs D, a 70-year-old European lady with a history of depression and obesity and a long-term heavy smoker, has not complied with taking her antidepressant medication and has not slept well for the past month. Her family noted that Mrs D has recently put on additional weight, is spending much time ruminating, watching television and eating convenience snacks. Her daughter was about to suggest that Mrs D should visit her GP to have a check up when Mrs D sustained very severe chest pain. She vomited once, late one evening. Mrs D managed to call her daughter, just saying 'HELP ... my chest...' before she collapsed. Her daughter contacted the emergency services who responded promptly and a neighbour gave the ambulance paramedics access to Mrs D's house. The paramedics found Mrs D in a shocked state, barely conscious, with rapid, shallow breathing, thready pulse with tachycardia and very low blood pressure. Mrs D was given oxygen and intravenous fluids and transferred to the city hospital emergency department.

On admission, Mrs D was extremely anxious and shocked, and had severe pain in her chest and left arm. The nurse in charge of her care introduced herself and told Mrs D she would be cared for immediately and her pain would be treated at the earliest opportunity. The nurse made Mrs D as comfortable as possible, checking her respirations and oxygen levels. The nurse fully assessed Mrs D's pain, noting location, factors which made the pain worse, pain quality (which in Mrs D's case was strong 'pressure, squeezing' pain), intensity, the time the pain started and pain pattern/temporality. The nurse regularly checked Mrs D's respirations, pulse, blood pressure and temperature, documenting Mrs D's vital signs, with pain as the fifth vital sign. The nurse noted Mrs D's colour as pale and skin temperature as cool. The nurse commended a fluid intake and output chart for Mrs D, documenting the intravenous fluid intake. When Mrs D's daughter arrived at the emergency department, she gave the nurse Mrs D's full medical and biosychosocial history and lifestyle, indicating, when asked, that Mrs D had never had a heart attack. The nurse worked with the emergency department physician, who prescribed oxygen and medication interventions. The nurse and physician worked with the emergency department team to care for Mrs D.

Q1. What is Mrs D's suspected diagnosis and how is Mrs D's nursing care prioritized immediately on arrival to the emergency department?

A: Mrs D has the symptoms of a acute myocardial infarction, which will be confirmed using a 12-lead electrocardiogram to be read within 10 minutes. Monitoring is initiated as soon as possible to confirm the diagnosis of acute myocardial infarction though elevated ST segment of more than 1 mm in contiguous leads, together with the laboratory test confirmation of raised serum cardiac enzymes and biomarkers.

Q2. The ECG confirms an elevated ST segment on two contiguous ECG leads, which is indicative of an acute myocardial infarction associated with cardiac muscle injury. With a confirmed diagnosis of STEMI and blood specimens confirmed as positive by laboratory tests for increased cardiac troponin I, T and C, creatine-kinase-MB and myoglobin, how does Mrs D's initial nursing management proceed?

A: The immediate priority is to bring Mrs D's pain under control and to continue with oxygen. Morphine is administered as the preferred drug of choice to reduce pain and anxiety, together with aspirin to prevent platelet aggregation, nitroglycerin, a potent vasodilator which helps to relieve chest pain by improving cardiac blood flow, and a beta blocker, all of which preserve the myocardial tissue from further necrosis. The nurse administers the medications as prescribed, and documents and monitors their effectiveness in bringing Mrs D's pain under control. The nurse helps her to be more restful and comfortable, reducing her fear and anxiety, the latter of which are associated with the stress response, which puts further pressure on her myocardial oxygen requirement.

There are many other causes of acute pain that are unaddressed in this chapter. Venous thromboembolism (VTE) is one of the most frequent, highly preventable, causes of inhospital patient deaths. VTE presents as deep vein thrombosis (DVT), possibly with the potentially fatal complication of pulmonary embolism (PE). Critically ill patient groups and patients with stroke have the highest incidence. However, many patients are at risk, especially post-operative patients and patients with limited mobility. Preventative thromboprophylaxis is underutilised. The nurse has a major role in the prevention of venous thromboembolism and each nurse needs to be aware of the signs and symptoms of DVT and PE, and their prevention and management (Morrison, 2006).

## Chapter summary

- Topical analgesia is strongly supported for children undergoing skin-penetrating procedures, and care should be taken regarding allergy. Systemic absorption of prilocaine is a risk factor for some infants. EMLA should be removed quickly following procedures.
- Pharmacological interventions for children require careful selection because of the potential side-effects. Immediate post-operative pain is treated with opioids. Patient-controlled analgesia is suitable for children who are able to understand cause and effect.
- Post-tonsillectomy pain requires careful, informed management. The nurse has a major role in educating the child and parent in coping and in mastering skills for the post-tonsillectomy two-week recovery period using pharmacologic and nonpharmacologic interventions.
- Acute abdominal pain has many causes and may be vascular, from blood supply occlusion to the intestines, comprised of visceral pain due to obstruction or distension of the capsules of the visceral organs, inflammatory and/or somatic pain from the parietal peritoneum.
- All acute pain can potentially result in shock, a clinical syndrome of hypoperfusion of tissues, hypermetabolism and activation of the inflammatory and stress responses. These symptoms must be addressed early, when the blood pressure is within normal limits for patient survival.
- The nurse, as a member of the multidisciplinary team, holistically assesses the patient with acute pain. The nurse measures, observes, documents and monitors the patient's five vital signs, body fluid intake and output and excreta, communicating status changes to the acute care team. Peri- and post-operative opioid medication requires careful monitoring.
- The misdiagnosis of appendicitis is one of the most litigious occurrences in emergency medicine. A biopsychosocial history is essential to preclude social causes of pain and to support the clinical examination and additional test findings, which, together, inform diagnosis.
- Acute coronary syndrome is an international problem. Early diagnosis with ECG and serum enzyme and cardiac biomarkers of STEMI enhances appropriate interventions and patient recovery. Psychological and lifestyle factors contribute to etiology and prevention. The nurse has a major role to play in venous thromboembolism prevention.

## Reflective exercise

Consider how biopsychosocial pain assessment contributes to more effective care of the patient with acute pain.

## Recommended reading

Bromley, L. and Brander, B. (2010) *Acute Pain*. Oxford: Pain Management Library.
Cayley, W.E. (2005) 'Diagnosing the cause of chest pain', *American Family Physician*, 72: 2012–2021.
Hinkle, J.L. and Cheever, K.H. (eds) (2014) *Brunner and Suddarth's Textbook of Medical–Surgical Nursing* (13th edn). Riverwoods, IL: Wolters Kluwer/Lippincott Williams and Wilkins. (For chapters on pain and pre-operative, intra-operative and post-operative nursing management.)
Morrison, R. (2006) Venous thromboembolism: scope of the problem and the nurse's role in risk assessment and prevention. *Journal of Vascular Nursing*, 24 (3): 82–90.

## Websites relevant to this chapter

American Heart Association: www.heart.org/HEARTORG/
American Society for Preventative Cardiology: www.aspconline.org/
ANZCA Acute Pain Management Scientific Evidence (2010): www.anzca.edu.au/resources/college-publications/pdfs/Acute%20Pain%20Management/books-and-publications/acutepain.pdf
European Society of Cardiology: www.escardio.org/Pages/index.aspx
National Institute for Health and Clinical Excellence Guidelines: www.nice.org.uk/

# References

Allister, L., Bachur, R., Glickman, J. and Horwitz, B. (2011) Serum markers in acute appendicitis. *Journal of Surgical Research*, 168: 70–75.

Alvarado, A. (1986) A practical score for the early diagnosis of acute appendicitis. *Annals of Emergency Medicine*, 15: 557–564.

Atef, A. and Aly Fawaz, A. (2008) Peritonsillar infiltration with tramadol improves pediatric tonsillectomy pain. *European Archives of Otorhinolaryngology*, 265: 571–574.

Brownfield, E. (2001) Pain management. Use of analgesics in the acute abdomen. In: *Making Health Care Safer: A Critical Analysis of Patient Safety Practices. Evidence Report/Technology Assessment*, No 43. AHRQ Publication No 01-E058. Rockville (MD): Agency for Healthcare Research and Quality. pp. 396–400. Available at: www.ahrq.gov/clinic/ptsafety/. (accessed 13 July 2014).

Davis, T., Bluhm, J., Burke, R., Iqbal, Q., Kim, K., Kokoszka, M., Larson, T., Puppala, V., Setterlund, L., Vuong K. and Zwank, M. (2012) *Diagnosis and treatment of chest pain and acute coronary syndrome (ACS)*. Bloomington, MN: Institute for Clinical Systems Improvement (ICSI).

Dhingra, B. and Mishra, D. (2011) Immediate versus as-needed acetaminophen for post-immunisation pyrexia. *Annals of Tropical Paediatrics*, 31: 339–344.

Di Cesare, A., Parolini, F., Morandi, A., Leva, E. and Torricelli, M. (2013) Do we need imaging to diagnose appendicitis in children? *African Journal of Pediatric Surgery*, 10 (2): 68–73.

Dressler, D.K. and Weitmann, K. (2014) Management of patients with coronary vascular disorders. In J.L. Hinkle and K.H. Cheever (eds), *Brunner and Suddarth's Textbook of Medical–Surgical Nursing* (13th edn). Riverwoods, IL: Wolters Kluwer/Lippincott Williams and Wilkins.

Edmondson, D., Richardson, S., Falzon, L., Davidson, K.W., Mills, M.A., et al. (2012) Posttraumatic stress disorder prevalence and risk of recurrence in acute coronary syndrome patients: a meta-analytic review. *PLoS One*, 7 (6): e38915 (doi:10.1371/journal.pone.0038915).

Edwards, B., Washington, I., Pretlow, L., Passmore, G., Dias, J. and Wise, S. (2013) Sequential assessment of troponon in the diagnosis of myocardial infarction. *Clinical Laboratory Science*, 26: 95–99.

Ergul, E. (2006) Importance of family history and genetics for the prediction of acute appendicitis. *The Internet Journal of Surgery*, 10 (1): 1–6.

FDA (2013) Drug Safety Communications (02/20/2013). *Safety Review Update of Codeine Use in Children; New Boxed Warning and Contraindication on Use after Tonsillectomy and/or Adenoidectomy.* Available at: www.fda.gov/downloads/Drugs/DrugSafety/UCM339116.pdf (accessed 13 July 2014).

Flynn Makie, M.B. (2014) Shock and multiple organ dysfunction syndrome. In J.L. Hinkle and K.H. Cheever (eds), *Brunner and Suddarth's Textbook of Medical–Surgical Nursing* (13th edn). Riverwoods, IL: Wolters Kluwer/Lippincott Williams and Wilkins.

Gottschalk, A. and Ochroch, E.A. (2013) Thoracic pain. In S.B. McMahon, M. Koltzenburg, I.Tracey and D.C. Turk (eds), *Wall and Melzack's Textbook of Pain* (6th edn). Philadelphia, PA: Elsevier Saunders.

Greco, C. and Berde, C.B. (2010) Acute pain management in children. In S.M. Fishman, J.C. Ballantyne and J.P. Rathmell (eds), *Bonica's Management of Pain* (4th edn). Riverwoods, IL: Wolters Kluwer/Lippincott Willliams and Wilkins.

Hall, J.E. (2011) *Guyton and Hall Textbook of Medical Physiology*. Philadelphia, PA: Elsevier Saunders.

Hinkle, J.L. and Cheever, K.H. (eds) (2014) *Brunner and Suddarth's Textbook of Medical–Surgical Nursing* (13th edn). Riverwoods, IL: Wolters Kluwer/Lippincott Williams and Wilkins.

Howard, D., Finn Davis, K., Phillips, E., Ryan E., Scalford, D., Flynn-Roth, R. and Ely, E. (2014) Pain management for pediatric tonsillectomy: an integrative review through the perioperative and home experience. *Journal for Specialists in Pediatric Nursing*, 19: 5–16.

Howell, J.M., Eddy, O.L., Lukens, T.W., Thiessen, M.E. W., Weingart, S.D. and Decker, W.W. (2010) Clinical policy: critical issues in the evaluation and management of emergency department patients with suspected appendicitis. *Annals of Emergency Medicine*, 55: 71–116.

Ingraham, A.M., Cohen, M.E., Bilimoria, K.Y., Pritts, T.A., Ko, C.Y. and Esposito, T.J. (2010) Comparison of outcomes after laparoscopic versus open appendectomy for acute appendicitis. *Surgery*, 148(4): 625–637 (doi:10.1016/j.surg.2010.07.025).

Kennedy, L. (2014) Preoperative, intraoperative and postoperative nursing management. In J.L. Hinkle and K.H. Cheever (eds), *Brunner and Suddarth's Textbook of Medical–Surgical Nursing* (13th edn). Riverwoods, IL: Wolters Kluwer/Lippincott Williams and Wilkins.

Kumar, P. and Clark, M. (eds) (2012) *Clinical Medicine* (8th edn). Philadelphia, PA: Saunders Elsevier.

Kwan, K.Y. and Nager, A.L. (2010) Diagnosing pediatric appendicitis: usefulness of laboratory markers. *American Journal of Emergency Medicine*, 28: 1009–1015.

Macaluso, C.R. and McNamara, R.M. (2012) Evaluation and management of acute abdominal pain in the emergency department. *International Journal of General Medicine*, 5: 789–797.

Maybin, J. and Serpell, M.G. (2012) Neuropathic pain. In L.A. Colvin and M. Fallon (eds), *ABC of Pain*. Chichester: Wiley-Blackwell.

Mayer, E.A., Gupta, A. and Yu Wong, H. (2013) A clinical perspective on abdominal pain. In S.B. McMahon, M. Koltzenburg, I.Tracey and D.C. Turk (eds), *Wall and Melzack's Textbook of Pain* (6th edn). Philadelphia, PA: Elsevier Saunders.

Mindermann, T. and Maurer, D. (2013) Delayed diagnosis of myocardial infarction due to deep brain stimulation. *Acta Neurochirurgica*, 155: 1679–1680.

Morrison, R. (2006) Venous thromboembolism: scope of the problem and the nurse's role in risk assessment and prevention. *Journal of Vascular Nursing*, 24 (3): 82–90.

Pasero, C. and McCaffery, M. (2011) *Pain Assessment and Pharmacologic Management*. St Louis, MO: Elsevier Mosby.

Santillanes, G., Simms, S., Gausche-Hill, M., Diament, M., Putnam, B. Renslo, R., Lee, J., Tinger, E. and Lewis, R.L. (2012) Prospective evaluation of a clinical practice guideline for diagnosis of appendicitis in children. *Academic Emergency Medicine*, 19: 886–893.

Sertel, S., Herrmann, S., Greten H.J., Haxsen, V., El-Bitar, S., Simon, C.H., Baumann, I. and Plinkert, P.K. (2009) Additional use of acupuncture to NSAID effectively reduces post-tonsillectomy pain. *European Archives of Otorhinolaryngology*, 266: 919–925.

Snyder, J.S., Gurevitz, S.L., Rush, L.S., Mc Keague, L.C. and Greenlea Houpt C. (2012) Appendicitis review. *Clinician Reviews*, 22 (1): 23–28.

Stanko, D., Bergesio, R., Davies, K., Hegarty, M. and von Ungern-Sternberg, B. (2013) Postoperative pain, nausea and vomiting following adeno-tonsillectomy: a long-term follow-up. *Pediatric Anesthesia*, 23: 690–696.

Sutters, K.A., Savedra, M.C. and Miaskowski, C. (2011) The pediatric PRO-SELF Pain Control Programme: an effective educational programme for parents caring for children at home following tonsillectomy. *Journal for Specialists in Pediatric Nursing*, 16 (4): 280–294.

Sylvester, D.C., Rafferty, A., Bew, S. and Knight, L.C. (2011) The use of ice-lollies for pain relief post-paediric tonsillectomy: a single-blinded, randomised, controlled trial. *Clinical Otolaryngology*, 36: 566–570.

Thygesen, K., Alpert, J.S., Jaffe, A.S., Simoons, M.L., Chaitman, B.R. and White, H.D. (2012) Third universal definition of myocardial infarction. *European Heart Journal*, 33: 2551–2567.

# 9

# Chronic non-malignant pain

---

## Learning objectives

The learning objectives of this chapter are to:

- recognize the socio-economic and quality-of-life issues associated with chronic pain
- know that chronic pain requires a biopsychosocial approach to diagnosis, treatment and care
- understand the nurse's role in the care of patients of all ages living in the community with chronic pain
- recognize how the different roles of the multidisciplinary team contribute to maximizing the patient's rehabilitation and function

---

## Introduction

This chapter discusses:

- types of chronic non-malignant pain experienced across the lifespan;
- the nurse's role as part of the multidisciplinary team giving interdisciplinary care to relieve symptoms and suffering;
- care systems for patients with chronic non-malignant pain.

Chronic pain of non-malignant origin is generally referred to as chronic pain. Cancer pain, which is pain of malignant origin, is discussed in Chapter 10.

# A systems approach to the management of chronic pain

Australia leads the way in recognizing chronic pain as a disease in its own right, and other countries are in the process of enacting similar legislation to recognize chronic pain in this way and to regard the adequate treatment of pain as a human right (National Pain Strategy (Pain Australia), 2010) (see Chapter 14). Professor Hans Kress, President of The European Federation of IASP Chapters (EFIC), stated that 'chronic pain poses a substantial burden on the individual and also on society, including an enormous economic burden on health care systems' (Kress, 2012). The EFIC symposia in 2010 and 2011 produced *The Societal Impact of Pain: A Road Map for Action* (Treede et al., 2011), which promotes the monitoring of progress across Europe on a set of eleven indicators. These indicators focus on the implementation of:

1. Chronic pain care plans, with adequate wait times and financing.
2. A high-level working group on pain care to monitor progress.
3. An educational programme on pain pathophysiology for the general public ('Pain is Real').
4. Government endorsement of pain research as a priority in national research road maps that address the societal impact of pain and the burden of chronic pain on the health, social and employment sectors.
5. Ensured patient access to pain care (early diagnosis, treatment and medication; secondary prevention).
6. The introduction of mandatory pain medicine and care as teaching subjects in the curricula for nurses, physicians, psychologists and other healthcare professionals.
7. The installation of a network within the national health system for pain management.
8. Pain care as a top priority for the national statutory healthcare authorities.
9. A recognition by the authorities of the right of every citizen to have access to adequate pain care (demonstrated by a regulation or policy).
10. A National Action Plan against pain.
11. A policy to monitor outcomes of pain care.

In the USA, the Joint Commission on Accreditation of Healthcare Organizations (JCAHO) (2012) has identified eight critical components of a successful pain management programme:

1. Use of national pain standards
2. Commitment of a senior leader champion

3. Consistent oversight of a pain project manager
4. Collaboration of the interdisciplinary team
5. Provision of a systematic performance improvement methodology
6. Provision of a pain management infrastructure
7. Promotion of the patient's continuous learning
8. Transition of care for all stakeholders.

## Access to chronic pain services

Access to chronic pain services should be available for patients of all ages across the life-span. A comprehensive chronic pain service has in place optimal community-based primary care services. These comprise the General Practitioner and Practice Nurse/Community Health Nurse being educated in pain management and providing services to patients with chronic pain on an individualized care regimen. The patient's biopsychosocial care regimen includes pharmacological and nonpharmacological interventions so that pain is fully controlled or stabilized in order to optimize the patient's quality of life. If pain eruptions occur, and when these episodes cannot be managed by primary care community services, there should be in place a rapid referral system to a multidisciplinary pain centre of excellence. Here, the patient's case will be reviewed, treatment can be revised and a rehabilitation plan for the patient is put in place in conjunction with primary care services. The patient should also have referral access to physiotherapy, complementary therapies, social and psychological services, advice on diet and a healthy lifestyle, and health promotion advice such as smoking cessation and weight reduction. For a subset of patients with chronic pain, referral options for pain and addiction services may be required.

Chronic non-malignant pain, often known as persistent pain, is both a personal and socio-economic problem, affecting people of all ages. People with chronic pain must be viewed within their social and cultural context since cultural and social factors contribute to both the etiology and the experience of chronic pain. People with chronic pain mostly either live in the wider community or in nursing homes and long-term care facilities. Therefore, many chronic pain consultations (and follow-ups) take place initially (and after) with General Practitioners/Primary Care Physicians either in the patient's homes or in the patient's place of residence or the primary care provider's office (Joint Commission on Accreditation of Healthcare Organizations, 2012). Because degenerative conditions are primarily associated with older age, as people live longer, they may live with more than one disease, known as comorbidities, which are each frequently accompanied by pain symptoms. For example, a person may suffer bouts of angina pain from cardiovascular disease as well as the regular pain of arthritis.

# Control of chronic pain is about relieving pain and distress

Chronic pain can be classified as localized, regional or widespread, and many chronic pain conditions present initially as musculoskeletal pain, while a percentage of people suffer from chronic widespread pain, for which there is, as yet, no universally accepted definition. Chronic widespread pain is associated with pain involving multiple body regions. Chronic widespread pain appears to involve a set of central nervous system processes associated with central sensitization and includes fibromyalgia, irritable bowel syndrome and interstitial cystitis and somatization. Chronic widespread pain massively reduces the sufferer's quality of life, imposing symptoms of multifocal pain, fatigue, insomnia, memory difficulties and mood disorders, as well as many functional problems associated with activities of daily living. These types of pain condition, known as central pain conditions, often respond more to the central nervous system neural modulating agents, particularly antidepressants and anticonvulsants, in contrast to the acute and peripheral pain states, which respond more to non-steroidal anti-inflammatory drugs and opioid medication (Sarsi-Puttini et al., 2011).

Research has yet to fully clarify the exceptionally challenging intricacies of neuropsychobiology and genetics of chronic pain. Improved technology, particularly functional MRI scanning, is helping to clarify specific pain-related activity in multiple brain regions, which currently remains only crudely identified (Apkarian et al., 2011). One research hypothesis is that the pain sufferer's genetically determined pain sensitivity may combine with neuroplastic changes that increase pain transmission, making the pain sufferer more susceptible to hyperalgesia or allodynia (Sarsi-Puttini et al., 2011).

Relief of suffering and pain aims to change the activity within the brain's neuronal circuits from activity underpinning the experience of pain, distress and arousal to neuronal activity underpinning a sense of improved coping, of feeling 'in control' and thus reducing the experience of pain and distress. Activity in brain neuronal circuits has currently unknown meaning, although this may be understood when technology is sufficiently developed. Figure 9.1 shows the brain circuitry in the transition from acute to chronic pain and the complexity of the neuronal interactions (Apkarian et al., 2011; Sarsi-Puttini et al., 2011).

Persistent pain is associated with neuronal plasticity leading to changes in the central nervous system. These changes include long-term changes in neurons in the anterior cingulate cortex which contribute to the maintenance and exacerbation of pain. Also, increased pain sensitivity experienced by people expecting pain is accompanied by increased activity in the anterior cingulate cortex. Imaging studies are beginning to highlight the neurobiology underpinning the role of social and psychological factors in pain (Lumley et al., 2011).

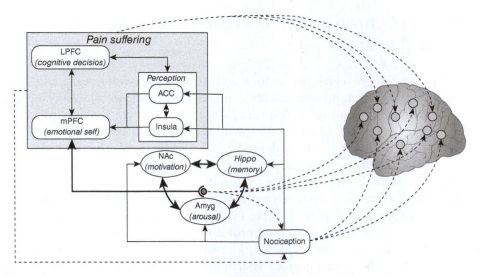

**Figure 9.1**   A model regarding brain circuitry involved in the transition from acute to chronic pain

A model regarding brain circuitry involved in the transition from acute to chronic pain. Nociceptive information, perhaps distorted by peripheral and spinal cord sensitization processes, impinges on limbic circuitry (Hippo, hippocampus; NAc, nucleus accumbens; and Amyg, amygdala). The interaction of limbic circuitry with prefrontal processes determines the level at which a certain pain condition transitions to a more emotional state.

Source: Apkarian, A.V., Hashmi, J.A., Baliki, M.N. (2011) Pain and the brain: specificity and plasticity of the brain in clinical chronic pain. *Pain*, 152: S49–S64. Copyright (2011). The figure has been reproduced with permission of the International Association for the Study of Pain® (IASP). The figure may NOT be reproduced for any other purpose without permission.

## The nurse's role in the care of the community-living patients with chronic pain

The nurse has a major role in facilitating patient education, lifestyle adjustment and access to social support, such as chronic pain patient support groups which offer patient education and coping skills acquisition programmes. When required, the nurse empowers the patient to access appropriate psychological and support services to learn new coping skills both to manage to live with chronic pain and to help bring pain under control. As with all types of pain, chronic pain requires a multidisciplinary team approach, giving interdisciplinary care for an effective patient outcome regarding pain control and management. The nurse and the patient are both part of that care team (Flor and Turk, 2011; Joint Commission on Accreditation of Healthcare Organizations, 2012; Sarsi-Puttini, et al., 2011).

For the person with chronic pain living in the community, the Community Health Nurse or Practice Nurse may be the patient's first point of contact with medical services, and the health professional who refers them to the General Practitioner/Primary Care Physician. In primary care, the role of the General Practitioner/Primary Care

Physician is helping the community-living patient to maintain an optimal standard of health and quality of life. Health systems care provision varies from country to country. In many countries, the General Practitioner/Primary Care Physician and the Practice Nurse and/or Community Health Nurse share a role in patient history-taking, pain assessment, treatment, documentation, treatment monitoring and follow-up, patient education and support, all of which require optimal patient-centred communication skills. When patients with chronic pain are newly discharged from hospital, all details of patient care, including details of their analgesic regimens (which may include complex epidural and peripheral catheters) for chronic pain, should be sent either with the patient or directly from the hospital to the General Practitioner/Primary Care Physician. Continuity between and within care settings requires thorough and complex information and a specific care pathway, giving clear indication who is responsible for the patient's care. Communication giving details of ongoing analgesic and other medications and treatment requirements is an important aspect of this information, so that potentially adverse interactions can be prevented and unplanned readmissions avoided (Joint Commission on Accreditation of Healthcare Organizations, 2012).

# The nurse's role in optimizing the control of chronic pain

Included in the information on the patient's discharge to community care should be the level of pain that the patient finds comfortable on a Number Rating Scale of 0–10. Ideally, the patient's pain will be at zero. However, in chronic pain this is not always achievable and frequently the aim is to bring the patient's pain to the point where they feel comfortable and they can tolerate the pain as 'mild discomfort' (often scored as 3–4 on a Number Rating Scale of 0–10). During and following pain flare-ups, community-living patients are strongly encouraged to maintain a pain diary so that the effectiveness of their analgesic and nonpharmacological pain treatments can be monitored over time and their pain brought back under control. Chronic pain can rapidly become problematic when it is out of control. As with all pain, it is important to bring and maintain the pain under control early, not to regularly wait until the pain becomes 'so bad I have to take medications'. This latter behaviour incurs spikes – peaks and troughs – in analgesic drug–blood plasma levels, which renders the analgesic medication ineffective.

The Practice Nurse/Community Health Nurse has a major role in educating the patient to take analgesic medication as prescribed on an 'at the clock' basis in order to maintain steady state blood plasma drug levels and avoid peaks and troughs. The treatment regimen should be written out in full for the patient, with the reason, dose and time for each medication. A common reason for patients suffering needless, out-of-control chronic pain is a lack of compliance with the treatment regimen, sometimes through a lack of patient education and/or due to fear of addiction. In such cases, the blood plasma level does not maintain a steady state and analgesic medication is therefore ineffective. When the patient's pain is brought under control and kept under control, over time, with review, the analgesic 'at the clock' dosage may be reduced or discontinued if no longer required.

Optimal chronic pain management requires maintaining a blood plasma steady state level of the appropriate analgesic drug for type of pain, patient age and physical status. For all patients, and especially older, frail patients, many analgesic medications, especially opioids, can induce feelings of drowsiness and dizziness, increasing the risk of falls' injuries. For these patients pain treatment may commence with lower doses of carefully selected opioid medications taken on an 'as needed' (PRN) basis, combined with a non-opioid taken 'at the clock' (ATC); for example, paracetamol taken at the clock by the older person, with oral morphine taken 'as needed' (PRN) and medication adjusted to a combination of 'at the clock' non-opioid and weak opioid if required. Vigilant monitoring of side effects is required.(For the WHO Stepwise regimen for opioid administration, see Chapter 10; for a flexible, non-stepwise approach to chronic pain management, see Chapter 7.) Patients should be encouraged to discuss with their primary care physicians the risks associated with driving when taking certain medications.

Sometimes, additional medication, on an as-needed (PRN) basis, may be required, particularly for anticipated very painful procedures, such as wound care or skin debridement, or painful catheter, prosthetic care, or wound dressing changes. Medication should be given before the painful procedure, having been discussed with the Practice Nurse/Community Health Nurse and prescribed by the General Practitioner, and should be compatible with and not interfere with the patient's regular prescribed medication. The Practice Nurse/Community Health Nurse should utilize a pain intensity measure before and after the painful procedure.

## The nurse's role in patient education

The role of Practice Nurse/Community Health Nurse includes educating the patient about how to complete a pain diary routinely. If the patient has any memory deficit, or requires support for compliance with maintaining the diary, family support can be very helpful. Many patients with chronic pain now belong to chronic pain support groups, some of which offer members an online pain diary which the patient can complete on their own computer. For regular Primary Care Physician visits or for home visits from the Community Health Nurse, the patient and their close others can download the logged diary information between dates, as required. This will facilitate monitoring the effectiveness of the patient's pain medication and other pain management interventions, and allow early intervention and problem solving.

# The role of the nurse in the community care of people with chronic non-malignant pain

This nursing role includes liaising with the primary care (General Practitioner/ Primary Care Physician) and secondary care (hospital) multidisciplinary care team in ensuring that patient care information is correct, and checking any unclear details (Lyons and Coleman, 2009). Increasingly, patient records are computerized, and access codes for the multidisciplinary care team make access to and transfer of patient information for interdisciplinary care easier (Joint Commission on Accreditation of Healthcare Organizations, 2012). However, this is not yet routinely available.

For the nurse providing patient education for community-living patients, important aspects of patient education in the context of managing chronic pain are as follows:

- Teaching patients how to check their pain levels according to a 0–10 Numbers Rating Scale, supported with a Verbal Rating Scale to describe how the pain feels.
- At times of pain flares and ongoing bouts of chronic pain, encouraging the patient to maintain a regular pain diary, with at least daily completion, using both a Number Rating Scale and a Verbal Rating Scale, with support of their close others if required. A pain diary is helpful in monitoring the effectiveness of pain management interventions and facilitating the early identification and treatment of pain problems.
- Indicating to the patient that their pain diary should also contain the name of their prescribed analgesic medications and the dosage regimen. The diary should also note nonpharmacological interventions that the patient uses as complementary therapies for pain management, such as heat or cold applications, the use of acupuncture, biofeedback or relaxation techniques, and the patient should document when these are used.
- Indicating to the patient that if the patient needs to access emergency services because of a sudden onset of severe pain (7 or higher on a Number Rating Scale of 0–10), then it is useful for the patient and family to bring the patient's pain diary to the emergency department.

The nurse's role also includes acting to address the patient's analgesic requirements within the scope of nursing practice, and to refer on to the General Practitioner/ Primary Care Physician, or appropriate multidisciplinary team member, if there are changes in the patient's pain levels. Precautions are required for all opioid medications regarding the risks of sedation, respiratory depression, nausea and vomiting, and pruritus. A preventative approach to constipation is always required for patients on opioid medications; stimulant laxatives should be prescribed. Nurses should always consult the National Formulary of their country, together with a drug guide with nursing considerations, such as *Mosby's Drug Guide for Nursing Students* (Skidmore, 2013).

Comfort provision and pain prevention is central to optimal nursing care: for instance, checking on the effectiveness of and possible side-effects associated with medication, giving wound care and changing dressings, checking the positioning of immobile patients and checking their pressure areas, and checking optimal functioning of all catheters. When working with the palliative care team for severely ill patients cared for in the community and patients at the end of the life, nurses need to liaise with the palliative care nurse regarding nursing requirements and work on a team basis to ensure that the patient's care needs are met and that families are supported. This may include providing patient care, for example in routine personal hygiene, washing, shaving, mouth care, care of hair, hands and feet, changing the patient's position and prevention of pressure sores.

# Children's response to chronic pain

Children vary in their response to chronic pain. Children who are more impaired by the pain experience are more likely to seek medical help. For these children, the pain experience is associated with a broad range of psychosocial issues that negatively impact on their quality of life, including problems with family and peer relationships, and academic difficulties. The challenge for pain practitioners, particularly the Primary Care Physician, is in distinguishing between the child with an undiagnosed, progressive disease process which requires direct treatment and the child with a chronic pain syndrome, for whom the focus is the treatment of their pain.

Children with chronic pain syndrome have usually been evaluated by many practitioners from multiple disciplines, but have received no conclusive diagnosis. When this point is reached, one of the most critical aspects of the evaluation of the child is the acceptance by the child, his or her family and provider that medical investigation indicates that the focus now needs to be on the management of the pain. When the Primary Care Physician is examining the child with pain, there are red flags that suggest ongoing progressive disease as well as specific questions associated with each chronic pain condition. If red flags show that further investigation is warranted, the parents and child are informed. Otherwise, the child and family are informed that the child most likely has a chronic pain syndrome (Schechter et al., 2010).

# The management of chronic pain in children

In managing chronic pain in children, symptom monitoring is vital to check on the effectiveness of treatment as well as the possible emergence of new symptoms that may indicate an unrecognized disease process. A pain diary should be completed on at least a daily basis, using either a Number or Faces Rating Scale and a Verbal Rating Scale, as well as noting the impact of interventions on aspects of function and quality of life. The primary aim is to help the child return to optimal functioning and quality of life as soon as possible, through a multicomponent treatment plan and by adopting a rehabilitation approach.

Pharmacological treatment is aimed at reducing central sensitization so gabapentin and amitriptyline are often prescribed. Nortriptyline is recommended as a first-line tricyclic for children with neuropathic pain. Non-steroidal anti-inflammatory drugs (NSAIDs) are associated with rebound headache and abdominal pain in children, but are the mainstay of chronic inflammatory disorders. Aspirin is contraindicated. Opioids are given with great caution in children with chronic pain, and only if other medications are not effective, as long-term side-effects such as opioid hyperalgesia can be especially hazardous, with a more rapid onset in children compared with adults. Acetaminophen, an NSAID or codeine or dihydrocodeine is given for the pain of sickle cell disease. An NSAID drug is given together with morphine in sickle cell disease crisis, which potentiates the analgesia and may allow a lower analgesic dose to be effective. All drugs should begin with low doses and be escalated gradually, with frequent reassessment. Opportunities for immediate phone help, if required by the child's parents, should be available (British National Formulary (BNF), 2014a, 2014b; Schechter et al., 2010).

Special precautions are required for morphine and all opioids, with prevention of respiratory arrest and respiratory depression being a priority. Bowel care is vital, and stimulant laxatives should be prescribed. Nurses should always consult the National Formulary of their country and a drug guide with nursing considerations, such as *Mosby's Drug Guide for Nursing Students* (Skidmore, 2013), which explains drug dosages, the side-effects of each drug, nursing considerations, and patient and family educational information (BNF, 2014b; Skidmore, 2013).

The success of a chronic pain management programme for children is measured in terms of improved child function and family functioning, as well as the child's optimal sleep patterns and regular school attendance (Schechter et al., 2010). School can be seen as a major stressor for adolescent children in pain, and distraction can be a helpful coping strategy (Forgeron and McGrath, 2008). Cognitive behavioural therapies and complementary therapies have a major role in the child's rehabilitation, along with, and potentially instead of, analgesia. There is robust evidence for biofeedback for recurrent headaches, particularly with behavioural management strategies, being effective pain management complementary therapies (Schechter et al., 2010; Tsao et al., 2008).

# The impact of fear-related inactivity for adults and children

Pain-related disability in children and adults may be incurred through fear-related inactivity. Children and adults who have high levels of anxiety and pain catastrophizing tend to react to pain by hypervigilance and hyperarousal, which increases their psychological need to escape or avoid the pain – the stress 'flight' response, which is often demonstrated by inactivity. The resultant disuse of musculoskeletal structures is associated with further pain and disability. For this reason, physio-therapy and appropriate graded exercise, together with cognitive behaviour therapies to reduce stress and enhance coping skills, have an essential place, along with appropriate analgesia, in pain rehabilitation for patients with pain of all ages (Fuss et al., 2011).

## Chronic pain in adults and older adults

Brain imaging studies in adults have shown that fibromyalgia, irritable bowel syn-drome and low back pain support the existence of central pain augmentation and may represent biological amplification of all sensory stimuli. Strong evidence shows that drugs that block some types of neurotransmitters or augment the activity of others will typically be the most effective treatment for this spectrum of central pain states. Figure 9.2 shows the level of evidence for appropriate pharmacological therapies and their associated effect on neurotransmitters impacting central pain states (Phillips and Clauw, 2011).

Adult patients with fibromyalgia often have chronic fatigue syndrome, a complex ill-ness characterized by prolonged debilitating fatigue and multiple non-specific symptoms of headaches, recurrent sore throats, fever, muscle and joint pain, and neurocognitive complaints. Patients with chronic fatigue syndrome often have depression and may use

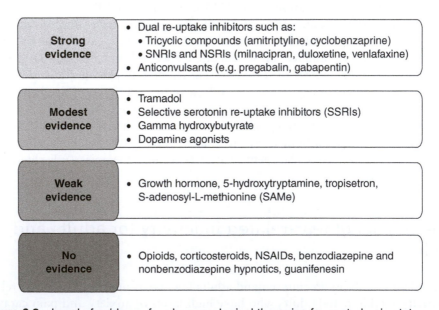

**Figure 9.2**   Level of evidence for pharmacological therapies for central pain states

maladaptive coping behaviours, such as catastrophizing and fear avoidance, which, through modulation of the descending pain pathways, influence their pain perception and are associated with pain amplification (Meeus and Nijs, 2007).

The biopsychosocial model is highly relevant to irritable bowel syndrome (IBS), which is part of the larger group of functional gastrointestinal disorders (FGIDs). FGIDs share disturbances in the regulation of peripheral, spinal and central pain pathways that are not yet fully understood. IBS is characterized by recurrent abdominal pain, which is associated with altered bowel habits although there are no obvious structural abnormalities. The physiological abnormalities of IBS are closely associated with stress. The combination of gastrointestinal motor, sensory and central nervous system activity impact the development of IBS. The bi-directional and integrated system of the neural pathways between the gastrointestinal tract and the brain (the brain–gut axis) may impact the dysregulation of the central and enteric nervous system which induces dysmotility and visceral sensitivity, modified by psychosocial processes. Psychological therapies such as cognitive behavioural therapy (CBT) are often appropriate for patients with IBS. CBT helps patients to learn new ways of thinking and behaving to control symptoms, cope with emotional anxieties and improve illness behaviour (see Table 9.1) (Tanaka et al., 2011; van Oudenhove and Aziz, 2009).

# Emotions, cognition and multidisciplinary chronic pain rehabilitation

Emotions modulate the pain experience by influencing cognitions and behaviours. The brain generates and organizes psychological and social experience. With psychological help, the person with pain can understand his or her feelings and motivations and work with them. Counselling, psychotherapy, cognitive behavioural therapies and similar psychological therapies allow access to the primary emotions of anger, loss and grief, as well as to positive emotions (Lumley et al., 2011). Recognition of the important role of emotions and cognitions in pain perception has facilitated the development of multidisciplinary pain rehabilitation programmes, where the psychologist is a key part of the pain rehabilitation process (Roth et al., 2012). The biopsychosocial model of chronic pain has promoted the rehabilitation model of care, where controlled exercise leads to reduced pain, distress and illness behaviour (Waddell, 1987) (see Table 9.1).

# Osteoarthritis in older age: biopsychosocial etiology and treatment approach

The preservation of cognitive function and mobility are a major concern to older people in maintaining their quality of life and independence. Chronic pain conditions

**Table 9.1** Outline of pain types with responsiveness to and inhibition by therapies (each individual with pain has potential for variation in pain processing mechanisms; their pain experience may comprise possible combinations of pain types)

| Type of pain | Responsive to procedural interventions | Medication responsive | Pain facilitators/cause | Pain inhibitors |
|---|---|---|---|---|
| Nociceptive | Yes (cause and context dependent) | Paracetamol NSAIDs Opioids | Pro-inflammatory cascades peripherally and centrally associated with Inflammation and /or mechanical damage in all tissues eg. Trauma, cancer pain, osteoarthritis; | Drugs which work centrally and peripherally/ nonpharmacological interventions to increase descending inhibition TENS/Relaxation and other CAM therapies/ Rehabilitative and strengthening physical therapies and exercise as advised during and following recovery to retrain and strengthen weakened tissues and structures/ prevent development of chronic pain; health promoting interventions |
| Neuropathic | Yes (cause and context dependent) | Anticonvulsants Tricyclic antidepressants/ SNRIs/SSRIs Capsaicin/ cream Local anaesthetics Cautious and appropriate use of selected opioids | Damage to or pathological changes in the peripheral and/or central nervous system: e.g. Peripheral and central nerves (post herpetic neuralgia) Trigeminal neuralgia nerve entrapment( many types: eg carpal tunnel compression/ traumatic cause/ cancer disease and treatment /central nerve damage of spinothalamocortical pathways (eg stroke; phantom limb pain; spinal cord injury/ multiple sclerosis spasticity. | Drugs which work centrally and peripherally/ Spinal drug delivery systems/ Nonpharmacological interventions to increase descending inhibition TENS/SCS Relaxation and other CAM therapies Appropriate physical therapies, rehabilitation and exercise, especially yoga, T'ai chi, walking, swimming and stretching as advised; health promoting interventions. |
| Central (non-nociceptive) | Yes (cause and context dependent) | Dual uptake inhibitors: Tricyclic antidepressants SNRIs/SSRIs/ Tramadol Anticonvulsants pregabalin and gabapentin | Disturbances in central pain processing mechanisms e.g. irritable bowel syndrome; fibromyalgia; low back pain; tension headache; pelvic pain and endometriosis | Drugs which reduce facilitation and increase activity in descending antinociceptive pathways Especially duloxetine, venlafaxine and tramadol/SNRIs and SSRIs TENS/SCS/Biofeedback/relaxation and other CAM therapies/Appropriate physical therapies, rehabilitation and exercise, especially yoga, T'ai chi, walking, swimming and stretching as advised; health promoting interventions. |

Adapted from Phillips, K. and Clauw, D.J. (2011) 'Central pain mechanisms in chronic pain states-maybe it is all in their head', *Best Practice & Research Clinical Rheumatology*, 25: 141–154 and Bennett, M.I. (2010) *Neuropathic Pain*. 2nd Ed. Oxford Pain Management Library.

can readily disturb the balance of maintaining the muscle mass, strength and general vigour required to prevent disability, which can potentially result in a person's loss of independence. Approximately 75% of older people (over the age of 75 years) have musculoskeletal symptoms, which may be indicative of more than one disorder. When an older patient requests a medical consultation regarding musculoskeletal symptoms, accurate diagnosis may be difficult, depending on the complexity of the patient's medical and biopsychosocial history.

Osteoarthritis is the most common joint disorder worldwide and is a major cause of pain and disability in older people. Once considered a degenerative disease and an inevitable consequence of older age, osteoarthritis has more recently been construed as an age-related disorder involving joint mechanics. With improving knowledge of the mechanisms of joint ageing, this condition may be treatable in the future.

While osteoarthritis manifests as a degradation and loss of articular cartilage, affected joints have living cells which respond to mechanical stimulation and function. Ageing contributes to arthritis as the biggest single risk factor for the development of osteoarthritis in susceptible joints, but age on its own does not cause osteoarthritis.

The American College of Rheumatology osteoarthritis criteria are frequently used for diagnosing osteoarthritis. These require a biopsychosocial approach to clarify the relationship between age factors and additional osteoarthritis risk factors. Figure 9.3 outlines the interaction of ageing changes in joint function and tissues, with additional

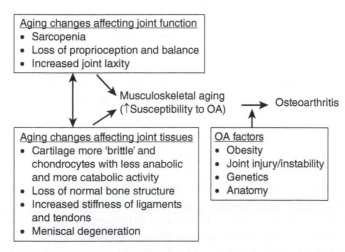

**Figure 9.3** Relationship between musculoskeletal ageing and the development of osteoarthritis

Copyright (2009). Source: *Hazzard's Geriatric Medicine and Gerontology* (6th edn), Halter, J.B., Ouslander, J.G., Tinetti, M.E., Studenski, S., High, K.P. and Asthana, S. (eds), Chapter 112: Aging of the muscles and joints, Figure 112–5; p. 1360. McGraw Hill Medical. Copyright. Republished with permission of McGraw Hill (2009).

risks factors of obesity, joint injury, and genetic and anatomical factors. Osteoarthritis can best be thought of as the result of excessive mechanical stress applied in the context of systemic susceptibility (Anderson and Loeser, 2010; Hunter, 2011; Loeser and Delbono, 2009).

## Osteoarthritis of the knee

Between 10% and 12% of adults have symptoms of osteoarthritis. While osteoarthritis manifests most commonly in the hip, knee and hand joints, for people aged 65 years and over osteoarthritis of the knees has a greater risk of limiting mobility in terms of being able to climb stairs or walk independently than that imposed by any other disease. Osteoarthritis of the knee represents mechanical failure of the synovial joint as a result of an imbalance between the repair and breakdown of joint tissue, often in situations where the load on the knee joint exceeds the stress capacity of the joint's tissues to bear that load, leading to equilibrium imbalance. Joint cells themselves destroy cartilage by an imbalance between anabolic and catabolic activity. Osteoarthritis is a process involving cartilage inflammation characterized by local production of cytokines and inflammatory mediators (Hunter, 2011; Loeser and Delbono, 2009).

The context of systemic susceptibility is also important, so that the risk of developing the disease of osteoarthritis increases if the person has a positive family history (genetic predisposition), is female, of older age and obese. Obesity is the greatest of all risk factors for osteoarthritis. Stress to the knee joint is drastically increased by additional body weight; each extra kilogramme of body weight imposes four times that much load on the knee joint. An engineering model of stress considers how much stress-induced pressure can be applied to a hard material before that material 'gives way' or destructs. The hard material of human bone is a living, cellular substance. Knee joint destruction is characterized by progressive cartilage loss, subchondral bone remodelling at the joint articular surface, osteophyte (bone spur) formation and synovial (smooth joint lining) inflammation (Anderson and Loeser, 2010; Hunter, 2011).

The prevalence of osteoarthritis increases with age. Women over 55 years are more commonly affected than men of the same age range. The patient may present with joint pain, transient morning joint stiffness and have functional limitation. Joint failure may lead to disablement and loss of quality of life. The patient's full medical and biopsychosocial history is obtained, including their history of past injuries (especially injuries from weight-bearing sport), or previous meniscal or cruciate ligament tear. A family history is a strong risk factor. The presence of osteoporosis is inversely related to a risk of osteoarthritis. To elicit the patient's comprehensive musculoskeletal and biopsychosocial history, questions include asking the patient about their own general health now and previously, age, race and ethnicity, past medical history, family history, their pain now and previously, general sensations related to stiffness, swelling, their medications, psychosocial and occupational history, and the extent and impact of their current disability. Biological, psychological and social factors all play a significant role in the experience of pain for the person with osteoarthritis (Hunter, 2011).

# Diagnosis of osteoarthritis of the knee

A diagnosis of osteoarthritis of the knee is based on the following:

- X-ray radiographic features which are graded according to disease severity, particularly joint space narrowing due to cartilage thinning, subarticular sclerosis, and the presence of subchondral cysts and osteophytes;
- MRI scans show cartilage injury, meniscal tears and subchondral bone marrow changes;
- blood tests may be carried out if the diagnosis is not clear for the patient's history and clinical examination. There are no specific blood tests which can predict osteoarthritis. Erythrocyte sedimentation rate (ESR) is normal, but C-reactive protein (CRP) may be raised.

# The nurse's role in the management of the patient with osteoarthritis

The treatment of symptoms and disability is the priority in osteoarthritis, to reduce and limit the risk of further joint destruction. Patient education and health promotion are key factors in helping the patient to comply with treatment and reduce pain and distress.

**Pain management** involves pharmacological and nonpharmacological interventions to help reduce swelling and stiffness and regain and increase mobility. All interventions should be designed for the individual, with nonpharmacological interventions particularly aimed at reducing risk, focusing on weight reduction, and addressing altered alignment and muscle weakness. Obesity is the greatest risk factor for disease onset, with mechanical factors dominating risk of disease progression (Hunter, 2011).

The patient may find the application of hot or cold packs to the knee reduces swelling and stiffness. Acupuncture is often found to be useful as an adjuvant therapy by patients with knee osteoarthritis (Abdulla et al., 2013). Patients may find local topical application of NSAIDs or capsaicin preparations useful; these should be used as directed and applied 3–4 times daily, according to and using the manufacturer's instructions. Treatment is reviewed after a week. The patient is warned about possible photosensitivity of the affected area, which should not be exposed to sunlight. Intra-articular corticosteroid injections may help to relieve pain in knee osteoarthritis in the short term (Abdulla et al. 2013).

Acetaminophen is effective for osteoarthritis and is the medication of choice, prescribed before NSAIDs for older people who are more likely to suffer side-effects from NSAIDs or coxibs, especially gastric bleeding and cardiotoxicity. Medications should be taken 'at the clock' during painful bouts of osteoarthritis (which is frequently asymptomatic) to maintain a blood plasma steady state. Asking and educating the patient to keep a pain diary is strongly recommended, so that the Practice Nurse/Community Health Nurse can monitor the effectiveness of pharmacological and nonpharmacological interventions for pain relief. Analgesic medications taken 'at the clock' generate a blood plasma steady state so that analgesia 'peaks and troughs' are eliminated, and pain is more consistently controlled. If opioid medication is required for severe pain, a weak opioid medication, tramadol, is advised. Tramadol has fewer side-effects of constipation and respiratory depression, and a reduced addiction potential than strong opioids. A pain diary is absolutely essential if patients are taking opioid medications. Vigilant monitoring for adverse events and anticipated prevention of side effects is essential for older people taking NSAID and opioid medication, with the lowest dose possible prescribed. A proton pump inhibitor is required for patients taking NSAIDs. To reduce risk of constipation a combination of stimulant laxatives and stool softeners is essential for older patients throughout opioid therapy (Abdulla et al., 2013).

**Rehabilitation – weight loss and exercise**: a multidisciplinary team care approach is required to establish a rehabilitation care plan. The physiotherapist will advise on a suitable exercise regimen, aiming to build muscle strength to limit further degenerative loss of skeletalmuscle mass (sarcopenia), increase the strength of the patient's quadriceps (the large muscle group comprising the rectus femoris and three vasta muscles which extend the knee) and to increase their calorific expenditure. The nutritionist will advise on the constituents and amounts of a healthy diet, increasing fibre, fruit and vegetable intake and reducing foods which contribute to weight gain and obesity. The interaction between exercise activity, calorie intake and expenditure, and types of foods ingested is critically important in aiming for weight loss. Knee replacement surgery may be recommended. The real need is preventative focus on health promotion of obesity prevention and treating potentially reversible changes of earlier disease, rather than watching and waiting, which can result in loss of life (Hunter, 2011).

CLINICAL EXAMPLE

## Potential for opioid addiction in all types of chronic pain

**Hazard: Chronic pain can act as a 'bully'** Seeking negative reinforcement, the bully's behaviour is rewarded by an action, which, in the context of chronic pain, is the person taking medication to 'stop the bully'. Addiction is more likely when opioid medication is taken PRN for moderate to severe chronic pain in a situation when a blood plasma non-opioid analgesic steady state is not already established because of a lack of or under-medication with non-opioid analgesia. When a patient takes opioid analgesic medication 'PRN' without any other regular non-opioid analgesia 'at the clock', a potentially dangerous and addictive situation can easily arise. The patient feels the onset of mild pain; non-opioid analgesia has not built up to steady state in the patient's blood plasma; the minor pain is interpreted by the brain as signalling something that is 'going to get much worse' so the patient takes opioid medication; the patient repeats these actions; opioid medications are taken PRN for mild pain and the patient may become addicted.

## During pain flare-ups

There are certain rules to follow in the case of pain flare-up:

> **Rule 1:** ALWAYS insist that the community-living patient keeps a pain diary for opioid medication.
>
> **Rule 2:** Do not prescribe opioid analgesia alone. ALWAYS include a non-opioid analgesia, especially acetaminophen, which acts centrally as an opioid-sparing medication. Educate and instruct the patient to take both medications as prescribed, and keep a record in the pain diary, along with all interventions used to control pain.
>
> **Rule 3:** When the patient complies with analgesic schedules, their pain intensity rating is more like to reduce. Regular review is strongly advocated. When the patient's pain score is lowered to 4 or less on a Number Rating Scale and the patient considers their pain as mild, opioid medication should be gradually reduced and discontinued. Acetaminophen can then be taken 'at the clock' when the pain intensity rating is 4 until the pain intensity rating reduces to less than 4, when acetaminophen can be taken 'PRN'. Pain intensity ratings should be reviewed in the context of the patient's functionality.

Chronic pain is a major public health issue. An increasingly aged global population will require expert nursing knowledge and patient care to help people optimally manage and prevent pain associated with chronic diseases.

## Chapter summary

- Governments in the United States, Europe and Australia aim to address chronic non-malignant pain through legislation, the development of National Pain Strategies, local policies and initiatives to improve the quality of and access to multidisciplinary pain services for people with chronic pain, and research and teaching in pain.
- Chronic non-malignant pain is both a personal and socio-economic problem which affects people of all ages. The person with chronic non-malignant pain must be viewed within his or her cultural context. A biopsychosocial care model addresses the multifactorial issues associated with the disease and interdisciplinary care.

*(Continued)*

*(Continued)*

- The multidisciplinary pain team offers interdisciplinary care. For the person with chronic pain living in the community, the Community Health Nurse or Practice Nurse may be the patient's first point of contact with primary care and the General Practitioner/Primary Care Physician.
- Patient-centred communication skills are required for history taking, assessment, treatment monitoring, patient education and support. When patients are discharged from hospital to the community, extra care is required to check that treatments, including pain treatments, are correct.
- An important role for the Community Nurse in chronic non-malignant pain management flare-ups is in ensuring patients are educated to take prescribed pain medications 'at the clock' to maintain a blood plasma steady state. It is strongly advised to teach the community-living patient to complete a pain diary.
- Children with chronic pain syndrome have usually been evaluated by many practitioners. When this point is reached, one of the most critical aspects of the evaluation of the child is the acceptance by the child, his or her family and provider that medical investigation indicates that the focus now needs to be on the management of the pain.
- Emotions are increasingly seen to have a role in the pain experience, modulating the pain experience by influencing cognitions and behaviours. Cognitive behavioural and other psychological therapies allow access to primary emotions and the development of adaptive coping skills.
- Osteoarthritis is the most common cause of pain and disability, which has a higher prevalence in older age. Causative factors are intrinsic and extrinsic, with the extrinsic factor of obesity being modifiable by diet and exercise. A biopsychosocial approach is required. The nurse therefore has a major role in patient care.

## Reflective exercise

Consider your own views about prescribing opioid medication for community-living people with chronic non-malignant pain. Do you think a stepwise analgesia approach with non-opioid and opioid medication and careful monitoring is warranted?

## Recommended reading

Cervero, F. (2012) *Understanding Pain: Exploring the Perception of Pain.* Cambridge, MA: MIT Press.

Flor, H. and Turk, D.C. (2011) *Chronic Pain: An Integrated Biobehavioural Approach.* Seattle, WA: International Association for the Study of Pain.

Schofield, P. (ed.) (2007) *The Management of Pain in Older People.* Chichester: Wiley.

Schofield, P. and Merrick, J. (eds) (2008) *Pain in Children and Youth.* New York: Nova Science.

## Websites relevant to this chapter

European Federation of IASP Chapters (EFIC): http://efic.org/

Joint Commission on Accreditation of Healthcare Organizations on the safe use of opioids in hospitals: www.jointcommission.org/sentinel_event_alert_safe_use_of_opioids_in_hospitals/

Joint Commission on Accreditation of Healthcare Organizations, *Pain Management: A Systems Approach to Improving Quality and Safety* (2012): www.jcrinc.com/pain-management-a-systems-approach-to-improving-quality-and-safety/

American College of Rheumatology, for information on arthritis and rheumatic diseases: www.rheumatology.org/Search.aspx?SearchText=osteoarthritis

# References

Abdulla, A., Adams, N., Bone, M., Elliott, A.M., Gaffin, J., Knaggs, R., Martin, D., Sampson, L. and Schofield, P. (2013) Guidance on the management of pain in older people. *Age and Ageing*, 42: i1–i57.

Anderson, A.S. and Loeser, R.F. (2010) Why is osteoarthritis an age-related disease. *Best Practice and Research: Clinical Rheumatology*, 24: 15–26.

Apkarian, A.V., Hashmi, J.A., Baliki, M.N. (2011) Pain and the brain: specificity and plasticity of the brain in clinical chronic pain. *Pain*, 152: S49–S64.

British National Formulary (2014a) *BNF 66 for Adults September 2013–March 2014*. London: Pharmaceutical Press.

British National Formulary (2014b) *BNF for Children July 2013–July 2014*. London: Pharmaceutical Press.

Flor, H. and Turk, D.C. (2011) *Chronic Pain: An Integrated Biobehavioural Approach*. Seattle, WA: International Association for the Study of Pain (IASP).

Forgeron, P. and McGrath, P.J. (2008) Self-identified needs of youth with chronic pain. In P. Schofield and J. Merrick (eds), *Pain in Children and Youth*. New York: Nova Science.

Fuss, S., Pagé, M.G. and Katz, J. (2011) Persistent pain in a community-based sample of children and adolescents: sex differences in psychological constructs. *Pain Research and Management*, 16 (5): 303–309.

Hunter, D.J. (2011) Osteoarthritis. *Best Practice and Research: Clinical Rheumatology*, 25: 801–814.

Joint Commission on Accreditation of Healthcare Organizations (2012) *Pain Management: A Systems Approach to Improving Quality and Safety*. Joint Commission Resources. Washington, DC: JCAHO.

Kress, H.G. (2012). Introduction. In: European Federation of IASP, *Reflection Process on Chronic Diseases in the EU: The Role of Chronic Pain. Systematic Literature Report*. Belgium: EFIC.

Loeser, R.F. and Delbono, O. (2009) Aging of the muscles and joints. In J.B. Halter, J.G. Ouslander, M.E. Tinetti, S. Studenski, K.P. High and S. Asthana, *Hazzards's Geriatric Medicine and Gerontology* (6th edn). New York: McGraw-Hill Medical.

Lumley, M.A., Cohen, J.L., Borszcz, G.S., Cano, A., Radcliffe, A.M., Porter, L.S., Schubiner, H. and Keefe, F.J. (2011) Pain and emotion: a biopsychosocial review of recent research. *Journal of Clinical Psychology*, 67 (9): 942–968.

Lyons, W.T. and Coleman, E.A. (2009) Transitions. In J.B. Halter, J.G. Ouslander, M.E. Tinetti, S. Studenski, K.P. High and S. Asthana, *Hazzards's Geriatric Medicine and Gerontology* (6th edn). New York: McGraw-Hill Medical.

Meeus, M. and Nijs, J. (2007) Central sensitisation: a biopsychosocial explanation for chronic widespread pain in patients with fibromyalgia and chronic fatigue syndrome. *Clinical Rheumatology*, 26: 465–473.

National Pain Strategy (Pain Australia) (2010), www.painaustralia.org.au/images/pain_australia/NPS/National%20Pain%20Strategy%202011.pdf (accessed 9 February 2014).

Phillips, K. and Clauw, D.J. (2011) Central pain mechanisms in chronic pain states – may be it is all in their head. *Best Practice and Research: Clinical Rheumatology*, 25: 141–154.

Roth, R.S., Geisser, M.E. and Williams, D.A. (2012) Interventional pain medicine: retreat from the biopsychosocial model of pain. *Translational Behavioral Medicine*, 2 (1): 106–116.

Sarzi-Puttini, P., Atzeni, F. and Mease, P.J. (2011) Chronic widespread pain: from peripheral to central evolution. *Best Practice and Research: Clinical Rheumatology*, 25: 133–139.

Schechter, N., Palermo, T.M., Walco, G.A. and Berde, C.B. (2010) Persistent pain in children. In S.M. Fishman, J.C. Ballantyne and J.P. Rathmell (eds), *Bonica's Management of Pain* (4th edn). Riverwoods, IL: Wolters Kluwer/Lippincott Williams and Wilkins.

Skidmore, L. (2013) *Mosby's Drug Guide for Nursing Students* (10th edn). St Louis, MO: Elsevier Mosby.

Tanaka, Y., Kanazawa, M., Fukudo, S. and Drossman, D.A. (2011) Biopsychosocial model of irritable bowel syndrome. *Journal of Gastroenterology and Motility*, 17: 131–139.

Treede, R.D. and van Rooij, N., with Alon, E., Kress, H.G., Langford, R., Krcevski Skvarc, N.,Varrassi, G., Vissers, K.C.P. and Wells, J.C.D. (2011) *The Societal Impact of Pain: A Road Map for Action*. Belgium: European Federation of IASP Chapters (EFIC)/Societal Impact of Pain (SIP).

Tsao, J.C.I., Lu, Q. and Zeltzer, L.K. (2008) Beyond traditional cognitive-behavioural therapy: novel psychological and alternative approaches to pediatric pain. In P. Schofield and J. Merrick (eds), *Pain in Children and Youth*. New York: Nova Science.

van Oudenhove, L. and Aziz, Q. (2009) Gastro-intestinal pain. In M.A. Giamberadino (ed.), *Visceral Pain: Clinical, Pathophysiolgical and Therapeutic Aspects*. Oxford: Oxford University Press.

Waddell, G. (1987) New clinical model for the treatment of low back pain. *Spine*, 12 (7): 632–644.

# 10

# Cancer pain

## Learning objectives

The learning objectives of this chapter are to:

- recognize the extent of the global problem of under-treated cancer pain
- know the major domains of cancer pain which require assessment
- recognize the importance of measuring pain as the fifth vital sign and distress as the sixth vital sign in cancer care
- understand the five phrases of the WHO Analgesic Ladder and the implications of each for optimal cancer pain relief

## Introduction

Cancer pain often massively reduces the patient's quality of life, and the quality of life of his or her close others, and impacts negatively on the socio-economic aspects of every country. The need for the comprehensive addressing of cancer pain is recognized by many governments, and has resulted in the publication of guidelines in the USA, Europe and individual countries globally, including the first National Pain Strategy by Pain Australia (2010). This chapter discusses the assessment and management of cancer pain in the context of these guidelines.

## The personal impact of cancer pain

Research shows that severe pain continues to be a common reality for many patients with cancer (Breivik et al., 2009). Approximately 70% of patients with cancer experience severe pain at some time during their illness. Up to 75% of patients with advanced cancer experience pain and 50% of patients at end of life experience moderate to severe pain (Breitbart et al., 2010).

Cancer pain is acknowledged to be under-treated and a major public health problem, despite World Health Organization recommendations regarding the Analgesic Ladder for pain relief, which was introduced in 1986, upgraded in 1996 and is accepted worldwide (World Health Organization, 1996). A systematic review of the prevalence of pain in patients with cancer by van den Beuken-van Everdingen et al. (2007) showed that of the patients with pain, more than one-third graded their pain as moderate or severe.

The European Pain in Cancer (EPIC) survey (Breivik et al., 2009) sought to increase understanding of cancer-related pain and treatment across Europe. According to the Breivik et al. (2009) survey, which was conducted in 11 European countries and Israel during 2006–2007, of 5,084 patients contacted, 56% suffered moderate to severe pain at least monthly. Of the 573 patients selected for the second survey phase, 69% reported pain-related difficulties with everyday activities and 50% believed their healthcare provider did not consider their quality of life a priority (Breivik et al., 2009). While a higher percentage of cancers are now curable, many people live long term with metastatic cancer due to more effective treatments. This has major implications for maintaining quality of life by ensuring optimal symptom control and functionality.

Although cancer is experienced by people of all ages, it is more frequently a disease of older age. An older patient's subjective experience of cancer pain may worsen the pain they already experience from a pre-existing comorbid condition, for example pain from arthritis or osteoporosis (Fitzgibbon and Loeser, 2010; Mantyh, 2013).

## Cancer pain is comprised of elements of acute and chronic, malignant pain

The disease of cancer is invasive and mechanical. An advanced, spreading cancer disease may move body organs out of place as well as invade all types of body tissue, organs and structures. While a separate classification of cancer pain, as distinct from acute and chronic pain, may not be advocated by some clinicians, it is important to realize the potential severity of cancer-related pain, which is sometimes referred to as pain of malignant origin (Turk and Okifuji, 2010).

Chronic pain caused by cancer is best thought of as acute pain persisting over time caused by the concurrent involvement of different anatomical structures, as well as a constantly evolving local tumour progression and metastatic spread (Shipton, 1999). Many cancer and associated cells cause cancer pain. Tumour, tumour-associated stromal cells and immune cells produce many algogenic mediators (for example, prostaglandins, adenosine triphosphate, cytokines, endothelins and bradykinin), some of which have receptors on peripheral terminals and can activate nociceptors. As a result of these mechanisms, cancer pain can arise at the original tumour site or through metastatic disease (i.e. the spread of cancer cells). The most common cancer types frequently metastasize to bone, liver and lung (Mantyh, 2013).

# The impact of cancer treatments on the pain experience

Surgery, chemotherapy and radiation are the primary types of cancer treatment. Successful treatment for cancer is strongly associated with patient survival. While the aim of surgery, radiation and chemotherapy is to remove or destroy the cancer tumour and associated cells, the treatment side-effects of each of these modalities may compound the pain experience. Post-surgical complications and pain syndromes may arise due to central sensitization, inadequate analgesia peri-operatively and possible nerve or structural injury during surgery, infections, haemorrhage, cardiovascular and pulmonary and other systemic complications. Radiation and certain chemotherapies (particularly taxanes, platinum-based compounds, vinca alkaloids and proteasome inhibitors) can cause peripheral nerve neurotoxicity, leading to neuropathic pain and sensory disturbances (Fitzgibbon and Loeser, 2010; Mantyh, 2013; Murtagh and Higginson, 2010).

# Cancer-related 'breakthrough' or severe 'incident pain'

Cancer 'breakthrough' or severe 'incident pain' is defined as 'pain that is a transitory exacerbation of pain that occurs in addition to otherwise stable persistent pain' in patients on opioid medication (Fitzgibbon and Loeser, 2010; Portenoy and Hagen, 1990). Breakthrough pain is by nature unpredictable, acute and may be severe to the point of debilitation, and difficult to control.

Breakthrough pain can have rapid onset, be of short duration and significant intensity, and may be:

- Incident-related breakthrough pain: this is directly related to an event or activity, such as weight-bearing, turning in bed or a bowel movement. If the pain can be anticipated, analgesia should be given in advance.
- End of dose failure: this is when too much time has elapsed between doses of analgesia and the patient's medication requirement. Appropriate time-contingent doses of analgesia and associated monitoring of the patient's symptoms can prevent this type of breakthrough pain.
- Spontaneous breakthrough pain: this is unpredictable and often fleeting. While adjunctive analgesia may provide effective relief, longer-lasting breakthrough

pain requires rapid onset analgesia. Frequent incidences of spontaneous breakthrough pain require re-titration of opioid medication, adjustment of adjunctive medications and careful monitoring of the side-effects (Fitzgibbon and Loeser, 2010; Portenoy and Hagen, 1990).

# Bone pain in cancer

Bone pain in cancer may be due to either cancer spread to the bone, known as metastatic bone pain, or to pain due to bone cancer. Both types are especially serious for potential of loss of bone strength and reduction in functionality and quality of life, and both require early identification and specific treatment. Animal models of metastatic bone cancer pain for the major cancers have been developed that show similarities and differences in the way different tumours drive bone cancer pain. These models indicate that multiple factors are involved in generating and maintaining bone cancer pain (Sabino et al., 2003).

Cancer cells usually have a more acidic environment than that of normal cells. Bone metastases are associated with an abnormal proliferation of osteoclasts – cells which resorp bone – and there is an increased potential for bone fracture. The capsaicin receptor TRPV1, together with the acid-sensing ion channel 3 (ASIC3), respond to the more acidic environment and osteoclastic function to further drive bone cancer pain (Mantyh, 2013). Changes unique to specific cancer cell types lead to neurochemical changes similar to the peripheral and central sensitization of other pain states, suggesting a potential for the development of new pharmacological treatments for bone cancer pain (Sabino et al., 2003). Bisphosphonates – drugs which help to prevent further loss of bone mass in patients with low bone mineral density – are now increasingly used to alongside anti-cancer treatments to help relieve bone pain and, in some patients, may modify and disrupt the process of metastatic cancer spread (Coleman and McCloskey, 2011).

Half body radiation theory has been used since the 1970s as effective palliation for bone pain from widespread metastatic cancer. A recent technological advance is helical tomotherapy, a combination of spiral CT scanning and intensity-modulated radiation therapy. It uses hundreds of slim pencil beams of radiation, spirally rotating around the tumour, focusing from all directions, and allows precision-delivered radiation to the exact shape of each patient's tumour. The result is reduced damage and fewer side-effects to adjacent body organs and structures. A recent study, using half body irradiation with helical tomotherapy in 13 patients diagnosed with breast cancer and multiple painful bone metastases to the lower body, resulted in pain relief for 85% of the group. Six patients stopped analgesic drug consumption, and there was an especially marked reduction in the frequency of diarrhoea compared with conventional lower half body irradiation due to the reduced dose of radiation to the intestine (Furlan et al., 2014).

# Impact of cancer pain on quality of life

Patients with cancer-related breakthrough and uncontrolled cancer pain make more pain-related hospital and emergency department visits and incur greater treatment costs. Family relationships can be impaired, anxiety and depression can reduce psychological quality of life and functionality may be reduced with the impairment of physical activities, sleep and the activities of daily living (Fitzgibbon and Loeser, 2010).

Pain interacts with the other symptoms that are frequently associated with cancer, particularly fatigue, nausea, constipation, dyspnoea, weakness, impaired cognition and psychological distress (Breitbart et al., 2010). Inadequate pain assessment and under-treatment of cancer pain are both due to a myriad of causes, some of which include:

- a lack of a defined policy or standard in acute care settings to enforce pain assessment as obligatory in patient care;
- inadequate patient–healthcare professional communication;
- a patient's reluctance to report or disclose their real pain experience for fear of being 'a nuisance', not being believed or causing distress to their close others;
- a lack of staff training and time for pain management (Fitzgibbon and Loeser, 2010; Somers et al., 2010).

Pain is the greatest cause of fear for the person who has been diagnosed with cancer. Patients are concerned about disease progression and the possibility of accompanying unbearable pain. Patients have found that, in locations where pain is not routinely measured, their pain experience may not be routinely enquired about. In resource-restricted services, delivery healthcare professionals may come under social pressure to judge 'deservingness' about resource allocation in terms of spending budgets on opioid and other expensive treatments. This restriction, together with a cynicism towards the patient's pain report, increases the risk of under-treatment of pain (Williams and Gessler, 2010).

# Domains requiring assessment in cancer-related pain

An expert group conference on cancer pain assessment and classification (Kaasa et al., 2011) agreed that:

- pain intensity;
- breakthrough pain;
- neuropathic pain; and
- psychological distress

are the key domains which require assessment, particularly with patients having moderate to severe pain, as these domains interact with each other.

## Pain intensity in cancer

The expert group (Kaasa et al., 2011) reached a consensus to use a Number Rating Scale (NRS) to measure pain intensity in adults with cancer pain, with zero being 'no pain' and 10 being 'pain as bad as you can imagine'. A pain intensity scale can also be used to measure breakthrough pain and neuropathic pain (Knudsen et al., 2012). The National Comprehensive Cancer Network (NCCN) Distress Thermometer is the recognized scale to measure psychological distress in cancer (Holland and Bultz, 2007). In addition to the regular experience of cancer pain, breakthrough pain and psychological distress are salient features of cancer and support the rationale for an holistic approach to the care of the person with cancer (Holland and Bultz, 2007; Institute of Medicine, 2007; Klepstad et al., 2011).

When assessing cancer pain, the pain intensity measurement is pivotal in indicating the patient's medication requirement. Pain quality helps to identify the pathophysiology. For example, superficial somatic, nociceptive pain is well localized and often described as sharp or burning, whereas deep somatic pain is less well localized and can be cramping, pressing or throbbing. Visceral pain may be described as crampy, diffuse or gnawing when caused by the cancer obstructing a hollow viscus, or, if an organ capsule is involved, may be aching, sharp or throbbing. Visceral pain is accompanied by autonomic signs of nausea, vomiting and sweating, and is associated with emotional anxiety and distress. Neuropathic pain may be described as burning, tingling or lancinating (Cherny, 2013).

# Non-opioid and opioid analgesia and the WHO Analgesic Ladder for Pain Relief

The principles of optimal pain relief and comprehensive pain management are similar for all people, regardless of age, gender, race and ethnicity. However, consideration of age and cognitive ability informs the choice of pain assessment tool. Very great care needs to be taken to check appropriate medications and doses for children and frail older people with renal, cardiac and/or hepatic impairment, as, in these population groups, drug side-effects and inappropriate doses may cause harm and possibly prove fatal.

## The World Health Organization's three-step Analgesic Ladder for cancer pain relief

Tables in the Appendix refer to the World Health Organization's three-step Analgesic Ladder for cancer pain relief (World Health Organization (hereafter WHO), 1996) (see Figure 10.1). The WHO ladder provides the type of analgesic medication required according to the experience of the patient's pain intensity, as mild, moderate or severe. Cancer pain is often at least moderate pain, and requires treatment with a combination of opioid and non-opioid analgesic medications taken with non-analgesic medications, known as adjuvant medications (see Tables in Appendix). For patients with chronic cancer pain living in the community there are usually certain protocols to follow when selecting the appropriate WHO Analgesic Ladder step, for either beginning or adjusting the patient's analgesic medications.

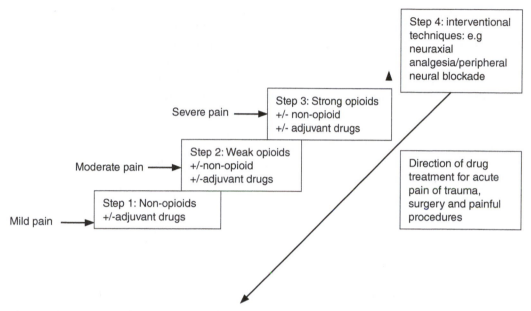

**Figure 10.1** A four-step Analgesic Ladder

Note: At the time of writing the World Health Organization Analgestic Ladder (which the first three steps are based on) the is currently under upgrade review. Readers are advised to check the www.who.int for the latest guidance.

Source: The World Health Organization Analgesic Ladder is currently under upgrade review; Figure redrawn with reference to Sinatra, R.S. (2011) A stepwise approach to pain management in R.S. Sinatra, J, S. Jahr and J.M Watkins-Pitchford (eds) *The Essence of Analgesia and Analgesics*. Cambridge: Cambridge University Press.

In the event that a non-specialist setting does not have the legal authority to pre-scribe opioid medication, the patient may need urgent referral to a pain specialist centre or palliative care team.

## Effectively relieving cancer pain

The WHO (1996) recommends relieving cancer pain through the administration of anal-gesic medication using a method tested in the 1980s and summarized by five phrases: 'by mouth', 'at the clock', 'by the ladder', 'for the individual', and 'attention to detail'.

For patients starting pain management treatment with strong opioids, Step 3 of the WHO Analgesic Ladder recommends that the preferred route for morphine drug administration is **by mouth,** with immediate release liquid morphine.

The **initial** oral morphine dose depends on the severity of the patient's pain, his or her previous medication doses, age, level of frailty, and whether his or her medical history includes renal or liver impairment. Patients who either have not taken morphine (a) before or (b) for a long time are referred to as, respectfully, 'opioid naïve', which means that they require careful observation for possible opioid side-effects and need to begin treatment with a lower dose, which is then titrated up to an analgesic effect. The WHO Analgesic Ladder (1986, 1996) for pain relief titration recommendation is to 'start low, go slow'. **Opioid titration** is the process of gradually increasing the analgesic dose until the patient is comfortable. The next dose is given before the effect of the previous one has worn off. The recommenced oral morphine starting dose for 'opioid naïve' **adult** patients is 20–30 mg **daily** oral morphine divided into four-hourly doses of 5 mg = 2.5 ml. Strength is usually adjusted so that the dose volume is 5 ml or 10 ml. For most patients, pain is controlled with doses of 10–30 mg every four hours. To achieve a drug steady state and obtain optimal pain relief the drug must be taken '**at the clock**' (atc), that is, with regular time intervals (WHO, 1996, 1986). For appropriate starting dosages for differently aged patients, **check** dosages in relevant latest edition of the National Formulary of your country and *Mosby's Drug Guide for Nursing Students* (Skidmore, 2013).

In the **acute care hospital setting**, following a comprehensive biopsychosocial pain assessment, the patient is commenced on a medication dose that meets his or her pain requirement. Boundaries between numbers and the verbal descriptors of mild, moderate and severe need to be considered in the context of the patient's function, alongside their pain intensity. For instance, pain that is described as '4' by the patient may be mild if their behaviour and demeanour agrees with their description, or may be moderate according to how the pain is impacting on function. Analgesic medication is given '**by the ladder**'. If the patient's pain is mild, they may start on Step 1 of the WHO Analgesic Ladder with a non-opioid medication. Frequently in the case of cancer pain, the patient describes their pain as at least moderate, with a Number Rating Scale (NRS) score of 5–6, and, more often, as severe, with an NRS score of 7 or more, with indications that pain is impacting on function. Pain that is mild to moderate, with an NRS score of about 5, may be treated with a mild opioid such as tramadol, in addition to the non-opioid medication. When an opioid for mild-to-moderate pain in combination with a non-opioid fails to relieve the pain, an opioid for moderate-to-severe pain should be substituted. Only one drug from each of the non-opioid and opioid groups should be used at the same time (WHO, 1996). More often, the patient has severe pain with an NRS score of 7 or more, and needs to go straight to Step 3 of the WHO Analgesic Ladder.

While the oral route is preferred, the patient's initial dose of morphine may be required intravenously, to avoid first-pass metabolism, and titrated upwards to achieve a blood plasma steady state more rapidly. An antiemetic is especially required if morphine is given intravenously to bring severe pain under control. When the patient's pain is under control and concordant with the patient's functional status, oral morphine at the appropriate dose and type should be given 'at the clock', along with a non-opioid.

Analgesia is provided '**for the individual**', that is, each patient has individual analgesic requirements based on their cancer diagnosis, treatment side-effects and biopsychosocial pain assessment. The correct dose is the dose that works for the individual patient, so there are no standard doses for opioid drugs. For cancer pain, the use of morphine should be dictated by the intensity of pain and not by life expectancy (WHO, 1996). Adjuvant medication, such as the benzodiazepine diazepam (nursing safety note: CAUTION with side-effects: shorter acting benzodiazepines may be preferred for patients with hepatic impairment), may be required to relieve anxiety, particularly for severe cancer pain, depending on the level of anxiety and distress. Adjuvant medications are given for specific indications. These are:

- to treat the adverse effects of analgesics, particularly nausea and constipation;
- to enhance pain relief;
- to treat concomitant psychological disturbances, such as insomnia, anxiety and depression (WHO, 1996).

Usually patients develop a tolerance to opioid side-effects, except constipation. Anti-emesis medication may be required in the early stages of taking morphine and a less sedating phenothiazine, for example prochlorperazine (nursing safety note: CAUTION, check all potential drug interactions with a reliable online drug checker, such as: http://reference.medscape.com/drug-interactionchecker) is usually the drug of choice.

**Constipation** is a very serious and unpleasant side-effect of opioid medication and, of itself, causes pain and distress and possible abdominal complications. Patients taking opioid medications MUST have laxatives prescribed to avoid an otherwise potentially serious reduction in their quality of life. A proactive, pre-emptive approach is required to prevent opioid-induced constipation. Patients need to take regular stool softeners and stimulant laxatives, such as senna or biscodyl, which increases bowel motility. Patients already on a laxative regime may still suffer intermittent exacerbations of constipation and require osmotic laxatives.

# Patient education regarding opioid analgesia for patients with cancer living in the community

Patients with cancer living in the community should have their drug regimen written out in full, with '**attention to detail**' regarding all drug names (of non-opoids, opioids and adjuvant medications), and reason for taking them, as well as the dosages. Patients should have their questions answered and have access to further instructions with a liaison nurse if required. It is important to emphasize the need to take each medication on a regular 'at the clock' basis, as prescribed, so very basic instructions about keeping drug levels steady in the blood plasma and taking the medication at set times (usually 10.00 am, 14.00 pm and 18.00 pm), linking the first and last doses to the patient's waking and bedtime hours, is essential. The patient should be warned about possible adverse drug effects and know how to get appropriate professional help quickly, with a readily contactable name and contact number (WHO, 1996).

It is very strongly recommended that patients with cancer living in the community keep a pain diary to observe the effectiveness or otherwise of the analgesic treatment regimen and to be able to adjust the regimen early if required. In addition to advising on medically appropriate and adequate fluid (water) intake, appropriate physical activity and a diet with adequate fibre, the nurse needs to ensure that the patient (or their close other as support) is educated to pay special attention to taking laxatives as part of the daily drug regimen to avoid constipation. If a constipation problem arises, the patient should be advised to seek medical attention as soon as possible (American Pain Society, 2008).

Dosages given in Tables in the Appendix are estimates only. Each nurse should have immediate access to the drug formulary used in their country and to a nursing drug guide with nursing teaching points, for example, *Mosby's Drug Guide for Nursing Students* (Skidmore, 2013). It is also strongly recommended that online guidance (from the NCCN, NICE or an equivalent organization) is consulted regularly, in conjunction with the recommended formulary because best-practice indicators in pain management for various cancers (as medication recommendations) may differ according to cancer type and stage and are regularly updated.*

## Titration of opioid medication

Titration refers to dose adjustment in which a measured amount of one medicinal compound is given following a previous known dose of the same compound already taken by/administered to the patient, until the required pain relief for the patient is attained. Titration builds on the concept of drug blood plasma steady state and increasing steady state blood plasma concentration levels of a drug compound to levels that give effective pain relief.

Non-opioid analgesics are very helpful for controlling pain caused by soft tissue and muscle infiltration and NSAIDs block prostaglandin biosynthesis in metastatic bone cancer. However, of vital importance is the recognition that a 'ceiling effect' is achieved with increasing doses of non-opioid medications. Therefore, there is a limit to the analgesic effect which can be achieved by increasing the non-opioid drug dose (as well as potentially very serious side-effects of larger doses than those recommended). When pain is not relieved by a non-opioid, an opioid should be added (WHO, 1996). Morphine does not have a ceiling effect and can be titrated up to the patient's pain relief requirements, or until adverse side-effects occur.

---

*Always have the opioid antagonist Naloxone available in the acute setting in case of the adverse effect of respiratory depression following opioid administration.

This makes morphine the gold standard for cancer pain. The most life-threatening side-effect of morphine and other opioid medication is respiratory depression, which is the rationale for:

- close observation of opioid side-effects;
- having the opioid antidote Naloxone always available;
- regular patient pain intensity measurement to check the effectiveness of the increased opioid dose;
- switching to a different opioid if dose titration incurs adverse side-effects or does not give required pain relief.

## Titration of oral morphine for cancer-related breakthrough pain

If cancer-related breakthrough pain occurs between regular doses of morphine, an additional rescue dose should be given. The standard dose for breakthrough pain is one-sixth of the regular total 24-hour (**daily**) dose, which equates with one four-hourly dose, so that a patient prescribed oral morphine sulfate 30 mg **daily** divided into four-hourly doses six times a day of 5 mg would receive a breakthrough dose of 5 mg. The rescue dose can be repeated two–four-hourly if required. The amount of medication given by rescue doses should not exceed one-third to one-half of the total **daily** dose. In the event that further rescue doses are required, the **daily** dose should be adjusted (titrated). For example, a patient with cancer pain prescribed 30 mg **daily** of oral morphine sulphate, that is, 5 mg taken four-hourly, who has also required three rescue doses of 5 mg oral morphine sulphate in the past 24 hours for breakthrough pain, requires dose titration. Titration is as follows: the DAILY dose (30 mg) is added to the total rescue dose requirement for the past 24 hours (3 × 5 mg = 15 mg), to give 30 mg + 15 mg = 45 mg, which becomes the new DAILY dose given in four-hourly doses = 45 mg ÷ 6 = 7.5 mg every four hours.

The same process is repeated until the patient obtains pain relief and is comfortable, or if adverse side-effects occur, in which case consideration of opioid switching or other medications is required. Morphine is titrated against the patient's pain, which, when controlled, may allow for a gradual reduction of medication to a lower dose to prevent withdrawal symptoms (BNF, 2014a; Fallon and McConnell, 2007; Pasero and McCaffery, 2011).

## Adverse effects of opioid analgesia

People respond differently to medication for individual physiological and genetic reasons. Too strong a starting dose, or titrating up too rapidly with stronger doses, can result in side-effects of opioid analgesia which include, but are not limited to: possible coma, respiratory depression, shock, tachycardia, nausea and vomiting and pinpoint pupils, urinary retention, severe constipation. Opioids may cause drowsiness, confusion, sedation and may impair driving. Morphine crosses the placenta, so caution is advised in pregnancy and in breast-feeding mothers. Morphine interacts with alcohol, anti-psychotic medications, sedatives relaxants and hypnotics to increase their central nervous system depression side-effect. With certain herbs there may be an increase in central nervous system depression. Cranberry juice and oats reduce the effect of morphine.

**Important nursing considerations** include **comprehensive** pain assessment before drug administration, giving opioid medication before pain becomes extreme, regular monitoring of pain intensity, monitoring and recording all vital signs (with pain as the fifth vital sign), monitoring for opioid adverse side-effects, particularly respiratory depression, nausea and vomiting, and drowsiness, checking fluid balance intake and output and observing for possible urinary retention, and particularly checking and preventing constipation by increasing fluid intake, using stimulant laxatives and/or by adding bulk in the patient's diet (BNF, 2014a; Pasero and McCaffery, 2011; Skidmore, 2013).

## Genetics and opioid analgesia metabolism

Opioids are metabolized by two major enzyme systems in the liver: the CYP450 and the glucuronosyltransferases (UGTs). Drugs interact with the CYP450 system as a substrate, an inhibitor or an inducer. There are many CYP450 enzyme types, with enzymes CYP2D6 and CYP3A4 being highly relevant to opioid metabolism. Patients may lack these enzymes genetically or these enzymes may be required to metabolize more than one drug at any given time, placing a burden on the enzyme requirement. Hydromorphone, morphine and oxymorphone are mostly metabolized by the UGTs. Other and different opioids act as substrates for (are metabolized by) CYP2D6 and CYP3A4 enzymes. Other drugs being metabolized at the same time as certain opioids may acts as inhibitors, slowing the enzymes or inducers that boost enzyme activity.

Certain populations of patients have one of four differing CYP2D6 phenotypes, by which patients are either poor, intermediate, extensive or ultra rapid metabolizers. However, the pro drug codeine requires 2D6 to convert to morphine. Slow metabolizers may not respond well to codeine, while ultra rapid metabolizers may have a toxic response to codeine (Pasero and McCaffery, 2011).

## Neuropathic cancer pain

An international survey of patients with cancer pain indicated that up to 40% of cancer pain can be neuropathic. The most frequent causes of chronic neuropathic pain are:

- direct tumour infiltration of a peripheral nerve;
- tumour infiltration of a nerve plexus: the site varies with cancer type – in breast cancer the tumour can spread to the brachial plexus;
- radiculopathy: the tumour spreads to involve dorsal spinal roots;
- post-surgical pain syndromes: the most common examples are post-mastectomy, post-thoracotomy, post-radical neck dissection and phantom limb pain;
- neuropathic pain is often a side-effect of chemotherapy and radiation therapies.

The mechanisms of cancer pain are frequently mixed, so all of the above should be considered as possible causes when trying to identify neuropathic cancer pain. The same is true for intense or distressing persistent or severe pain which does not respond to useful treatment and if the cancer tumour location is known or the pain is likely to be from nerve compression.

A Number Rating Scale can be used to assess pain intensity of neuropathic pain. In addition, the location, quality and pattern of the pain give valuable information regarding the source of the pain. The Leeds Assessment of Neuropathic Symptoms and Signs (LANSS) (Bennett et al., 2005) is a simple diagnostic assessment tool to identify neuropathic pain. In addition to the sensation of burning or lancinating pain, possible abnormal sensations of crawling, pricking, itching or tingling, allodynia, hyperalgesia, skin colour changes and numbness should be checked for. Neuropathic pain in cancer is often severe, highly complex in origin and may require an opioid trial monitored carefully for side-effects and titrated until pain control is optimal.

Careful and empathic explanation needs to be given to the patient and his or her family to maintain their trust and help them cope with possible changes in therapeutic regimen. Achieving maximum pain control may be a prolonged process, involving opioid switching, and can be very psychologically challenging for the patient and his or her family. Morphine may interact synergistically with other drugs given as co-analgesics, which are very effective for neuropathic pain, such as the antiepileptic gabapentin, so careful observation and appropriate morphine dose reduction may be required. Tricyclic antidepressants are effective as co-analgesics, but cardiotoxity is a potential problem. Venlafaxine may be the antidepressant adjuvant of choice in the older, frailer patient. All possible side-effects need to be considered and the patient monitored appropriately (Murtagh and Higginson, 2010).

## Spinal cord compression

This is an oncological emergency that is most commonly caused by compression of the spinal cord and nerve roots by a metastatic paravertebral tumour extending into the epidural space, bone collapse and displacement due to metastases, or primary spinal cord malignancy (Stern, 2014). Pain is the symptom most commonly experienced by patients experiencing spinal cord compression. Ambulant patients may feel limb weakness, as if the limb has 'gone to sleep', have difficulty in walking and or have 'pins and needles' in their legs and feet, and/or tingling down the leg to the foot.

CLINICAL EXAMPLE

## NICE guidelines for the early detection of metastatic spinal cord compression

Inform patients at high risk of developing bone metastases, patients with diagnosed bone metastases, or patients with cancer who present with spinal pain about the symptoms of metastatic spinal cord compression (MSCC). Offer information (for example, in the form of a leaflet) to patients and their families and carers which explains the symptoms of MSCC, and which advises what to do if patients develop these symptoms. Contact the MSCC coordinator urgently (within 24 hours) to discuss the care of patients with cancer and any of the following symptoms, which are all suggestive of spinal metastases:

- pain in the middle (thoracic) or upper (cervical) spine
- progressive lower (lumbar) spinal pain
- severe unremitting lower spinal pain
- spinal pain aggravated by straining (for example, at stool, or when coughing or sneezing)
- localized spinal tenderness
- nocturnal spinal pain preventing sleep.

Contact the MSCC coordinator immediately to discuss the care of patients with cancer and symptoms suggestive of spinal metastases who have any of the following neurological symptoms or signs suggestive of MSCC, and view them as an oncological emergency: neurological symptoms, including radicular pain, any limb weakness, difficulty in walking, sensory loss or bladder or bowel dysfunction (NICE, 2014).

## Procedural pain in cancer

For adults and older-aged adults, when 'as needed' (PRN) analgesic medication is required for an anticipated painful procedure, the analgesic medication should be given at a time prior to the procedure to allow for the PRN analgesic dose to reach peak effect to coincide with the most painful time of the procedure. The analgesic onset of oral morphine is rapid. The peak effect of morphine is one to two hours after dosage, depending on the route of administration. If a patient with cancer already has substantial cancer pain that is well controlled with morphine, consideration of a painful procedure analgesic requirement that is sufficient to prevent the patient's well-controlled background pain from becoming exacerbated is very important and will vary according to individual patient requirements (Fallon and McConnell, 2007).

Wound pain may be a combination of acute nociceptive, inflammatory and neuropathic pain from tissue damage, infection and ischaemia, with sensitized nociceptors giving rise to hyperalgesia. The patient may experience anticipatory anxiety from memories of previous painful dressing changes, lowering the patient's pain threshold, especially if the previous dressing changes resulted in psychological distress for the patient and traumatized skin prolonging healing time. The patient's pain intensity should be measured before the dressing change, followed by selected analgesic dosage, according to the patient's requirement to reach peak effect before dressing removal. If the combination of non-opioids with a weak opioid has been shown to be ineffective, a strong opioid should be given prior to the procedure (at least 30–60 minutes prior) to allow for peak effect at the point of old dressing removal, as wound procedure pain is most intense at this point. Dressings that have adhered to the wound and surrounding skin area have the potential to traumatize both the patient's wound and the patient if not carefully soaked and removed very carefully. Silicone-based and other atraumatic wound dressings help to reduce wound pain because the dressing does not adhere to the skin or wound surface. Pain intensity should be measured again following the dressing change completion. Some patients find distraction techniques helpful during wound dressing procedures; optimal nurse–patient communication can identify relaxation and distraction methods to help the patient cope better with the procedure, with fewer adverse psychological consequences (Edwards, 2013; Solowiej and Upton, 2012; WUWHS, 2008).

Many procedures in cancer care are repeated at regular, sometimes frequent intervals, which involve venepuncture, lumber puncture and biopsy. While a rare event, pre-term and newborn babies who have immaturely developed systems do have cancers and require chemotherapy and analgesic interventions, posing challenges for paediatric oncologists in calculating humane, effective and accurate chemotherapeutic and analgesic dosage. Higher plasma concentrations of morphine are required to produce analgesic effect, because morphine clearance is lower and half life is longer compared with a 2–6-year-old child (Veal and Boddy, 2012).

In children, while the venepuncture procedure may not be classified as 'very painful', when the procedure happens almost daily there may be fear and distress, especially for children and the parents of children, both at the time of the invasive needle procedure event and in anticipating the event, exacerbating the pain and causing increased pain intensity. For cancer care to be humane and compassion shown to the patient, care needs be taken to reduce the patient's anxiety preceeding, during and following the procedure(s) as well as his or her pain experience. Minor venepuncture procedures can be treated with EMLA provided there are no contraindications. The EMLA topical anaesthesia is applied according to the directions (see BNF (2014b) for children for recommended pre-intervention times to apply EMLA topical anaesthesia) prior to the procedure so that a maximum analgesic peak effect may coincide with the invasive procedure. Distraction techniques are very helpful for children for needle invasive procedures. Each child's opinion of their preferred video, colouring book or activity should be ascertained and the child engaged with the process through gentle explanation before and during the procedure.

# Clinical hypnosis and procedural pain

In a randomized clinical trial to assess the benefits of self-hypnosis to control venepuncture-induced pain and anxiety in children with cancer and parental anxiety during the procedures, 45 patients (ages 6–16 years) were randomized to one of three groups: local anaesthetic (EMLA), local anaesthetic plus hypnosis, and local anaesthetic plus attention. Results indicated the increased benefits of the local anaesthetic plus hypnosis group, compared with the other two groups (Liossi et al., 2009).

A controlled trial by Liossi and Hatira (2003) of 80 children with cancer undergoing regular lumbar punctures assigned the children to one of four groups: direct hypnosis with standard medical treatment, indirect hypnosis with standard medical treatment, attention control with standard medical treatment and standard medical treatment alone. Direct and indirect hypnosis were equally effective and more effective than standard medical treatments (Liossi and Hatira, 2003). A recent review concluded that hypnosis is an effective pain-control technique for cancer-related procedure pain and chronic pain in children. Further studies are warranted in this area (Tomé-Pires and Miró, 2012).

# The measurement of cancer-related psychological distress as the sixth vital sign

The British Pain Society's *Cancer Pain Management* guideline document endorses the biopsychosocial model as the best standard of care for patients with cancer pain (British Pain Society, 2010). The BPS guidelines state that '**psychological distress increases with the intensity of cancer pain**' (British Pain Society, 2010).

Guidelines by the US National Comprehensive Cancer Network® (NCCN®) advocate the use of the term 'distress' to avoid labelling and stigmatizing patients and to help reduce barriers to care. They recognize that all patients with cancer deal with issues that cause some level of distress at some stage during their cancer illness experience (Holland et al., 2014; see also Holland and Bultz, 2007). The International Psycho-Oncology Society (IPOS), British Pain Society, NICE, NCCN® and the Institute of Medicine (IOM) all recommend routine screening for distress as the sixth vital sign, which is defined as:

> a multifactorial unpleasant emotional experience of a psychological (cognitive, behavioural, emotional) social and/or spiritual nature that may interfere with the ability to cope effectively with cancer, its physical symptoms and its treatment. Distress entends along a continuum ranging from common normal feelings of vulnerabilty, sadness and fears to problems that can become disabling, such as depression, anxiety, panic, social isolation and existential and spiritual crises. (Holland et al., 2014)

The (NCCN) Distress Thermometer (DT) (see Figure 10.2) is an effective tool for detecting clinical evidence of moderate to severe distress, which is indicated by a score of 4 or more on the DT. By using the problem checklist, issues of major concern to the patient can be identified and an initial problem-solving discussion with the appropriate interdisciplinary healthcare professional, often the Clinical Nurse Specialist, may help to resolve some issues for the patient. The DT has been validated for populations with cancer in several countries; studies agree that referral to psychological or psychiatric services (as appropriate) is recommended in patients with DT scores of 4 or more (Ryan et al., 2011).

Anxiety can overwhelm the patient by reducing his or her sense of mastery and coping and problem-solving ability. Younger-age, female gender, being separated, divorced, widowed and having lower socio-economic status are associated with increased anxiety in patients with cancer (Levin and Alici, 2010; Valentine, 2006). The patient's belief about the meaning of their pain (for example, if a new pain signifies disease progression), as well as a level of psychological well-being and mood, are contributing factors to the patient's subjective pain experience. In patients with cancer, as for all patients, it is essential to believe the patient's pain report (Breibart et al., 2010).

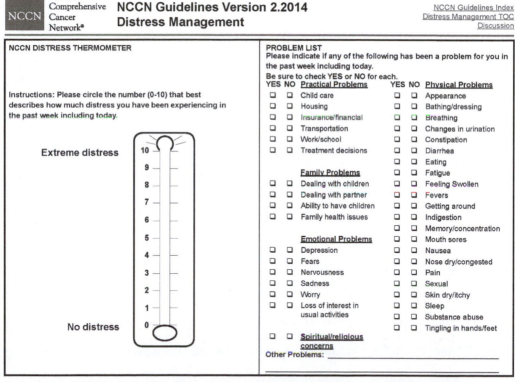

**Figure 10.2** Screening tools for measuring distress

# Chapter summary

- Government and professional recognition of the need to address the widespread under-treatment of cancer pain has led to the publication of guidelines and quality standards that aim to alleviate cancer pain and associated suffering.
- An expert group conference on cancer pain assessment has agreed that domains which require assessment are pain intensity, breakthrough pain, neuropathic pain and psychological distress.
- The Number Rating Scale is recommended to measure cancer pain intensity as the fifth vital sign and the Distress Thermometer to measure distress as the sixth vital sign. An assessment of pain and distress in cancer should be written into local policies.
- Pain intensity scores can be interpreted together with Verbal Rating Scales and patient functionality in differentiating between mild, moderate and severe pain and deciding whether the patient requires non-opioid or opioid medication.
- Patients with moderate to severe pain either begin with or progress to Step 3 of the WHO Analgesic Ladder to an opioid, with non-opioid and with adjuvant medication. An opioid trial and opioid switching may be required to identify the most effective opioid medication.
- For effective cancer pain relief, a nurse–patient relationship is required based on trust, communication and explanation with the patient and his or her close family about how the patient's interdisciplinary care will achieve optimal pain relief.
- Vigilance is required to prevent adverse effects for patients taking opioid medication. Patients need to be asked about and monitored for possible side-effects. The antagonist Naloxone must always be available.
- Spinal cord compression is an oncological emergency encountered in patients with a range of cancer types and stages. The nurse should seek immediate intervention according to local protocols for patients with signs and symptoms of spinal cord compression.

# Reflective exercise

If you were a patient with severe cancer pain and your GP referred you, as a patient in a distressed state, to a cancer centre of excellence as an emergency admission, what qualities would you hope for in the nurse in charge of your care?

# Recommended reading

Bennett, M.I. (ed.) (2010) *Neuropathic Pain* (2nd edn). Oxford: Pain Management Library.

Davies, A. (2007) *Cancer-Related Bone Pain*. Oxford: Pain Management Library.

Davies, A. (2012) *Cancer-Related Breakthrough Pain* (2nd edn). Oxford: Pain Management Library.

Forbes, K. (ed.) (2007) *Opioids in Cancer Pain*. Oxford: Pain Management Library.

Paice, J.A., Bell, R.F., Kalso, E.A. and Soyannwo, O.A. (eds) (2010) *Cancer Pain: From Molecules to Suffering*. Seattle, WA: International Association for the Study of Pain.

## Websites relevant to this chapter

World Health Organization (1996) *Cancer Pain Relief* (2nd edn). Geneva: WHO. Available at: http://apps.who.int/iris/bitstream/10665/37896/1/9241544821.pdf?ua=1

For clinical practice guidelines in oncology (including supportive care and distress): www.nccn.org/default.aspx

International Psycho-oncology Society: www.ipos-society.org/

Recommended drug interaction checker: http://reference.medscape.com/drug-interactionchecker

National Institute for Health and Care Excellence (NICE): www.nice.org.uk

# References

American Pain Society (2008) *Principles of Analgesic Use in the Treatment of Acute Pain and Cancer Pain: Research, Education, Treatment, Advocacy* (6th edn). Chicago, IL: APS.

Bennett, M.I. (2012) Treatment of cancer pain. In I. Tracey (ed.), *Pain 2012: Refresher Courses: 14th World Congress on Pain*. Seattle, WA: International Association for the Study of Pain (IASP).

Bennett, M.I., Smith, B.H., Torrance, N. and Potter, J. (2005) 'The S-LANSS score for identifying pain of predominantly neuropathic origin: validation for use in clinic and postal research', *Journal of Pain*, 6: 149–158.

Breitbart, W.S., Park, J. and Katz, A.M. (2010) Pain. In J.C. Holland, W.S. Breitbart, P.B. Jacobsen, M.S. Lederberg, M.J. Loscalso and R. McCorkle (eds), *Psycho-Oncology* (2nd edn). Oxford: Oxford University Press.

Breivik, H., Cherny, N., Collett, B., de Conno, F., Filbet, M., Foubert, A.J., Cohen, R. and Dow, L. (2009) Cancer-related pain: a pan-European survey of prevalence, treatment, and patient attitudes. *Annals of Oncology*, 20: 1420–1433.

British National Formulary (2014a) *BNF 66 for Adults September 2013–March 2014*. London: Pharmaceutical Press.

British National Formulary (2014b) *BNF for Children July 2013–July 2014*. London: Pharmaceutical Press.

British Pain Society (2010) *Cancer Pain Management*. January, p. 49.

Cherny, N.I. (2013) Cancer pain assessment and syndromes. In S.B. McMahon, M. Koltzenburg, I. Tracey, D.C. Turk, *Wall and Melzack's Textbook of Pain* (6th edn). Philadelphia, PA: Elsevier Saunders.

Coleman, R.E. and McCloskey, E.V. (2011) Bisphosphonates in oncology. *Bone*, 49: 71–76.

Edwards, J. (2013) Dealing with wound-related pain at dressing change. *Journal of Community Nursing*, 27 (4): 36–42.

Fallon, M. and McConnell, S. (2007) Principles of opioid titration. In K. Forbes (ed.), *Opioids in Cancer Pain*. Oxford: Pain Management Library.

Fitzgibbon, D.R. and Loeser, J.D. (2010) *Cancer Pain: Assessment Diagnosis and Management*. Riverwoods, IL: Wolters Kluwer/Lippincott Williams and Wilkins.

Furlan, C., Trovo, M., Drigo, A., Capra, E. and Trovo, M.G. (2014) Half-body irradiation with tomotherapy for pain palliation in metastatic breast cancer. *Journal of Pain and Symptom Management*, 47: 174–180.

Holland, J.C. and Bultz, B.D. (2007) National Comprehensive Cancer Network (NCCN). The NCCN guidelines for distress management: a case for making distress the sixth vital sign. *Journal of the National Comprehensive Cancer Network*, 5: 3–7.

Holland, J.C., et al. (2014) NCCN Clinical Practice Guidelines in Oncology (NCCN Guidelines®) for *Distress Management* V.2.2014. © National Comprehensive Cancer Network, 2014.Available at: NCCN.org (accessed 3 July 2014).

Institute of Medicine (2008) *Cancer Care for the Whole Patient: Meeting Psychosocial Health Needs*. Washington, DC: The National Academies Press.

Kaasa, S., Aplone, G., Klepstad, P., et al. (2011) An expert conference on cancer pain assessment in classification, the need for international consensus: working proposals on international standards, *BMJ: Support for Palliative Care*, 1: 281–287. Cited in A.K. Knudsen, P. Klepstad, C. Brunelli, N. Aass, A. Caraceni and S. Kaasa (2012) Classification and assessment of cancer pain. In I. Tracey (ed.), *Pain 2012: Refresher Courses 14th World Congress on Pain*. Seattle, WA: International Association for the Study of Pain.

Klepstad, P., Fladvad, T., Skorpen, F., et al. (2011) Influence from genetic variability on opioid use for cancer pain: a European genetic association study of 2,294 cancer pain patients. *Pain*, 152: 113–145. Cited in A.K. Knudsen, P. Klepstad, C. Brunelli, N. Aass, A. Caraceni and S. Kaasa (2012) Classification and assessment of cancer pain. In I. Tracey (ed.), *Pain 2012: Refresher Courses 14th World Congress on Pain*. Seattle, WA: International Association for the Study of Pain.

Knudsen, A.K., Klepstad, P., Brunelli, C., Aass, N., Caraceni, A. and Kaasa, S. (2012) Classification and assessment of cancer pain. In I. Tracey (ed.), *Pain 2012: Refresher Courses 14th World Congress on Pain*. Seattle, WA: International Association for the Study of Pain.

Levin, T.T. and Alici, Y. (2012) Anxiety disorders. In J.C. Holland, W.S. Breitbart, P.B. Jacobsen, M.S. Lederberg, M.J. Loscalso and R. McCorkle (eds), *Psycho-Oncology* (2nd edn). Oxford: Oxford University Press.

Liossi, C. and Hatira, P. (2003) Clinical hypnosis in the alleviation of procedure-related pain in pediatric oncology patients. *International Journal of Clinical and Experimental Hypnosis*, 51 (1): 4–28.

Liossi, C., White, P. and Hatira, P. (2009) A randomised clinical trial of a brief hypnosis intervention to control venepuncture-related pain of pediatric cancer patients. *Pain*, 142: 255–263.

Mantyh, P.W. (2013) Cancer pain: causes, consequences and therapeutic opportunities. In S.B. McMahon, M. Koltzenburg, I. Tracey and D.C. Turk, *Wall and Melzack's Textbook of Pain* (6th edn). Philadelphia, PA: Elsevier Saunders.

Murtagh, F.E. and Higginson, I.J (2010) Cancer neuropathic pain. In M.I. Bennett (ed.), *Neuropathic Pain* (2nd edn). Oxford: Pain Management Library.

National Institute for Health and Care Excellence (NICE) (2014) *Metastatic Spinal Cord Compression Overview*. Available at http://pathways.nice.org.uk/pathways/metastatic-spinal-cord-compression?fno=1#content=view-node%3Anodes-symptoms-suggestive-of-spinal-metastases

National Pain Strategy (Pain Australia) (2010), www.painaustralia.org.au/images/pain_australia/NPS/National%20Pain%20Strategy%202011.pdf (accessed 9 February 2014).

Pasero, C. and McCaffery, M. (2011) *Pain Assessment and Pharmacologic Management.* St Louis, MO: Elsevier Mosby.

Portenoy, R.K. and Hagen, N.A. (1990) Breakthrough pain: definition, prevalence and characteristics. *Pain,* 41: 273–281.

Ryan, D.A., Gallagher, P. ,Wright, S. and Cassidy, E.M. (2011) 'Sensitivity and specificity of the Distress Thermometer and a two-item depression screen (Patient Health Questionnaire-2) with a 'help' question for psychological distress and psychiatric morbidity in patients with advanced cancer', *Psycho-Oncology,* 21 (12): 1275–1284.

Sabino, M.A., Luger, N.M., Mach, D.B., Rogers, S.D., Schwei, M.J. and Mantyh, P.W. (2003) Different tumors in bone each give rise to a distinct pattern of skeletal destruction, bone-related cancer pain behaviours and neurochemical changes in the central nervous system. *International Journal of Cancer,* 104: 550–558.

Shipton, E.A. (1999) *Pain: Acute and Chronic.* London: Arnold.

Skidmore, L. (2013) *Mosby's Drug Guide for Nursing Students* (10th edn). St Louis, MO: Elsevier Mosby.

Soloweij, K. and Upton, D. (2012) 'Painful dressing changes for chronic wounds: assessment and management', *British Journal of Nursing,* 21(20): S20–S25.

Somers, T.J., Keefe, F.J., Kothadia, S. and Pandiani, A. (2010) Dealing with cancer pain: coping, pain catastrophising and related outcomes. In J.A. Paice, R.F. Bell, E.A. Kalso and O.A. Soyannwo (eds), *Cancer Pain: From Molecules to Suffering.* Seattle, WA: IASP, p. 232.

Stern, C.L. (2014) Nursing management in cancer care. In J.L. Hinkle and K.H. Cheever, *Brunner and Suddarth's Textbook of Medical–Surgical Nursing.* Riverwoods, IL: Wolters Kluwer/Lippincott Williams and Wilkins.

Tomé-Pires, C. and Jordi Miró, J. (2012) Hypnosis for the management of chronic and cancer procedure-related pain in children. *International Journal of Clinical and Experimental Hypnosis,* 60 (4): 432–457.

Turk, C. and Okifuji, A. (2010) Pain terms and taxonomies of pain. In S.M. Fishman, J.C. Ballantyne and J.P. Rathmell (eds), *Bonica's Management of Pain* (4th edn). Riverwoods, IL: Wolters Kluwer/Lippincott Williams and Wilkins.

Valentine, A.D. (2006) Common psychiatric disorders. In J.C. Holland, D.B. Greenburg and M.K. Hughes (eds), *Quick Reference for Oncology Clinicians: The Psychiatric and Psychological Dimensions of Cancer Symptom Management.* Charlottesville, VA:: IPOS Press.

van den Beuken-van Everdingen, M.H., de Rijke, J.M., Kessels, A.G., Schouten, H.C., van Kleef, M. and Patijn, J. (2007) Prevalence of pain in patients with cancer: a systematic review of the past 40 years. *Annals of Oncology,* 18: 1437–1449.

Veal, G.J. and Boddy, A.V. (2012) Chemotherapy in newborns and preterm babies. *Seminars in Fetal and Neonatal Medicine,* 17: 243–248.

Williams, A. C. de C. and Gessler, S. (2010) Empathy in cancer pain. In J.A. Paice, R.F. Bell, E.A. Kalso and O.A. Soyannwo (eds), *Cancer Pain: From Molecules to Suffering.* Seattle, WA: IASP.

World Health Organization (1996) *Cancer Pain Relief (with a guide to opioid availability)* (2nd edn). Geneva: WHO (1st edn, 1986).

WUWHS (World Union of Wound Healing Societies) (2008) *Principles of Best Practice: Diagnostics and Wounds: A Consensus Document.* London: MEP.

# 11

# Pain management in palliative care and at end of life

## Learning objectives

The learning objectives of this chapter are to:

- know the definition, rationale for and goals of palliative care across the life span
- recognize that palliative care relieves pain and suffering for patients with malignant and non-malignant incurable diseases
- understand that optimal communication skills and symptom control are the core principles of palliative care
- understand the role of nursing in addressing patient and family care needs

## Introduction

This chapter discusses palliative and end-of-life care for all chronic, incurable diseases, malignant and non-malignant, which have proven resistant to curative treatment. The term 'palliative' is derived from the latin 'palliare', meaning 'to cloak'; the verb 'palliate' is based on the noun 'pallium', 'a cloak'. As populations live to an older age globally, increasing numbers of people suffer varying types of incurable chronic conditions. The primary aim of palliative care is to achieve optimal pain and symptom control for the patient to allow maximum quality of life to the end of his or her life (Gamondi et al., 2013a).

# The global need for palliative care services

Palliative care is no longer just synonymous with end-of-life care because there have been important changes in the last two decades in the patient population to whom palliative care is delivered. As well as patients with cancer, patients with serious debilitating non-cancer-related chronic diseases require, and increasingly receive, care according to palliative care principles. Globally, mortality in high-income countries is, mostly, the result of ischaemic cardiac disease, cerebrovascular disease and cancer, while 60% of deaths globally are due to chronic diseases, especially cardiovascular disease, diabetes, cancer and chronic respiratory disease, all diseases associated with an aging population. As pharmacological and nonpharmacological treatments improve (and cures remain elusive), patients with any of these diseases are likely to live longer, sometimes with symptoms which require long-term palliation to maintain optimal quality of life and functionality (Paice, 2010; van Mechelen et al., 2012). Globally, there is a very significant unmet need for palliative care. There is currently a global population of about 600 million people aged 60 years or older. With at least two family members involved in each patient's care, palliative care could improve the quality of life of more than 100 million people annually worldwide. Palliative care is especially necessary for patients with cancer and/or AIDS. The World Health Organization has pioneered a public health strategy for integrating the provision of easily accessible palliative care services into each country's healthcare system (Sternswärd et al., 2007).

# The World Health Organization's definition of palliative care

The World Health Organization (2002) states that:

> palliative care improves the quality of life of patients and families who face life-threatening illness, by providing pain and symptom relief, spiritual and psychosocial support from diagnosis to the end of life and bereavement.

WHO definitions of palliative care for adults and children are available at: www.who.int/cancer/palliative/definition/en/.

# The role of nursing in palliative care

Dame Cicely Saunders, called the Mother of Palliative Care, stated that 'palliative care stems from the recognition of the potential at the end of life for discovering and for giving, a recognition that an important dimension of being human is the lasting dignity and growth that can continue through weakness and loss. No member of the interdisciplinary team is more central to making these discoveries possible than the nurse' (Saunders, 1976). The basic assumption of palliative nursing is 'a whole person philosophy of care implemented across the lifespan and across diverse settings, where the patient and the family is the unit of care' (Ferrell and Coyle, 2006: ix).

## Internationally recognized goals of palliative nursing

The internally recognized goals of palliative nursing are as follows:

- To promote quality of life along the illness trajectory through the relief of suffering, including care of the dying and bereavement;
- To follow up for the family and significant others in the patient's life;
- To relieve suffering and enhance quality of life, including providing effective pain and symptom management;
- To address the psychosocial and spiritual needs of the patient and family;
- To incorporate cultural values and attitudes into the plan of care;
- To support those who are experiencing loss, grief and bereavement;
- To promote ethical and legal decision-making;
- To advocate for personal wishes and preferences;
- To use therapeutic communication skills;
- To facilitate collaborative practice (Coyle, 2006).

These learning goals for nurse education in palliative care are endorsed by the International Association for Hospice and Palliative Care (IAHPC) and the European Association for Palliative Care (EAPC) Task Force on Palliative Nurse Education (De Vlieger et al., 2004). The core competencies in palliative care education were outlined in an EAPC White Paper in 2013 (Gamondi et al., 2013a, 2013b).

In January 2014, the World Health Organization adopted Palliative Care Resolution EB134.R7, entitled 'Strengthening of palliative care as a component of integrated treatment within the continuum of care', a paragraph of which states:

taking into account that the avoidable suffering of treatable symptoms is perpetuated by the lack of knowledge of palliative care and highlighting the need for continuing education and adequate training for all hospital and community based health care providers and other care givers ... the resolution urges member states to include palliative care as an integral component of ongoing education ... basic training and continuing education on palliative care should be integrated as a routine element of all undergraduate medical and nursing professional education. (World Health Organization, 2014: 2–4)

The WHO, IAHPC and EAPC recommend palliative care education at all levels of healthcare professional training and as an essential component of continuing healthcare professional education.

# Roles and functions of the palliative care team members

The nurse's role, together with the physician's role, comprises the core palliative care team. They provide access to the essential psychosocial services. A healthcare team can be described as *an identified collective in which members share common team goals and work interdependently in planning, problem solving, decision making and implementing and evaluating team related tasks* (Faksvåg Haugen et al., 2010).

The **Advanced Nurse Specialist (Practitioner)** in palliative care is the nurse clinician, educator, researcher and consultant to the interdisciplinary team and wider colleagial and social community.

The **Clinical Nurse Specialist/Palliative Care Nurse** educates and supports the nursing team in their roles with holistic patient and family care, acts as a resource for pain management and symptom control, and, along with the Advanced Nurse Practitioner, combines nursing science with ethics and philosophy to foster standards for best quality clinical practice in palliative care, contributes to education and research projects, and especially shows leadership in bringing hope to end-of-life care.

The **patient and family** are the focus of care, with interdisciplinary care aiming to meet their identified goals to alleviate physical, psychological, spiritual and social suffering imposed by disease and illness consequences.

The **Primary Care Physician** refers the patient and family to the palliative care physician and liaises with interdisciplinary team members to provide necessary patient medical and psychosocial information, and for care planning.

The **Palliative Care Physician** provides expertise, collaborating and communicating with the interdisciplinary team members, particularly with regard to pain management and treatment and care decisions.

The **Social Worker** provides supportive interventions for and refers families to social services if required.

The patient may require or seek referral to the **Psychologist** for cognitive behavioural therapy to facilitate coping and/or the **Psychiatrist,** depending on levels of distress, to alleviate depression and anxiety which lower quality of life and impact on the pain experience.

The **Pastoral Care Chaplain** assesses and helps the patient and family address spiritual issues relating to the meaning and purpose of life, offers comfort and solace to the patient with distress related to loss of hope and to the family in their adversity, and discusses troubling faith issues.

The **Bereavement Counsellor** provides bereavement counselling and referral services for families who have lost loved ones or family members who are anticipating the loss of a loved one.

The **Physiotherapist and Occupational Therapist** work with patients receiving palliative care to maximize functionality, quality of life and remaining time, with input as required from the **Pharmacist** and **Speech** and **Nutritional Therapists**.

**Complementary therapists** offer diverse therapies, such as massage, aromatherapy, reflexology, relaxation, art and music therapies, which patients often find helpful for reducing stress associated with pain, treatments and the illness experience.

**Volunteers** have a major role in the hospice setting, providing companionship and support for patients and families, and support for palliative care programmes. Volunteers are overseen, recruited and trained by the **Volunteer Coordinator**, and volunteer training involves the Palliative Care Nurse (Krammer et al., 2010).

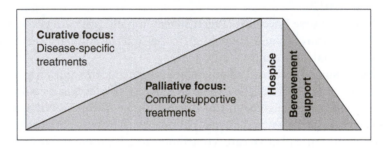

**Figure 11.1**   Proposed model for integration of palliative care

Copyright. Source: S.M. Fishman, J.C. Ballantyne and J.P. Rathmell (eds), *Bonica's Management of Pain* (4th edn). Riverwoods, IL: Wolters Kluwer/Lippincott Williams and Wilkins. Republished with permission of Lippincott Williams and Wilkins.

## Recommended integration of palliative care principles at an early stage of disease

Patients and families benefit greatly when palliative care is integrated into the patient's care plan early during the course of a disease (see Figure 11.1). If curative and palliative care are woven together, they facilitate prompt attention to pain, distress and other symptoms that cause suffering, and thereby enhance treatment benefits and maximize the patient's quality of life (Krammer et al., 2010; Paice, 2010).

Pain syndromes in palliative care may relate to underlying diseases and their treatment or may be discrete, such as pressure ulcers. People infected with human immunodeficiency virus (HIV) in the early stages and almost 100% of people in very advanced stages of infection experience pain. Pain associated with multiple sclerosis, amyotrophic lateral sclerosis, other neurological disorders, end-stage renal failure and heart failure can escalate at end of life, with disease progression and immobility (Paice, 2010; van Mechelen et al., 2012)

# Palliative care and cancer-related pain and suffering

There is a fundamental duty of care, based on ethics and human rights in palliative medicine, which asserts boldly and optimistically that even in the face of overwhelming illness, suffering can and must be relieved (Cherny, 2010). The aetiology of pain in advanced cancer is through tissue and/or nerve destruction as a consequence of tumour burden, treatment side-effects such as chemotherapy-induced neuropathic pain and metastases (Gordon-Williams and Dickenson, 2010; Vignaroli et al., 2012). Secondary bone metastases are a common pain problem in palliative care, along with secondary tumours of the lung and liver. Effective end-of-life palliative treatment of cancer-induced bone pain may require any of a combination of interventions comprised of corticosteroids, bisphosphonates, radiotherapy or radioactive isotopes, long-acting opioids and stabilization of the skeletal structure (Paice and Fine, 2010).

# Assessment in palliative care and at end of life

Comprehensive biopsychosocial assessment of the patient's pain and distress is essential at the first consultation, which may include the **McGill Short-Form Questionnaire** (SF-MPQ-2). Regular measurement of pain as the fifth vital sign, using patient-appropriate pain tools in hospital and hospice care settings, and asking the patient to keep a pain diary if he or she is living in the community contributes to quality care. Documentation and frequent communication among the interdisciplinary palliative care team help to ensure consistent standards of care, optimal pain control for the patient and prevent duplication of patient interviews (Paice, 2010).

## The Memorial Delirium Assessment Scale (MDAS)

Patients with advanced cancer may suffer from a diverse range of problems comprising pain, other symptoms and emotional distress, combined with delirium, and/or dementia and/or the neurological side-effects of cancer manifesting as changes in mental status, sensory and motor deficits, as well as treatment side-effects. **The Memorial Delirium Assessment Scale (MDAS)** is a 10-item clinician-administered assessment that evaluates the areas of cognition most sensitive to impairment with delirium. These are arousal, level of consciousness, memory, attention, orientation, disturbances in thinking and psychomotor activity. Scores range from 0 to 30, and a score of 13 or above suggests delirium (Breitbart et al., 1997; Pirl, 2006).

## The Brief Pain Inventory (BPI)

The relief of suffering and discomfort requires measurement to understand the impact on the patient. A numerical or verbal assessment can give pre- and post-pain treatment feedback and help with medication adjustment to achieve optimal pain control. The Brief Pain Questionnaire (Daut et al. 1983), now called the **Brief Pain Inventory (BPI)**, asks patients to circle a number from 0 to 10 that signifies the severity of their pain, with zero labelled as 'no pain' and 10 labelled 'pain as bad as you can imagine'. Following the pain ratings, patients are asked to report the medications or treatments they receive for pain, the percentages of relief these medications or treatments provide and patients' belief about the cause of their pain. Finally, patients are asked to rate how much pain interferes with mood, relations with other people, walking ability, sleep, normal work and enjoyment of life, using a Number Rating Scale (Bennett, 2009; Daut et al., 1983).

## Measurement of distress as the sixth vital sign

Routine screening for distress as the sixth vital sign is recommended. This is discussed in Chapter 10.

## The Hospital Anxiety and Depression Scale (HADS)

The **Hospital Anxiety and Depression Scale (HADS)** is a 14-item tool. Seven items assess anxiety and seven items assess depression. The severity of the symptoms suggests the possibility that the patient may have clinical depression or anxiety, which is then confirmed by clinical diagnostic interview by the trained palliative care physician or psychiatrist. The HADS may be the most widely used tool to assess mood disorders in patients with cancer (Pirl, 2006; Zigmund and Snaith, 1983).

# Communication at the end of life

Hope for the control of pain is a vital aspect of the relief of suffering which can be greatly increased if there is uncertainly about the relief of experienced pain. Suffering is linked also to the experience of despair, loneliness and vulnerability. The nurse has a central role as a member of the interdisciplinary care team in giving comfort to the patient and to his or her family caregivers who themselves may be distressed by the suffering experienced by their loved one and their own grief at their anticipated loss. Spiritual concerns about the meaning of life and death affect people with a religious or a non-religious worldview. Pastoral care may provide comfort, and help the patient to find meaning in their life experience and hope for a peaceful death with dignity. The role of the nurse in alleviating the suffering of dying patients and bereaved families is rooted in humanist, empathetic, quality care of the patient and his or close others (Witt Sherman, 2010).

At any stage of the cancer journey, and especially at the end of life, patients and their close others require emotional support and reassurance. Communications must be provided in a compassionate manner. Often patients and their families have to hear bad news over a series of days or weeks. How this news is given is crucially important to patients and families. Formal communication skills training is necessary to improve patient outcomes at end of life, as the cusp between life and death is emotionally complex. Interdisciplinary discussion on death and dying should be a predictable process, and should include discussions on limiting the use of invasive interventions, such as CPR, which burdens a dying person's suffering (Levin and Weiner, 2010).

Ultimately, people at the end of life need to be able to spend their remaining time meaningfully and to plan for loved ones before their death. Truthful imparting of information allows choice and dignity. Patients and caregivers mostly prefer honest and accurate information, provided with empathy and understanding. Healthcare professionals may be able to help patients cope with their terminal prognosis by exploring and fostering realistic forms of hope that are meaningful for each patient and his or her family (Clayton et al., 2008; Fallowfield, 2010; Fallowfield et al., 2002).

# The nurse's role in breaking bad news with the patient and family

Studies show that healthcare professionals, including nurses and physicians, are viewed as providers of emotional, informational and appraisal support for patients with cancer (Cobb, 1976; Galbraith, 1995). Social support can be construed as coping assistance (Thoits, 1986). A nurse who is competent in communications skills can help the patient and his or her close others to feel calm and less isolated before a difficult interview. The nurse can reassure them that expert help is available, that privacy will be respected and that the patient really is at the centre of care. Empathic listening is key. Checking how the patient feels before and after the interview and offering honest hope, giving the same information to both patient and family instills their confidence and trust towards the care team (Fallowfield et al., 2002).

The SPIKES anagram refers to a set of strategies for each member of the multidisciplinary care team to discuss bad news with the patient:

**Set up** the interview
Review the patient's **Perception** of their illness
Get an **Invitation** from the patient to deliver the news
Give the patient **Knowledge** and information
Respond to the patient's **Emotions**
**Summarize** the treatment plan and review all that has been communicated.
(Baile and Parker, 2010)

# Pain and symptom management in advanced cancer and at end of life

Morphine is the gold standard and pharmacological treatments are administered according to the World Health Organization's Analgesic Ladder for Pain Relief (WHO, 1986, 1996). In response to a request from the Cancer Control Program of the World Health Organization, the International Association for Hospice in Palliative Care (IAHPC) has developed a list of essential medicines for palliative care (available at: http://hospicecare.com/uploads/2011/8/iahpc-essential-meds-en.pdf).

Immediate-release morphine is the opioid of choice for moderate to severe pain (10 mg/5 ml orally), otherwise immediate-release (10–60 mg tablets) or sustained-release (10 or 30 mg tablets). The IAHPC states that government should not approve modified-release morphine, fentanyl or oxycodone without also guaranteeing widely available normal release morphine. In 2010 the IAHPC formed a working committee to determine the components of an opioid essential prescription package (OEPP) to be used when initiating prescription for the control of moderate to severe chronic pain. The OEPP consists of:

> Opioid:
> Morphine, oral, 5 mg every 4 hours
> Laxative:
> Combination of senna and docusate, oral, 8.6 mg/50 mg every 12 hours
> Or
> Bisacodyl, oral, 5 mg every 12 hours
> Antiemetic:
> Metoclopramide, oral, 10 mg every 4 hours OR as needed

In all cases, constipation is the most common adverse side-effect of opioids and laxative prophylaxis should be a priority when commencing and continuing opioid medication. Stimulant laxatives Bisacodyl (10 mg tablets), 10 mg rectal suppositories or senna (8.6 mg tablets) are recommended by the IAHPC. Generally, all patients receiving opioids require concurrent laxative. A review by

Twycross et al. (2012) is recommended for understanding the pathophysiology of opioid-induced constipation and mechanisms of action of commonly pre-scribed laxatives.

Resources for palliative care nursing and guidance on drug use and compatibili-ties are available elsewhere (for example, Ferrell and Coyle, 2006, 2010; Matzo and Witt Sherman, 2010; IAHPC, NICE, AHFS, BNF, NCCN). Some major hospice pharmacies offer a palliative medicine advice service by phone or email for health-care professionals working in palliative care.

## The syringe driver

The syringe driver is a recommended resource for continuous subcutaneous infu-sions in palliative care (Dickman and Schneider, 2011). During the last few weeks of life, patients frequently have a loss of appetite (anorexia), which gives rise to cachexia, a complex syndrome characterized by weight loss, wasting of muscle and severe debilitation. Pain may be widespread. The subcutaneous route is selected to deliver opioids, in conjunction with compatible drugs, to control symptoms which often accompany pain at the end of life.

. . . . . . . . . . . . . . . . . . . . . . . . . . . . . . . . . . . . . . . . . . . . . . . . . . . . . . . . . . . . . . . . . . . . . .

## Uncontrolled pain, distress and delirium in undiagnosed metastatic cancer

In the past month Mr D has experienced intermittent headaches, for which he has taken over-the-counter medication. In the past week he has vomited several times and his wife and son have noticed a change in his personality. In the past 24 hours Mr D has complained of very severe pain in his back. When his son contacted the General Practitioner's surgery he was advised to call an ambulance for direct admission to the hospital emergency department.

Asking Mr D's wife and son for their interpretation of Mr D's pain and distress, the emer-gency department nurse documented Mr D's vital signs, including pain as 10 on a Number Rating Scale as the fifth vital sign and distress as 10 on a Distress Thermometer as the sixth vital sign. Mr D showed signs of shock, with a lowered blood pressure, rapid respirations and dyspnoea, and cold clammy skin. Immediately oxygen was administered 4 L/min via a facial mask and the emergency department physician administered intravenous morphine 5 mg very slowly by intravenous injection to Mr D, having established from the nurse there was no known contraindication in Mr D's past medical history which was provided by his son and that Mr D was 'opioid naïve' (having not had any opioid medication recently). Fluids were administered intravenously and the nurse commenced a fluid intake and output chart for Mr D.

*(Continued)*

CLINICAL EXAMPLE

*(Continued)*

The nurse frequently monitored Mr D's vital signs, oxygen and fluid administration and communicated calmly and reassuringly to Mr D. The nurse, using a delirium screening checklist, confirmed the likelihood that Mr D had symptoms of delirium, characterized by an acutely changing or fluctuating mental status, inattention, disorganized thinking and altered level of consciousness with or without agitation. Anticipating a possible requirement for a pharmacological treatment regimen of several compatible drugs together to control pain and symptoms, the emergency department physician prescribed Haloperidol 1.5 mg subcutaneously PRN to treat Mr D's nausea and vomiting, delirium, restlessness and agitation.

Giving a biopsychosocial history on behalf of Mr D, when asked about a possible family history of cancer, Mr D's son confirmed that at least one person in their extended family had died from bowel cancer. The emergency department physician asked Mr D's wife and son for permission to carry out a bone scan for diagnostic purposes.

During the night Mr D was given slowly administered intravenous morphine 5 mg every four hours at the clock by the on-duty doctor and midazolam as a once only PRN dose of 0.5 mg slowly administered intravenously during the night when he became anxious and dyspnoeic. In the morning the bone scan procedure was explained to Mr D; he was informed that his son had signed consent forms on his behalf and the radioactive isotope tracer was administered to Mr D. The bone scan in the afternoon revealed widespread multiple metastases throughout Mr D's skeletal system. The hospital supported a palliative care two-bedded unit. A conference call was set up between the senior hospital physician responsible for Mr D's care, the palliative care nurse and the consultant palliative care physician at the hospice. The care team discussed Mr D's past medical and biopsychosocial history, findings of the current physical examination, his vital signs in the past 24 hours, pain and other symptoms, distress and delirium scores and laboratory and bone scan results. Immediate care decisions made for Mr D were:

- a brain scan urgently to check for brain metastases as a possible cause of intracranial pressure
- continuous subcutaneous infusion (CSCI) via a syringe driver of a combination of three compatible drugs diluted with NaCl, to be administered over 24 hours:

  - Oxycodone (strong opioid agonist with a ratio of 1:1.5 with morphine; sometimes the morphine to oxycodone ratio 2:1 is used, see Figure 11.2 Opioid Conversion Chart); as the patient had received 35 mg (7 × 5 mg) of morphine intravenously in past 24 hours, starting with oxycodone 15 mg to be titrated to pain, together with
  - B. Haloperidol 1.5 mg
  - C. Midazolam 10 mg
  - The three-drug combination to be administered by CSCI over 24 hours.

- A second separate continuous subcutaneous infusion, for refractory cancer-related bone pain, of 'burst' ketamine, 50 mg daily (reviewed daily, over three days) to block the influx of sodium and calcium ions by binding with the NMDA receptor as a receptor antagonist to glutamate, thereby reducing neuronal 'windup'. Ketamine has been found to be especially beneficial in refractory cancer pain at low or subanaesthetic doses, and is opioid sparing.

# Opioid Conversion Chart

There are differences in the literature regarding opioid conversion ratios. The conversion ratios listed below are the conversion ratios commonly used in practice at Our Lady's Hospice and Care Services (OLH&CS). The information outlined below is intended as a guide only. ALL OPIOID CONVERSIONS OUTLINED BELOW ARE APPROXIMATE ONLY. Therfore, all medication doses derived using the information below should be checked and prescribed by an experienced practitioner. The dosage of a new opioid is based on several factors including the available equi-analgesic dose data, the clinical condition of the patient, concurrent medications and patient safety. It is recommended that the new dose should be reduced by 30–50% to allow for incomplete cross-tolerance. The patient should be monitored closely until stable when switching opioid medications.

## GOLDEN RULE: WHEN CHANGING FROM ONE OPIOID TO ANOTHER ALWAYS CONVERT TO MORPHINE FIRST.

### ORAL MORPHINE TO ORAL OPIOIDS

| PO → PO | RATIO |
|---|---|
| Morphine → Oxycodone | 1.5:1 |
| Morphine → Hydromorphone | 5:1 |

### ORAL OPIOIDS TO PARENTERAL OPIOIDS

| PO → IV/SC | RATIO |
|---|---|
| Morphine → Morphine | 2:1 |
| Oxycodone → Oxycodone | 2:1 |
| Hydromorphone → Hydromorphone | 2:1 |

### PARENTERAL MORPHINE TO OTHER OPIOIDS

| IV/SC → IV/SC | RATIO |
|---|---|
| Morphine → Oxycodone | 1.5:1[a] |
| Morphine → Hydromorphone | 5:1 |
| Morphine → Alfentanil | 15:1 |

### TRANSDERMAL OPIOID TO ORAL MORPHINE

| TD → PO | RATIO |
|---|---|
| Buprenorphine → Morphine | 1:75 |
| Fentanyl → Morphine | 1:100 |

(Note: This table does not incorporate recommended does reductions of 30–50%.)

### MORPHINE
24 hour dose

| ORAL | IV/SC |
|---|---|
| 5mg | 2.5mg |
| 10mg | 5mg |
| 14.4mg | 7.2mg |
| 20mg | 10mg |
| 28.8mg | 14.4mg |
| 30mg | 15mg |
| 50mg | 25mg |
| 60mg | 30mg |
| 100mg | 50mg |
| 120mg | 60mg |
| 150mg | 75mg |
| 180mg | 90mg |
| 240mg | 120mg |

### OXYCODONE[b]
24 hour dose

A 2:1 ratio with morphine may also be used. See preparations outlined below.

| ORAL | IV/SC |
|---|---|
| 3.33mg | 1.66mg |
| 6.66mg | 3.33mg |
| 9.6mg | 4.8mg |
| 13.33mg | 6.66mg |
| 19.2mg | 9.6mg |
| 20mg | 10mg |
| 33.33mg | 16.66mg |
| 40mg | 20mg |
| 66.66mg | 33.33mg |
| 80mg | 40mg |
| 100mg | 50mg |
| 120mg | 60mg |
| 160mg | 80mg |

### HYDROMORPHONE
24 hour dose

| ORAL | IV/SC |
|---|---|
| 1mg | 0.5mg |
| 2mg | 1mg |
| 2.88mg | 1.44mg |
| 4mg | 2mg |
| 5.76mg | 2.88mg |
| 6mg | 3mg |
| 10mg | 5mg |
| 12mg | 6mg |
| 20mg | 10mg |
| 24mg | 12mg |
| 30mg | 15mg |
| 36mg | 18mg |
| 48mg | 24mg |

### FENTANYL

| TRANSDERMAL[a] | IV/SC |
|---|---|
| - | - |
| - | - |
| 6 micrograms/hour | - |
| | - |
| 12 micrograms/hour | - |
| | - |
| 25 micrograms/hour | - |
| | - |
| 50 micrograms/hour | - |
| | - |
| 75 micrograms/hour | - |
| | - |
| 100 micrograms/hour | |

### ALFENTANIL[b]
24 hour dose

| IV/SC |
|---|
| - |
| 0.3mg |
| 0.5mg |
| 0.7mg |
| 1 mg |
| 1.5mg |
| 2mg |
| 3.3mg |
| 4mg |
| 5mg |
| 6mg |
| 8mg |

### BUPRENORPHINE

| TRANSDERMAL[b] |
|---|
| - |
| 5 micrograms/hour[c] |
| - |
| 10 micrograms/hour[c] |
| 15 micrograms/hour[c] |
| 25 micrograms/hour[c] |
| 35 micrograms/hour[c] |
| 52.5 micrograms/hour[c] |
| 70 micrograms/hour[c] |

[a] National and International guidelines also support the use of a 2:1 ratio when switching between morphine and oxycodone.

[b] Oxycodone is available as immediate release capsules 5mg, 10mg and 20mg, liquid 1mg/ml or 10mg/ml and sustained release tablets 5mg, 10mg, 20mg, 40mg and 50mg. Oxycodone solution for injection is available is 10mg/ml and 50mg/ml strengths.

[c] See "The Use of Alfentanil in a Syringe Driver in Palliative Medicine' document available from the palliative Meds info webpages http://www.olh.ie/7-departments/166-palliative-meda-info/. Doses have been rounded to the nearest whole number or the nearest first decimal point.

[d] Transdermal Fentanyl and buprenorphine patches are prescribed in micrograms (mcg)/hour. Equivalent doses are based on the 24 hour dose of derdanyl or buprenorphine received from a patch. See product literature for further information.

[e] Based on buprenorphine to morphine ratio of 1:70–83

Prepared by: Palliative Meds Info. (See www.olh.ie for Terms and Conditions.)

Reviewed; January 2014   Review: January 2015

**Figure 11.2**  Opioid conversion chart

Source: Republished with permission of Our Lady's Hospice and Care Services Dublin.

(Continued)

*(Continued)*

- In addition, the care team decided to prescribe (glucocorticoid) dexamethasone for bone pain, nausea and vomiting; dexamethasone is compatible with ketamine and oxycodone but may not work well with midazolam, so the care team decided to prescribe dexamethasone 5 mg orally once daily, in the morning, to avoid disrupting the patient's sleep pattern. When oral medication is no longer feasible, dexamethasone may also be delivered via an additional syringe driver.
- A stimulant laxative and softening agent combined were also prescribed.
- All medications were to be monitored carefully for effectiveness and side-effects in the patient by the palliative care nurse and reviewed according to the patient's progressing care plan.

## Pharmacological interventions for dyspnoea

**Pharmacological interventions for dyspnoea** are directed at the cause (dosages are based on adult weights).

Morphine sulphate is the most effective medication for relieving dyspnoea. Morphine alters the patient's perception of his or her breathing experience by reducing respiratory drive and oxygen consumption; morphine increases blood plasma levels of carbon dioxide and decreases arterial pH. Decreasing the dose usually manages the morphine side-effect of somnolence. Patients already taking opioids require 50% of the usual dose to relieve dyspnoea. Opioid naïve adult patients should start on 5–10 mg PO, sublingually or subcutaneously, with dosages adjusted for other routes, repeated every two hours as needed (PRN).

## Nonpharmacological nursing management of dyspnoea

The calming, reassuring presence of the nurse with the patient can help to alleviate dyspnoea, as can helping the patient to find his or her most comfortable position. Distraction and relaxation exercises may reduce the patient's anxiety and distress. The nurse's aim is to reduce the patient's anxiety, distress and suffering and restore calmed breathing.

## Additional pharmacological interventions for dyspnoea

Short-acting benzodiazepine anxiolytics, for example, Lorezapam 0.5 mg PO or sublingually every four hours either ATC or PRN, may be helpful.

Anticholinergics: for example, hyoscine hydrobromide 1.2 mg every 24 hours is given subcutaneously to reduce respiratory secretions. Anticholinergics are effective for reducing secretion in the mouth and respiratory tract, which creates disturbing respiratory sounds known as the 'death rattle'.

Bronchodilators: for example, salbutamol 100 micrograms/metered dose inhalation at 10–20 minute intervals or 5 mg nebulized salbutamol at 20–30 minute intervals to reduce bronchospasm.

Corticosteroids: for example, dexamethasone 4–8 mg daily may reduce bronchospasm, inflammation and dyspnoea associated with advanced complex lung non-malignant diseases and cancers (lymphangitis carcinomatosis).

Where appropriate, antibiotics are given to relieve dyspnoea symptoms and provide comfort for patients near death who have signs and symptoms of an obvious upper respiratory tract infection. Further investigations should be avoided.

## Interdisciplinary interventions for dyspnoea

Interdisciplinary interventions for dyspnoea include chest physiotherapy and aids for expectoration.

## Pharmacological interventions for cough

Morphine 5 mg PO every four hours may relieve and suppress an intractable cough. Protussive expectoration aids may be contraindicated in debilitated patients. Moist inhalations of methol or eucalyptus may help. Sedatives Haloperidol 2.5 mg given subcutaneously and Levomepromazine 6.25 mg given subcutaneously may be especially useful at night, drying respiratory secretions through an anticholinergic effect and helping to calm the restless, confused patient.

## Nonpharmacological nursing management of cough

Calming reassuring presence by the nurse with the patient nursed in the position of most comfort for him or her.

## Nausea and vomiting

**Nausea and vomiting** occur frequently in patients receiving palliative care and at end of life. There are multiple causes for nausea and vomiting. Irritation in the upper gastrointestinal tract and obstruction of the gastrointestinal tract may result in vomiting, when any part of the upper digestive tract is irritated or over-distended, particularly the duodenum.

Vomiting signals are initiated from the pharynx to the upper part of the small intestines. Nerve impulses are transmitted by sympathetic and vagal nerve fibres to a collection of distributed nuclei in the medulla and pontine reticular formation, extending into the spinal cord. This is known as the **brain stem 'vomiting centre'**. Motor impulses travel from the vomiting centre via several cranial nerves to the upper gastrointestinal tract, via sympathetic and vagal nerves to the lower gastrointestinal tract and to the diaphragm and abdominal muscles via spinal nerves.

The **Chemoreceptor Trigger Zone (CTZ)** is a second vomiting zone located bilaterally on the floor of the fourth ventricle in the brain stem area postrema of the medulla. The CTZ is stimulated by nerve signals which arise when the CTZ is stimulated by the administration of specific drugs. Opioids are CTZ stimulants. Opioids act on the gastrointestinal tract and on the CTZ to promote nausea and vomiting (Hall, 2011: 804). An adult or child patient beginning opioid therapy, or switching from one opioid to a different opioid, requires an antiemetic medication which blocks emetic action at the CTZ (for example, domperidone). Metoclopramide is also a recommended first-line antiemetic.

The selection of antiemetic depends on the cause of the patient's symptoms, which should be carefully assessed from a biopsychosocial perspective. Situations which might precipitate the patient's nausea should be avoided. Tolerance to opioid medication-induced nausea usually develops within a few days. When they are no longer necessary, antiemetics should be discontinued in order to avoid unnecessary drug side-effects (for example, dystonic side-effects of metoclopramide). Interactions-caution is advised with children, young adults and older people (check the National Formulary of your country for dosages).

There are many drugs which may help to reduce nausea and vomiting through various mechanisms. Most have some adverse effects. Ondansetron and similar 5HT antagonists prevent vagal stimulation. However, side-effects include constipation, headache and hiccups. Therefore, drug selection has to be carefully matched with patient age, diagnosis, current health and palliative care status and medication requirement.

A patient experiencing nausea and vomiting on a daily or very regular basis should be prescribed antiemetics 'at the clock'. For patients with severe nausea and vomiting, pharmacists may compound medications into one lozenge, suppository or gel. For nausea and vomiting associated with increased intracranial pressure secondary to brain metastases, corticosteroids (for example, dexamethasone) are very effective.

The patient's self-report of nausea and vomiting and its impact on functionality is the most reliable guide. For patients living in the community, a daily diary of all symptoms, including nausea, is advised in order to ensure optimal management. Diaries can be completed with support from family members and/or caregivers.

In his book, *Mortally Wounded: Stories of Soul Pain, Death and Healing*, Dr Michael Kearney, the first Palliative Care Consultant in Ireland, states: 'we can make the process of dying easier by expertly controlling an individual's pain and other physical symptoms, while fostering open and honest communication with him or her and his or her family. This can transform what may have been a frightening and miserable existence into a time of continuing personal growth and completion' (Kearney, 1995: 3).

## Chapter summary

- The specialty of palliative care focuses on pain and symptom control for patients with incurable diseases, promoting access to palliative care services when needed, preferably at an early stage of the disease. The development of palliative care services continues.
- The World Health Organization has defined palliative care principles for adults and for children, focusing on the quality of life of patients and their families through the prevention and relief of suffering. It advocates the impeccable assessment and treatment of pain.
- The multidisciplinary palliative care team provides interdisciplinary care. Psychosocial services must be represented and the patient and his or her family members are all members of the palliative care team.
- Internationaly recognized goals and core competencies of palliative care nursing are endorsed by the IAHPC and EAPC. Palliative care education is an essential component of continuing healthcare professional development.
- Palliative care nursing and philosophy is patient- and family-centred. The nurse's role, combined with the physician's role, comprises the core palliative care team. They ensure access to essential psychosocial services.
- Communication and symptom control are the two core principles of palliative care. Communication skills training can improve nurse–patient communication, with implications for the quality of life of patients and families.
- Palliative care provision is based on an understanding of the impact of the patient's subjective experience of pain and distress. These components require comprehensive and ongoing measurement as the fifth and sixth vital signs.
- In palliative care, pain and symptom control is individualized. Opioids are selected and titrated to meet the patient's requirement for pain relief. CSCI is normally used as the route for the adminstration of multiple, compatible medications.

## Reflective exercise

Consider the skills, knowledge, personal and professional resources the nurse requires to provide high-quality, best-practice, palliative care nursing. Do you consider communication skills training to be important for your professional development?

## Recommended reading

Baile, W.F. and Parker, P.A. (2010) Breaking bad news. In D.W. Kissane, B.D. Bultz, P.M. Butow and I.G. Finlay (eds), *Handbook of Communication in Oncology and Palliative Care*. New York: Oxford University Press.

*(Continued)*

*(Continued)*

Clark, D. (2002) *Realising a Vision (1959–1967): Cicely Saunders – Founder of the Hospice Movement.* Oxford: Oxford University Press.

Kearney, M. (1995) *Mortally Wounded: Stories of Soul Pain, Death and Healing.* New York: Simon & Schuster.

Zighelboim, J. (2007) *To Health The New Humanist Oncology.* www.booksurge.com

## Websites relevant to this chapter

European Association for Palliative Care: www.eapcnet.eu/

The IAHPC's list of essential medicines for palliative care: http://hospicecare.com/uploads/2011/8/iahpc-essential-meds-en.pdf

Institute of Medicine (USA) (2002) *When Children Die: Improving Palliative and End of Life Care for Children and their Families.* Washington, DC: Institute of Medicine: www.iom.edu/reports/2002/when-children-die-improving-palliative-and-end-of-life-care-for-children-and-their-families.aspx

Institute of Medicine (USA) (2003) *Improving Palliative Care for Cancer.* Washington, DC: Institute of Medicine: www.iom.edu/reports/2003/improving-palliative-care-for-cancer.aspx

NICE (2012) *Opioids in Palliative Care: Safe and Effective Prescribing of Strong Opioids for Pain in Palliative Care of Adults.* UK Guidelines. London: NICE: http://publications.nice.org.uk/opioids-in-palliative-care-safe-and-effective-prescribing-of-strong-opioids-for-pain-in-palliative-cg140

World Health Organization's definition of palliative care: www.who.int/cancer/palliative/definition/en/

## References

Abu-Saad, H.H. (2001) *Evidence-Based Palliative Care: Across the Lifespan.* UK: Wiley Blackwell.

Addington-Hall, J.M., Bruera, E., Higginson, I.J. and Payne, S. (2007) *Research Methods in Palliative Care.* New York: Oxford University Press.

Baile, W.F. and Parker, P.A. (2010) Breaking bad news. In D.W. Kissane, B.D. Bultz, P.M. Butow and I.G. Finlay (eds), *Handbook of Communication in Oncology and Palliative Care.* New York: Oxford University Press.

Bennett, M.I. (2009) The Brief Pain Inventory: revealing the effect of cancer pain. *The Lancet Oncology,* 10 (10): 1020.

Breitbart, W.S., Rosenfeld, B., Roth, A., Smith M.J., Cohen, K. and Passik, S. (1997) The Memorial Delirium Assessment Scale. *Journal of Pain and Symptom Management,* 13: 128–137.

Caraceni, A., Hanks, G., Kaasa, S., Bennett, M.I., Brunelli, C., Cherny, N., Dale, O., De Conno, F., Fallon, M., Hanna, M., Haugen, D.F., Juhl, G., King, S., Klepstad, P., Laugsand, E.A., Maltoni, M., Mercadante, S., Nabal, M., Pigni, A., Radbruch, L., Reid, C., Sjogren, P., Stone, P.C., Tassinari, D. and Zeppetella, G. (2012) Use of opioid analgesics in the treatment of cancer pain: evidence-based recommendations from the EAPC. *The Lancet Oncology*, 13 (2): e58–e68.

Cherny, N.J. (2010) The problem of suffering and the principles of assessment in palliative medicine. In G. Hanks, N.I. Cherny, N.A. Christakis, M. Fallon, S. Kaasa, and R.K. Portenoy (eds), *Oxford Text Book of Palliative Medicine* (4th edn). Oxford: Oxford University Press.

Clayton, J.M., Hancock, K. and Parker, S. (2008) Sustaining hope when communicating with terminally ill patients and their families: a systematic review. *Psycho-Oncology*, 17: 641–659.

Cobb, S. (1976) Social support as a moderator of life stress. *Psychosomatic Medicine*, 38: 300–314.

Coyle, N. (2006) Introduction to palliative nursing care. In B.R. Ferrell and N. Coyle (eds), *Textbook of Palliative Nursing*. New York: Oxford University Press.

Daut, R.L., Cleeland, C.S. and Flanery, R.C. (1983) Development of the Wisconsin Brief Pain Questionnaire to assess pain in cancer and other diseases. *Pain*, 17: 197–210.

De Vlieger, M., Gorchs, N., Larkin, P.J. and Porchet, F. (2004) *A Guide for the Development of Palliative Nurse Education in Europe. Palliative Nurse Education: Report of the EAPC Task Force*. Milan: EAPC.

Dickman, A. and Schneider, J. (2011) *The Syringe Driver: Continuous Subcutaneous Infusions in Palliative Care* (3rd edn). New York and Oxford: Oxford University Press.

Doyle, D. and Woodruff, R. (2013) *The IAHPC Manual of Palliative Care* (3rd edn). Houston, TX: IAHPC Press.

Faksvåg Haugen, D., Nauck, F. and Caraceni, A. (2010) The core team and the extended team. In G. Hanks, N.I. Cherny, N.A. Christakis, M. Fallon, S. Kaasa and R.K. Portenoy (eds), *Oxford Textbook of Palliative Care* (4th edn). New York: Oxford University Press.

Fallowfield, L. (2010) Communication with the patient and family in palliative medicine. In G. Hanks, N.I. Cherny, N.A. Christakis, M. Fallon, S. Kaasa and R.K. Portenoy (eds), *Oxford Textbook of Palliative Care* (4th edn). New York: Oxford University Press.

Fallowfield, L.J., Jenkins, V.A. and Beveridge, H.A. (2002) Truth may hurt but deceit hurts more: communication in palliative care. *Palliative Medicine*, 16: 297–303.

Ferrell, B.R. and Coyle, N. (2006) Preface: For every nurse – a palliative care nurse. In B.R. Ferrell and N. Coyle (eds), *Textbook of Palliative Nursing* (2nd edn). New York: Oxford University Press.

Ferrell, B.R. and Coyle, N. (eds) (2010) *Oxford Textbook of Palliative Nursing* (3rd edn). New York: Oxford University Press.

Finlay, I.G. and Pease, N. (2010) Palliative medicine: communication to promote life near the end of life. In D.W. Kissane, B.D. Bultz, P.M. Butow and I.G. Finlay (eds), *Handbook of Communication in Oncology and Palliative Care*. New York: Oxford University Press.

Forbes, K. and Huxtable, R. (2006) Clarifying the data on double effect. *Palliative Medicine*, 20: 395–396.

Galbraith, M.E. (1995) What kind of social support do cancer patients get from nurses? *Cancer Nursing*, 18: 362–367.

Gamondi, G., Larkin, P. and Payne, S. (2013a) Core competencies in palliative care: an EAPC White Paper on palliative care education – part 1. *European Journal of Palliative Care*, 20 (2): 86–91.

Gamondi, G., Larkin, P. and Payne, S. (2013b) Core competencies in palliative care: an EAPC White Paper on palliative care education – part 2. *European Journal of Palliative Care*, 20 (3): 140–145.

Glass, E., Cluxton, D. and Rancour, P. (2006) Principles of patient and family assessment. In B.R. Ferrell and N. Coyle (eds), *Textbook of Palliative Nursing*. New York: Oxford University Press.

Gordon-Williams, R.M. and Dickenson, A.H. (2010) The management of pain: pathophysiology of pain in cancer and other terminal illnesses. In G. Hanks, N.I. Cherny, N.A. Christakis, M. Fallon, S. Kaasa and R.K. Portenoy (eds), *Oxford Textbook of Palliative Care* (4th edn). New York: Oxford University Press.

Hall, J.E. (2011) *Guyton and Hall Textbook of Medical Physiology* (12th edn). Philadelphia, PA: Elsevier Saunders.

Hanks, G.M., Cherny, N.I., Portenoy, R.K., Kaasa, S., Fallon, M. and Christakis, N. (2010) Introduction to the fourth edition: facing the challenges of continuity and change. In G. Hanks, N.I. Cherny, N.A. Christakis, M. Fallon, S. Kaasa and R.K. Portenoy (eds), *Oxford Textbook of Palliative Care* (4th edn). New York: Oxford University Press.

International Psycho-Oncology Society (IPOS) (July 2010) *Statement on Standards and Clinical Practice Guidelines in Cancer Care: Distress as the Sixth Vital Sign*. Charlottesville, VA: IPOS.

Kearney, M. (1995) *Mortally Wounded: Stories of Soul Pain, Death and Healing*. New York: Simon & Schuster.

Keltner, J.R., Vaida, F., Ellis, R.J., Moeller-Bertram, T., Fitzsimmons, C., et al. (2012) Health-related quality of life 'well-being' in HIV distal neuropathic pain is more strongly associated with depression severity than with pain intensity. *Psychosomatics*, 53: 380–386.

Krammer, L.M., Martinez, J., Ring-Hurn, E.A. and Williams, M.B. (2010) The nurse's role in interdisciplinary and palliative care. In M. La Porte Matzo and D. Witt Sherman (eds), *Palliative Care Nursing: Quality Care to the End of Life* (3rd edn). New York: Springer.

Levin, T. and Weiner, J.S. (2010) End-of-life communication training. In D.W. Kissane, B.D. Bultz, P.M. Butow and I.G. Finlay (eds), *Handbook of Communication in Oncology and Palliative Care*. Oxford: Oxford University Press.

Matzo, M. and Witt Sherman, D. (2010) *Palliative Care Nursing: Quality Care to the End of Life* (3rd edn). New York: Springer.

Morita, T., Chinone, Y., Ikenaga, M., Miyoshi, M., Nakaho, T., Nishitateno, K., Sakonji, M., Shima, Y., Suenaga, K., Takigawa, C., Kohara, H., Tani, K., Kawamura, Y., Matsubara, T., Watanabe, A., Yagi, Y., Sasaki, T., Higuchi, A., Kimura, H., Abo, H., Ozawa, T., Kizawa, Y. and Uchitomi, Y. (2005) Ethical validity of palliative sedation therapy: a multicenter, prospective, observational study conducted on specialized palliative care units in Japan. *Journal of Pain and Symptom Management*, 30 (4): 308–319.

Namisango, E., Harding, R., Atuhaire, L., Ddungo, H., Katabira, E., Muwanika, F.R., and Powell, R.A. (2012) Pain among ambulatory HIV/AIDS patients: multicenter study of prevalence, intensity associated factors and effect. *The Journal of Pain*, 13 (7): 704–713.

Paice, J. (2010) Pain Management at the end of life. In S.M. Fishman, J.C. Ballantyne and J.P. Rathmell (eds), *Bonica's Management of Pain* (4th edn). Riverwoods, IL: Wolters Kluwer/Lippincott Williams and Wilkins.

Paice, J.A. and Fine, P.G. (2010) Pain at the end of life. In B.R. Ferrell and N. Coyle (eds), *Textbook of Palliative Nursing*. New York: Oxford University Press.

Pirl, W.F. (2006) Screening instruments. In J.C. Holland, D.B. Greenberg and M.K. Hughes (eds), *Quick Reference for Oncology Clinicians: The Psychiatric and Psychological Dimensions of Cancer Symptom Management*. Charlottesville, VA: IPOS Press.

Saunders, C. (1976) Care of the dying. *Nursing Times,* reprint. London: Macxmillan.

Sternswärd, J., Foley, K.M. and Ferris, F.D. (2007) The public health strategy for palliative care. *Journal of Pain and Symptom Management*, 33 (5): 486–493.

Thoits, P.A. (1986) Social support as coping assistance. *Journal of Consulting and Clinical Psychology*, 54: 416–423.

Twycross, R., Sykes, N., Mihalyo, M. and Wilcock, A. (2012) Stimulant laxatives and opioid-induced constipation. *Journal of Pain and Symptom Management*, 43 (2): 306–313.

van Mechelen, W., Aertgeerts, B., De Ceulaer, K., Thoonsen, B., Vermandere, M., Warmenhoven, F., Van Rijswijk, E. and De Lepeleire, J. (2012) Defining the palliative care patient: a systematic review. *Palliative Medicine*, 27 (3): 197–208.

Vignaroli, E., Bennett, M.I., Nekolaichuk, C., De Lima, L., Wenk, R., Ripamonti, C.I. and Bruera, E. (2012) Strategic pain management: the identification and development of the IAHPC opioid essential prescription package. *Journal of Palliative Medicine*, 15 (2): 186–191.

von Roenn, J.H., Paice, J.A. and Preodor, M.E. (2006) Pain management in palliative care. In J.H. Von Roenn, J.A. Paice and M.E. Preodor (eds), *Current Diagnosis and Treatment of Pain*. New York: Lange.

Waldron, D., O'Boyle, C., Kearney, M., Moriarty, M. and Carney, D. (1999) Quality of life measurement in advanced cancers: assessing the individual. *Journal of Clinical Oncology*, 17: 3603–3611.

Wilcock, A. and Twycross, R. (2011) Ketamine. *Journal of Pain and Symptom Management*, 41 (3): 640–649.

Witt Sherman, D. (2010) Culture and spirituality as domains of quality of life. In M. Matzo and D. Witt Sherman (2010) *Palliative Care Nursing: Quality Care to the End of Life* (3rd edn). New York: Springer.

World Health Organization (1996) *Cancer Pain Relief (with a guide to opioid availability)* (2nd edn). Geneva: WHO (1st edn, 1986).

World Health Organization (2002) Definition of palliative care, available at: www.who.int/cancer/palliative/definition/en/ (accessed 17 July 2014).

World Health Organization (2014) *The Sixty-seventh World Health Assembly. Palliative Care Resolution EB 134.R7. Strengthening of Palliative Care as a Component of Integrated Treatment within the Continuum of Care*. Available at: http://apps.who.int/gb/ebwha/pdf_files/EB134/B134_R7-en.pdf (accessed 17 July 2014).

Zigmund, A.S. and Snaith, R.P. (1983) The Hospital Anxiety and Depression Scale. *Acta Anaesthesiologica Scandinavica*, 67: 361–370.

# 12

# Stress management and nonpharmacological interventions for pain

## Learning objectives

The learning objectives of this chapter are to:

- know the mechanisms of stress that are most relevant to human stress and illness
- understand the role of cognitive behavioural therapies in pain management
- recognize that relaxation therapies can be easily learned and taught by nurses
- be familiar with some evidence-based complementary therapies useful for pain management

## Introduction

This chapter looks at theories of stress and their relevance to pain and to nonpharmacological interventions for pain management. The rationale for nonpharmacological interventions in pain management (alongside prescribed pharmacological interventions) is to reduce distress and anxiety, increase comfort levels and the sense of control for the person with pain. Cognitive behavioural therapies equip patients with techniques to relieve stress and anxiety, and increase the patient's sense of self-esteem and mastery, which are often eroded by pain. Evidence based on nonpharmacological, complementary therapy interventions can also be very helpful for stress reduction for patients with pain.

# Definition and theories of stress

The word 'stress', derived from Latin, was used in the seventeenth century to mean 'hardship, straits, adversity or affliction'. The meaning evolved in the eighteenth century to denote 'force, pressure, strain or strong effort' regarding human organic or mental powers (Hinkle, 1973). In the twentieth century, sociobiological research began to investigate the effects of stress on the health and well-being of people. In 1910, for example, Sir William Osler assumed a causal relationship between hard work, stress and strain with his patients suffering from angina pectoris. For stress to occur, the consequences of failure must be important for the person concerned. Therefore, stress is linked to motivation. Almost all theories of motivation agree on the basic principle that action arises in an effort to improve conditions which are less than optimal (Welford, 1974).

# Three different viewpoints to stress

Historically, the psychological literature on stress has three different approaches: (1) an engineering or stimulus-based approach, treating stress as an external independent variable; (2) a medicophysiological or response-based approach, treating stress as a dependent variable; and (3) a dynamic, internal psychophysiological process, intervening between stimulus and response, which is mediated by a person's cognitions and has the potential to produce tension, mental strain and coping processes. In the current stress literature, the modernized medicophysiological, response-based and the dynamic, transactional psychophysiological approaches are highly relevant to understanding human stress.

# The psychophysiological view of stress

Stress in a human context is linked to the way each individual evaluates his or her relationships with the environment – a process termed 'cognitive appraisal' (evaluation) (Lazarus, 1966). What a person thinks and does to alter a troubled relationship with the environment changes either the relationship or the way it is appraised, thereby changing the emotions that flow from it (Lazarus, 1991). Coping can be defined as 'the person's constantly changing cognitive and behavioural efforts to manage specific external and/or internal demands that are appraised as taxing or exceeding the resources of the person' (Lazarus and Folman, 1984: 142). To say that someone is threatened is an evaluation limited to a particular encounter in which environmental conditions are appraised by a particular person who has his or her own set of psychological characteristics.

The transactional model views the person and the environment as being in a dynamic, mutually reciprocal, bi-directional relationship. A distressing event which is a result of a procedure or treatment can become a cause of anxiety for the future, known as anticipatory anxiety (Lazarus and Folkman, 1984). This is important for fear and pain perception in the context of illness. For example, if the outcome of a hospital procedure or treatment caused distress and suffering, anticipating the same event again can provoke anxiety as the patient worries whether the same level of unpleasant pain or related sensation will happen again. This type of anticipatory anxiety (rising to the level of fear) can be experienced following an unpleasant experience associated with change of wound dressings. It can be seen that this type of concern is linked to feelings of losing control of one's personal situation, which is a strong cause of distress and suffering, as well as a fear response, which can be both anticipatory and reactionary.

The relationship between pain and coping corresponds with the postulates of stress theory. The emotional responses to the pain experience of patients with advanced cancer include anxiety, depression and anger, along with the physiological and psychosocial effects and the meaning or significance of the pain experience being appraised as future threat, actual harm and/or challenge (Lazarus and Folkman, 1984). Arathuzik (1991a, 1991b) examined the relationships between the appraisal of pain and the coping strategies and behaviours used by patients with metastatic cancer to deal with their pain. Results indicated the overwhelming impact of the pain stressor, which interfered greatly with the patients' activities, causing them much anxiety and depression. Two patterns of correlations between the cognitive and affective pain appraisals emerged. These were associated with the coping behaviours and strategies used to manage the pain experience. Subjects who perceived pain as threatening or harmful, and as causing greater physiological and psychosocial effects, were withdrawn and very distressed, whereas subjects who were able to view their pain as challenging were able to devise and use a variety of strategies to deal with their pain, and this may have helped to reduce the emotional distress associated with their pain.

The medicophysiological, response-based approach to stress was defined by Selye (1956) as 'the nonspecific response of the body to any demand placed upon it' (Seyle, 1956: 75). Selye formulated a response-based approach to stress, based on the activation of the two neuroendocrine systems, the fast-acting SAM complex (Sympathetic-Adrenal Medullary system) and the slower acting HPA complex (Hypothalamic-anterior Pituitary-Adreno-cortical system). Selye (1956), who is viewed as the 'Father of Stress', considered that the stress response was triphasic in nature, involving an initial alarm stage, followed by a stage of resistance, which gives way, under some circumstances, to a final stage of exhaustion.

**The initial response to a stressor situation** is prompted by a neural message from the hypothalamus to the sympathetic nervous system to stimulate secretion of the catecholamines epinephrine (adrenaline) and norepinephrine (noradrenaline), both directly to target organs and from the adrenal medulla into the circulatory system.

**Table 12.1**  Changes in stress hormones related to emotions and behaviours (Gregson and Looker, 1996)

| Emotion: | Anger | Fear | Depression | Serenity | Elation |
|---|---|---|---|---|---|
| Behaviour: ➡<br>Stress<br>hormones<br>⬇ | aggressive<br>'fight' | withdrawn<br>'flight' | submissive<br>loss of control | relaxed<br>meditation | loving<br>supportive |
| Adrenaline | increase | large increase | no change | decrease | decrease |
| Noradrenaline | large increase | increase | no change | decrease | decrease |
| Cortisol | no change | increase | large increase | no change | decrease |

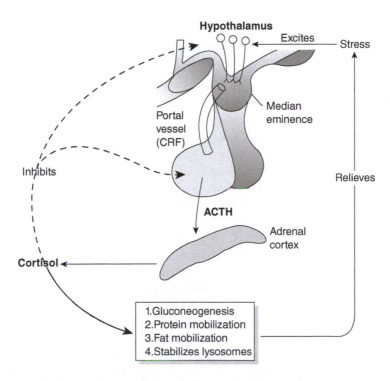

**Figure 12.1**  Mechanism for regulation of glucocorticoid secretion

Physiological effects of the sympathetic stimulation include increases in respiration, the rate and strength of cardiac contractions, peripheral vasoconstriction, increased blood to muscles, decreased gut lumen peristalsis, tone and gastric activity, stimulation of the sweat glands, pupillary dilation and increased mental alertness. This rapid mobilization of bodily resources was described by Walter B.

Cannon (1915) as preparing the body for 'fight or flight' (that is, for an immediate emergency or alarm reaction). Cannon was among the first to use the term 'stress' and to introduce stress terminology to the scientific community. Cannon developed the concept of homeostasis, the need for organisms to maintain a stable internal environment. Homeostasis is a dynamic oscillatory state by which the organism tries to maintain a balance between need and fulfilment and coping with stressors. Both Selye and Cannon used the term 'stress' in the body's 'physical reaction' sense (Rice, 1999). Table 12.1 shows that the two major emotions associated with the stress response are anger, associated with the urge to 'fight', and fear, promoting the urge to run and hide – 'flight'. Figure 12.1 shows the biological mechanicism of the stress response.

## The stress response and pain

Pain stimuli travel via the spinothalamic tract (and additional tracts) through the brain stem to the median eminence of the hypothalamus. Pain acts as a stressor, prompting the hypothalamus to release corticotropin–releasing factor (CRF) into the hypophysial portal system, which prompts the anterior pituitary gland to release adrenocorticotrophic hormone (ACTH). ACTH acts on the adrenal cortex to stimulate the production of large amounts of cortisol, which prompts release of glucose, protein and fat to relieve physiological stress. Initially, cortisol has a negative feedback effect, prompting the hypothalamus, according to a feedback system, to reduce the secretion of CRF and prompting the anterior pituitary gland to decrease the formation of ACTH, to regulate plasma cortisol levels. Stress can always break through the feedback control mechanism, so that stress stimuli can cause intermittent exacerbations of cortisol secretion or, when stress stimuli are ongoing, such as in the experience of unrelieved pain, prolonged cortisol secretion (see Figure 12.1) (Hall, 2011).

The hippocampus regulates cortisol level and is considered to play an important role in turning off the stress response. If cortisol levels remain high, the hippocampus become damaged and degenerates and the feedback mechanism of detecting blood cortisol levels and sending signals to the hypothalamus to reduce blood cortisol levels does not function. Prolonged secretion of cortisol compromises the immune system and underpins much physiological damage (Kolb and Whishaw, 2011: 275).

In teaching coping techniques, it is helpful to explain the basics of the relaxation response to the patient as most cognitive behavioural and complementary therapies aim to reduce the stress response and induce the relaxation response. In this way, sympathetic activity is reduced and parasympathetic activity increased. The stress response is quietened and the mind and body become relaxed (Gregson and Looker, 1996).

The relationship between emotion and coping has two major perspectives. According to an animal model, emotion and coping are viewed from a Darwinian phylogenetic perspective as drive, activation or arousal-motivated behavioural responses that enable the animal to protect itself and/or vanquish its enemy. It emphasizes learned behaviours that facilitate survival in the face of life-threatening dangers. According to a psychoanalytic ego psychology model, coping is defined as cognitive (thinking) processes, such as denial, repression, suppression and intellectualization, as well as problem-solving behaviours. These are invoked to reduce anxiety and other distressing emotional states. While the primary criterion of successful coping in the animal model is survival, the ego psychology model focuses on adaptive outcomes such as psychological well-being, somatic health and social functioning. Both the animal and ego psychology models view coping as a response to emotion; its function is the reduction of arousal or tension (Folkman and Lazarus, 1988). This is a vital point for pain management and is central to the rationale for nonpharmacological therapies which are designed to help the person to reduce their anxiety, reduce suffering and to be more comfortable.

Emotion both facilitates and interferes with coping. However, over time coping can also impact on emotional reaction (Folkman and Lazarus, 1988). Coping consists of cognitive and behavioural efforts to manage specific external and/or internal demands that are appraised as taxing or exceeding the resources of the person (Lazarus and Folkman, 1984). These cognitive and behavioural efforts are constantly changing as a function of continuous appraisals and reappraisals of the person–environment relationship, which is also always changing (Folkman et al., 1986).

## Coping

Coping has two major functions: to manage or alter the situation that is causing distress (problem-focused coping) and/or to regulate emotional responses to the problem, for example anger, anxiety and/or grief (emotion-focused coping). These functions work in conjunction with changes in the person that are a result of feedback about what has happened and from changes in the environment that are independent of the person (Folkman and Lazarus, 1988).

Coping has three main features. First, coping is a process. Coping is what the person thinks and does in a stressful encounter and how these thoughts and actions change as the situation unfolds. Second, coping is context-dependent and is influenced by the particular appraisal that initiates it and by the resources available to manage that encounter. Finally, coping refers to efforts to manage – not the success of those efforts – and as a process, coping should be defined independently of whether or not it was successful (Folkman et al., 1991; Lazarus and Folkman, 1984). Coping processes, which by definition are changeable, lend themselves to modification through education, counselling and psychotherapy (Folkman et al., 1991).

# Cognitive behavioural therapies as a coping tool for the person with pain

Many studies on the benefits of cognitive behavioural therapies have focused on the benefits for patients with cancer, partly because many patients with cancer are frequent health service users and participate in research programmes during or between treatment cycles. Patients with non-malignant chronic pain also have recognised need for supportive therapies. Cognitive behavioural therapy for chronic pain began in the 1960s and 1970s with the application of behavioural principles to the study of pain.

Cognitive behavioural therapies (CBT) for pain focus on pain-related cognitions and behaviours. Studies show that changing a patient's beliefs through cognitive behavioural therapy leads to changes in patient functioning. A person's behaviour or cognition changes by being replaced with a more rewarded behaviour or cognition. The feedback to the person is more rewarding (that is, the new behaviour or thought is reinforced). CBT especially focuses on changing catastrophizing, negative thinking, maladaptive coping and learned responses which are non-productive. The major focus is to enhance the person's perception of increased control over their pain, helping them to improve their mood to reduce negative thinking and replace maladaptive with adaptive behaviours, leading to improved function and sense of mastery and reduced pain experience (Sloman, 1995).

The International Association for the Study of Pain (IASP) recognizes that cognitive behavioural therapy for pain is an essential part of care. It states that all pain units should provide psychological and cognitive behavioural therapies for patients as part of their treatment plans. Psychological assessment by the clinical psychologist working in the specialist pain centre focuses on the suitability of cognitive behavioural therapy for the person with pain, particularly in terms of motivation and commitment. CBT skills need to be practised at home to be acquired and the person needs to be compliant with attending the CBT course. Patients with serious mental illness may need mental healthcare and treatment prior to participating in CBT for pain. The person's commitment to change is very much influenced by his or her social circumstances and the level of support available from their close others (Buenaver et al., 2010).

Most self-management therapies, cognitive behaviour therapies and stress management techniques focus on training patients to effectively cope with emotional reactions that interfere with daily functioning (Rosenbaum, 1993). Focusing on negative events and coping deficiencies is associated with a high level of arousal. Increasing coping behaviours helps to reduce anxiety, lower arousal and increase the person's sense of self-efficacy and sense of mastery (Bandura, 1977, 1986, 1992).

The role of nursing in patient education for stress management and cognitive behavioural therapies to cope with pain is regarded as a complementary therapy (that is, all therapies recommended here are intended for use alongside, and not instead of, analgesic medication). All types of cognitive behavioural therapies and stress management techniques emphasize self-management and share four common components: (1) education; (2) skills acquisition; (3) cognitive and behavioural rehearsal; and (4) generalization and maintenance.

## Stress management, cognitive behavioural and relaxation therapies in pain management nursing

Types of stress management and cognitive behavioural therapies that are relevant to pain management nursing include: breathing techniques, guided imagery, meditation, progressive muscle relaxation, self-hypnosis, biofeedback and autogenic training. Breathing techniques, guided imagery, meditation and progressive muscle relaxation can be easily learned by the nurse and by patients. Self-hypnosis, biofeedback and autogenic training require qualified therapist instruction over time. Somewhere in the region of 8–10 sessions, on the basis of one session weekly, with daily home practice are needed to acquire these techniques. Although they are not basic nursing interventions, they are often available in holistic care centres to which nurses can refer patients, once permission has been obtained from the patient's physician, GP or medical team (as appropriate).

**Relaxation techniques** are now regarded as basic nursing interventions. The nurse is advised to learn several relaxation techniques, by participating in classes in order to acquire a proficient level of expertise. Techniques include, for example, rhythmic breathing techniques, progressive muscle relaxation, meditation and visualization. Basic relaxation techniques are easy to learn and are useful interventions for helping patients with pain to feel calmer. With a basic repertoire of relaxation techniques the nurse can give tuition to patients with pain. The use of relaxation and imagery techniques by people with (cancer) pain and related emotional distress may help to increase their sense of control. These techniques, which people can initiate for themselves, help to reduce feelings of helplessness and hopelessness, divert attention away from the experience of pain and emotional reactions (associated with the diagnosis of cancer) and break the pain–anxiety–tension cycle, thereby facilitating pain relief through a calming effect. The techniques can be taught by nurses and readily learned by patients and provide a self-care strategy to help to improve quality of life and improve the patient's sense of control (Chen and Francis, 2010; Sloman, 1995). Patients are different and relaxation techniques have to be adjusted accordingly.

It must be emphasized that relaxation skills are complementary therapies and need to be used with analgesic medication. They are intended to help patients to reduce their stress response and increase their sense of control. Analgesics reduce pain to the level which allows the patient to focus on the relaxation technique.

Breathing and simple relaxation techniques are not effective in reducing pain without analgesia (Kwekkeboom and Gretarsdottir, 2006). Nurses should provide detailed information on each step of the body scan and the relaxation procedure. It is helpful to have instruction leaflets on hand to help remind patients of these relaxation techniques and to ask patients for their feedback about their effectiveness in inducing the relaxation response. The primary indicators are sensations of warmth (peripheral vasodilation) and heaviness (muscle relaxation).

For the patient in a hospital setting, pain should be measured immediately after the relaxation intervention; for the patient at home, it is helpful to make a pain diary entry immediately after the relaxation intervention (Kwekkeboom and Gretarsdottir, 2006). Patients need to find a relaxation technique that works for them and be motivated to practise daily and incorporate it into a daily routine to obtain the full health benefit. Providing and keeping a record of intervention effectiveness is one way of maintaining motivation.

In teaching patients how to elicit the relaxation response (Benson, 1975), which promotes the activity of the parasympathetic nervous system, the basic requirements are:

- a quiet environment (not essential);
- a mental device – as a focus or mantra;
- a passive attitude;
- a comfortable position (this is not always essential, but is advisable initially, when learning, or in a clinical setting).

It is helpful to adopt a sitting position and begin by instructing the patient how to carry out a quick body scan. This involves the patient checking for any tension or discomfort in their body, beginning with the feet and working upward through each muscle group, in order to be optimally comfortable before beginning the relaxation technique. Correctly taught, rhythmic, controlled breathing is an effective relaxation technique for calming anxious patients, and for use as a complementary therapy, alongside medication, before and during some painful procedures. Following a full body scan, starting at the feet, meditation uses rhythmic breathing with a mantra word, which is spoken on the regular slow exhalation. Jaw relaxation focuses on relaxing the organs of speech.

Progressive muscle relaxation (PMR) was developed by Jacobsen in 1929 and modified by Bernstein and Bokovec in 1973 (Kwekkeboom and Gretarsdottir, 2006). PMR is a systematic approach to relieving tension in the body and mind by tensing and relaxing the major muscle groups, starting from the feet and working systematically up to the head. The patients is instructed to focus on feelings of muscle tension while contracting each muscle group for 5–10 seconds and to experience the ensuing relaxing sensations of warmth and heaviness as they relax each muscle group. The patient is instructed to tense at increasing levels of contraction and then relax each muscle group three times and focus on the resulting sensations of relaxation (nursing safety note: CAUTION, PMR is contraindicated for patients with metastatic bone cancer due to the risk of sudden bone fracture on muscle clenching). PMR has been found to be beneficial for patients with arthritis, chronic low-back pain and leg pain related to pregnancy (Kwekkeboom and Gretarsdottir, 2006).

Autogenic training (AT) aims to enable the person, through passive concentration, to revert from a state of arousal associated with sympathetic activity of the autonomic nervous system to one of profound relaxation associated with parasympathetic activity (Luthe and Schultz, 1969). Alpha-waves, associated with calmness, relaxation and well-being, seem to increase with the practice of AT (Linden, 1990). At the beginning of the twentieth century, Johann Schultz, a German neurologist, observed that his hypnotized patients regularly reported two distinct sensations: 'a heaviness, especially in the limbs' and 'a sensation of warmth'. Through these findings, Schultz became convinced that 'hypnosis was an experience that the patient permitted to happen, the patient entering a trance through a "switch" which could be provoked and subsequently controlled by the patient' (Linden, 1990: 13). From these observations and further study, Schultz developed the system of AT, composed of six standard exercises for producing sensations of heaviness and warmth in the extremities, warmth in the epigastric region and coolness in the forehead and for regulation of heart rate and breathing.

Changes of a somatic nature are achieved by the basic AT methods, with advanced AT facilitating spiritual development. The term 'autogenic' also emphasizes that the patient is largely responsible for carrying out his or her own treatment by regular training that is focused on specific mechanisms (Luthe and Schultz, 1969). AT trainees can proceed safely to apply the method themselves and make it part of a health-promoting lifestyle (Carruthers, 1979). While research evidence of the benefits of autogenic training for helping patients with pain are limited by small sample sizes and few randomized controlled trials, studies indicate that 'Schultz type' autogenic training is an effective therapeutic approach that may lead to reduction in headache frequency and use of headache medication (Kanji, 2000; Zsombok et al., 2003). However, biofeedback and relaxation may be as effective as AT for tension-type headaches (Kanji et al., 2006). AT may help people with pain associated with irritable bowel syndrome (Shinozaki et al., 2010). A meta-analysis of clinical outcome studies shows that AT may have positive effects also for anxiety, depression and functional sleep disorders across a range of chronic, potentially painful diseases (Kanji, 2000; Stetter and Kupper, 2002), although more, large, controlled studies are required (Kanji and Ernst, 2000). A more recent review indicates that AT may be helpful in pregnancy by reducing anxiety prior to delivery (Marc et al., 2011). Autogenic training has potential benefits for use by nurses working in primary care settings and who care for patients with chronic and terminal illness. An AT qualification takes two years, following a qualification in a recognized healthcare profession, which is mandatory (Crowther, 2001).

Hypnosis, initiated in the West by Mesmer in the eighteenth century, and having declined in popularity in the nineteenth century, has recently gained popularity in healthcare. Hypnosis can be defined as 'a social interaction in which one person, designated the subject, responds to suggestions offered by another person, designated the hypnotist, for experiences involving alterations in perception, memory and voluntary action' (Patterson and Jensen, 2003: 495).

A recent study using fMRI technology to investigate the effect of hypnotic pain modulation on brain activity in patients with temporomandibular disorder (TMD) pain found that hypnotic hypoalgesia is associated with a pronounced suppression of cortical activity. The findings from this study were the first to describe hypnotic modulation of brain activity associated with nociceptive processing in chronic TMD pain patients (Abrahamsen et al., 2010). Studies show the efficacy of hypnosis for providing substantial pain relief in experimental pain conditions, with potentially useful clinical applications. Interest in hypnotic treatments for pain conditions is increasing (Patterson and Jensen, 2003). Studies have shown the benefits of hypnosis in the clinical setting for reducing procedural pain experience for children (Liossi and Hatira, 2003; Liossi et al., 2009). Studies have found the effects of self-hypnosis training on chronic pain to be similar to progressive muscle relaxation and autogenic training, both of which have a similar self-hypnosis component (Jensen and Patterson, 2006). In a comparison of self-hypnosis versus progressive muscle relaxation (PMR) in patients with multiple sclerosis and chronic pain, participants in the self-hypnosis training condition reported significantly greater decreases post-treatment compared to pre-treatment than participants in the PMR condition, and gains were maintained at three-month follow-up (Jensen et al., 2009).

## Safety issues in relaxation therapies

Once a person of any age understands the concept of a given complementary therapy, then they are suitable to participate, if there are no medical reasons against participation. Medical agreement has always to be sought for therapies other than the basic relaxation therapies. For instance, in autogenic training, patients with any one of several contraindicated long-term conditions (epilepsy, schizophrenia) are advised against taking the therapy. Safety must be taken into consideration with any complementary therapy. The relaxation response can be rapid and profound, and the nurse must ensure adequate care is taken to prevent sudden loss of blood pressure and potential resultant falls injuries, in both the clinical and community settings. It is necessary to educate the patient against this type of adverse event in the community setting by teaching him or her to pay attention to feelings of slight dizziness or lightheadedness when relaxing. A 'cancellation exercise', which is clenching the fists, bringing the clenched fists to the chin, stretching out the arms, breathing out and feeling the muscle tension in the arms, helps to counter the relaxation response. People with labile nervous systems should be warned to take extra care.

# Complementary therapies for pain which require basic technical equipment

## TENS: Transcutaneous Electrical Nerve Stimulation

The Gate Control Theory (Melzack and Wall, 1965) provided the rationale for electrical stimulation for pain modulation now referred to as TENS. TENS, or Transcutaneous Electrical Nerve Stimulation, is a useful adjuvant therapy, effective for many types of pain. The original rationale for the technique still applies. The Gate Control Theory (GCT) predicts that stimulation of large low-threshold Aβ afferents, which respond to touch and pressure, override and inhibit transmission from nociceptive C and Aδ afferents (Melzack and Wall, 1965). The large low-threshold Aβ afferents in peripheral nerves can be selectively stimulated by passing low-intensity electrical currents through the nerves. All nerves within about 4 cm below the surface of the skin can be stimulated by placing electrodes on the available skin surface areas, usually to stimulate the large nerves in the upper or lower arm, lower leg or any superficial skin nerves. Flexible non-toxic electrodes make contact with the skin through a conducting medium and the electrodes are connected to a pocket-sized battery-operated stimulator which emits a continuous series of electrical pulses, the frequency and duration of which can be varied by the user. TENS is thought to work by interrupting the neural propagation of pain.

More recent research has broadened the TENS technique to allow for different types of pain that may respond to electrical analgesia. Controlled human studies using TENS for pain management have shown TENS to be effective in pain associated with osteoarthritis, trigeminal neuralgia, migraine, phantom limb pain and peripheral neuropathies as well as shoulder pain secondary to stroke and for some types of post-operative pain (Allen and Wilson, 2010; Freynet and Falconz, 2010). TENS is recommended and may be helpful for pain reduction for women in labour (Dowswell et al., 2009; Jones et al., 2013).There are acknowledged variations in the effectiveness of TENS which may be due to variations in electrode placement, stimulation site and the time point when the analgesic effect is measured. 'TENS modes' have evolved to try to standardise parameters of clinical use (Chesterton et al., 2002).

**TENS sensory level stimulation** is used for immediate temporary relief of acute, chronic or post-operative pain. Also known as high-frequency or conventional TENS, sensory level stimulation delivers high-frequency (30–150pps), short-duration (50–19 μs) pulses at an amplitude just below the motor threshold, to produce comfortable paraesthesia in the area of the electrodes. Conventional TENS can be used during functional activities of daily living, exercise and work, after some 'learning time' by the patient to find their own maximally effective TENS electrode placement (Allen and Wilson, 2010).

**TENS motor level stimulation** is used for the management of chronic pain or to provide longer pain relief. Acupuncture-like TENS delivers low-frequency (2–4 PPS), longer duration (100–200 µs) pulses at an amplitude that causes muscle twitches. Acupuncture-like TENS controls pain by stimulating the production and release of endogenous opioids such as enkephalins and endorphins. The electrodes for acupuncture-like TENS are usually applied over a point near the painful region. Acupuncture-like TENS is not recommended for use during activities of daily living because of the muscle twitching (Allen and Wilson, 2010).

**Brief-intense TENS stimulation** is delivered at the highest tolerable intensity and causes both sensory and motor level stimulation. Brief-intense TENS is high-frequency (60–200 PPS), long-duration (150–500 µs) pulses at an amplitude which bring about strong paraesthesia, so is often recommended for use during painful procedures (Allen and Wilson, 2010).

**TENS is contraindicated** for people with pacemakers, cardiac arrhythmias or during pregnancy. People with electrical implants, cardiac or circulatory problems, particularly thrombosis or thrombophlebitis should not use TENS. Care is required to prevent possible skin irritation during prolonged TENS electrodes applications. Patients with movement control disorders, impaired cognition or a history of stroke or seizures, or who drive heavy machinery, are required to take special precautions (Allen and Wilson, 2010).


## Acupuncture

The intricacies of the mechanisms of acupuncture are still being debated. They are thought to involve the peripheral and central nervous system, possibly involving endorphin release, diffuse noxious inhibitory control and upregulation of certain receptors (TPRV1) of afferent pain fibres, which conduct pain signals to the central nervous system, in conjunction with cellular processes (Abraham et al., 2011; Lee and Ernst, 2011). Increasingly, healthcare providers are seeking value-for-money, nonpharmacological interventions that reduce the medication burden for patients, lower narcotic drug risks and expenditure, and effectively help to improve patients' health outcomes.

A study by McKee et al. (2013) looked at the benefits of acupuncture for a minority population, with an average age of 54 years, as an adjunct to the usual chronic pain treatment. Acupuncture was provided in 14 once-weekly sessions for either back pain or osteoarthritis. The acupuncture intervention was delivered in the community healthcare centre by student acupuncturists at no cost to patients. There was a significant reduction in pain severity and an improvement in physical well-being for the participants after treatment compared to baseline measures taken prior to the acupuncture treatments.

There are many reported adverse effects from acupuncture, particularly as a result of infections from unclean practices, so care is required to ensure the patient seeks a high standard of acupuncturist practitioner. A randomized controlled trial of 3,451 patient with chronic neck pain showed that acupuncture is a cost-effective treatment for patients with chronic neck pain (Ernst et al., 2011; Willich et al., 2006). Acupuncture may be more beneficial for certain types of chronic pains. An overview of Cochrane Reviews indicated that acupuncture is effective for osteoarthritis, migraine and tension-type headache, neck pain and low back pain (Lee and Ernst, 2011).

# Biofeedback

Biofeedback is a 'feedback loop' process in which information about the state of a biological process (via visual or aural feedback) increases a person's ability to voluntarily control physiological activities because they are provided with information about those activities. Usually the person is connected to an electronic instrument which can display feedback on a moment-to-moment basis, so that the person learns to control the physiological activity. Biofeedback requires the person to learn relaxation skills in order to be able to decrease muscle tension and, through feedback, reduce muscle tension and control heart rate and skin temperature.

The categories of biofeedback types have evolved and it is now possible to combine biofeedback with relaxation techniques to counteract sympathetic arousal associated with various disorders. Biofeedback is more commonly used for helping people to reduce headaches and is often used in conjunction with cognitive behavioural therapies, particularly relaxation-type therapies, which augment the treatment effect. The two most disabling and prevalent types of headaches – migraine and tension type headaches – respond well to biofeedback. For good effect, migraine headache is now usually treated with the combination of peripheral skin temperature feedback and electro-myographic feedback with relaxation. Electro-myographic feedback is directed at reducing pericranial activity and is especially beneficial for tension-type headaches.

Biofeedback is also useful for pediatric headache for both episodic and chronic headache types. Biofeedback for chronic headaches in children is associated with a better response than with other behavioural or pharmacological interventions. A review study found a positive association between the use of selective serotonin re-uptake inhibitors (SSRIs), ability to raise and maintain hand temperature and a positive outcome with biofeedback for children and adolescents with episodic (less than four headaches days per week) and chronic (four or more headache days per week) (Blume et al., 2012). Biofeedback without medication may be useful for headache sufferers who are pregnant or plan to become pregnant, or who prefer nonpharmacological interventions or who have found that medication aggravates symptoms. Biofeedback has been effective for sufferers of headaches compounded by medication overuse. Biofeedback, in general, is more effective than medication alone for headaches; biofeedback with medication may enhance outcome. However, not every person with headaches obtains relief and other behaviour approaches offer similar headache reduction for some patients. Studies show that biofeedback may help a particular subset of patients (Andrasik, 2010; Blume et al., 2012; Nestoriuc et al., 2008).

## Expectation, effectiveness and safety in complementary therapies

Expectation plays a role in complementary therapies, the placebo effect being integral to the impact. Patients' expectations can influence their health outcomes. Outcome expectations are the consequences that follow an intervention, whereas self-efficacy expectations refer to the patient's beliefs that they can perform actions to achieve valued outcomes. This effect has been found by Linde et al. (2007). In a study of 864 patients who were asked, at baseline, whether they considered acupuncture to be an effective therapy in general and what they expected from the treatment, a significant association was shown between better improvement and higher outcome expectations (Linde et al., 2007).

Safety is of paramount importance in selecting complementary therapies which will not negatively interact with or reduce the effectiveness of medications. The nurse has a role in educating patients about complementary therapies. However, there should be a choice component, as the placebo effect of patient expectation interacts with and impacts on intervention efficacy and thus on treatment outcome. Other evidence-based complementary therapies, such as T'ai Chi, yoga, reflexology and massage, may be very beneficial in improving function and areas of quality of life (for example, reducing fear and anxiety, improving sleep and mood, and improving mobility) for the person with chronic pain. In conjunction with an effective opioid-sparing medication treatment regimen in times of pain flares, complementary therapies can help to control pain. Medical advice should always be sought re suitability, to ensure safety and to optimise patient health outcome. The nurse is advised to educate the patient to use the complementary therapy (particularly relaxation/autogenic therapies) on a regular basis to maintain good health in pain-free times as well as at times of pain flares.

## Chapter summary

- Historically, the psychological literature on stress has three different approaches. The modernized medicophysiological, response-based approach and the dynamic, transactional psychophysiological approach are relevant to understanding the psychophysiology of human stress and illness.
- Stress can break through the psychophysiological feedback control mechanism. Stress stimuli can cause exacerbations of cortisol secretion or, when stress stimuli are ongoing, as in the experience of unrelieved pain, prolonged cortisol secretion. Prolonged cortisol secretion is very damaging.
- Coping resources represent characteristics of the person or of his or her environment. Coping responses are construed as adaptive cognitions (thoughts) and behaviours which the person facing the stressful situation uses as a repertoire to manage the perceived life stress or conditions.
- Cognitive behavioural therapies for pain focus on pain-related cognitions and behaviours. Changing the patient's beliefs through cognitive behavioural therapy

leads to changes in patient functioning, with maladaptive behaviours and cognitions being replaced with more rewarded behaviour or cognitions.

- Nurses have a major role in cognitive behavioural therapies and stress management for pain. Techniques emphasize self-management and have in common: (1) education; (2) skills acquisition; (3) cognitive and behavioural rehearsal; and (4) generalization and maintenance.
- Types of stress management and cognitive behavioural and therapies that are relevant to pain management include: breathing techniques, guided imagery, meditation, progressive muscle relaxation, self-hypnosis, hypnosis and autogenic training, TENS, acupuncture and biofeedback.
- The nurse is advised to learn several relaxation techniques, for example, rhythmic breathing techniques, progressive muscle relaxation, meditation and visualization. The nurse should participate in classes in order to achieve accuracy in the use of the technique. Basic relaxation techniques are easy to learn and useful.
- Medical agreement has always to be sought for therapies other than the basic relaxation therapies. Safety must be taken into consideration with any complementary therapy. The relaxation response can be profound and the nurse must teach adequate care to prevent sudden loss of blood pressure.

## Reflective exercise

Consider how, if a patient with chronic pain asked your advice, you would assist him or her to select a beneficial complementary therapy.

## Recommended reading

Benson, H. (1975) *The Relaxation Response*. New York: Morrow.
Rankin-Box, D. (ed.) (2001) *The Nurses' Handbook of Complementary Therapies* (2nd edn). London: Baillière Tindall/Royal College of Nursing.
Selye, H. (1956) *The Stress of Life*. New York: McGraw-Hill.

## Websites relevant to this chapter

American Hypnosis Association: www.hypnosis.edu/aha/
British Autogenic Society: www.autogenic-therapy.org.uk/about-bas/
Biofeedback instructions: www.bfe.org/protocol/pro08eng.htm

*(Continued)*

*(Continued)*

MyoTrac (TM) EMG portable unit: www.thoughttechnology.com/pdf/myotrac%20
  mar668.pdf
National Center for Complementary and Alternative Medicine (NCCAM):
  http://nccam.nih.gov/health/pain/chronic.htm

# References

Abraham, T.S., Chen, M.L. and Ma, S.X. (2011) TRPV1 expression in acupuncture points: response to electroacupuncture stimulation. *Journal of Chemical Neuroanatomy*, 41 (3): 129–136.

Abrahamsen, R., Dietz, M., Lodahl, S., Roepstorff, A., Zachariae, R., Østergaard, L. and Svensson, P. (2010) Effect of hypnotic pain modulation on brain activity in patients with temporomandibular disorder pain. *Pain*, 151: 825–833.

Allen, R.J. and Wilson, A.M. (2010) Physical therapy agents. In S.M. Fishman, J.C. Ballantyne and J.P. Rathmell (eds), *Bonica's Management of Pain* (4th edn). Riverwoods, IL: Wolters Kluwer/Lippincott Williams and Wilkins.

Andrasik, F. (2010) Biofeedback in headache: an overview of approaches and evidence. *Cleveland Clinic Journal of Medicine*, 77 (Suppl. 3): S72–S76.

Arathuzik, D. (1991a) The appraisal of pain and coping in cancer patients. *Western Journal of Nursing Research*, 13: 714–731.

Arathusik, D. (1991b) Pain experiences for metastatic breast cancer patients: unravelling the mystery. *Cancer Nursing*, 14: 41–48.

Bandura, A. (1977) Self-efficacy: towards a unifying theory of behaviour change. *Psychological Review*, 84: 191–215.

Bandura, A. (1986) *Social Foundations of Thought and Action: A Social Cognitive Theory*. Englewood Cliffs, NJ: Prentice-Hall.

Bandura, A. (1992) Exercise of personal agency through the self-efficacy mechanism. In R. Schwarzer (ed.), *Self-Efficacy: Thought Control of Action*. Washington, DC: Hemisphere.

Benson, H. (1975) *The Relaxation Response*. New York: Morrow.

Blume, H.K., Brockman, L.N. and Breuner, C.C. (2012) Biofeedback therapy for pediatric headaches: factors associated with response. *Headache*, 52: 1377–1386.

Bray, D. (2001) Biofeedback. In D. Rankin-Box (ed.) *The Nurses' Handbook of Complementary Therapies* (2nd edn). London: Baillière Tindall/Royal College of Nursing.

Buenaver, L.F., Campbell, C.M., Haythornwaite, J.A. (2010) Cognitive-behavioural therapy for chronic pain. In S.M. Fishman, J.C. Ballantyne and J.P. Rathmell (eds), *Bonica's Management of Pain* (4th edn). Riverwoods, IL: Wolters Kluwer/Lippincott Williams and Wilkins.

Cannon, Walter B. (1915) *Bodily Changes in Pain Hunger Fear and Rage: An Account of Recent Researches in to the Functional of Emotional Excitement*. USA: Appleton.

Carruthers, M. (1979) Autogenic training. *Journal of Psychosomatic Research*, 23: 437–440.

Chen, Y.L. and Francis, A.J.P. (2010) Relaxation and imagery for chronic nonmalignant pain: effects on pain symptoms, quality of life and mental health. *Pain Management Nursing*, 11 (3): 159–168.

Chesteron, L.S., Barlas, P., Foster, N.E., Lundeberg, T., Wright, C.C. and Baxter, G.D. (2002) Sensory stimulation (TENS); effects of parameter manipulation on mechanical pain thresholds in healthy human subjects. *Pain*, 99: 253–262.

Crowther, D. (2001) Autogenic training. In D. Rankin-Box (ed.), *The Nurses' Handbook of Complementary Therapies*. London: Baillière Tindall/Royal College of Nursing.

Downey, S. (2001) Acupuncture. In D. Rankin-Box (ed.), *The Nurses' Handbook of Complementary Therapies*. London: Baillière Tindall/Royal College of Nursing.

Dowswell, T., Bedwell, C., Lavender, T. and Neilson, J.P. (2009) Transcutaneous electrical nerve stimulation (TENS) for pain relief in labour. *Cochrane Database of Systematic Reviews* [Online], 2: CD007214.

Ernst, E., Lee, M.S. and Choi, T.-Y. (2011) Acupuncture: does it alleviate pain and are there serious risks? A review of reviews. *Pain*, 152: 755–764.

Folkman, S., Chesney, M., McKusick, L., Ironson, G., Johnson, D.S. and Coates, T.J. (1991) Translating coping theory into an intervention. In J. Eckenrode (ed.), *The Social Context of Coping*. New York: Plenum Press.

Folkman, S. and Lazarus, R.S. (1988) The relationship between coping and emotion: implications for theory and research. *Social Science and Medicine*, 26: 309–317.

Folkman, S., Lazarus, R.S., Dunkel-Schetter, C., Delongis, A. and Gruen, R.J. (1986) Dynamics of a stressful encounter: cognitive appraisal, coping and encounter outcomes. *Journal of Personality and Social Psychology*, 50: 571–579.

Freynet, A. and Falcoz, P.E. (2010) Is transcutaneous electrical nerve stimulation effective in relieving postoperative pain after thoracotomy? *Interactive CardioVascular and Thoracic Surgery*, 10: 283–288.

Gregson, O. and Looker, T. (1996) The biological basis of stress management. In S. Palmer and W. Dryden (eds), *Stress Management and Counselling: Theory, Practice, Research and Methodology*. London: Cassell.

Hall, J.E. (2011) *Guyton and Hall Textbook of Medical Physiology* (12th edn). Philadelphia, PA: Elsevier Saunders.

Hinkle, L.E. (1973) The concept of stress in the biological and social sciences. *Science, Medicine and Man*, 1: 31–48.

Jensen, M.R., Barber, J., Romano, J.M., Molton, I.R., Raichle, K.A., Osbourne, T.L., Engel, J.M., Stoelb, B.L., Kraft, G.H. and Patterson, D.R. (2009) A comparison of self-hypnosis versus progressive muscle relaxation in patients with multiple sclerosis and chronic pain. *International Journal of Clinical and Experimental Hypnosis*, 57 (2): 198–221.

Jensen, M.R. and Patterson, D.R. (2006) Hypnotic treatment of chronic pain. *Journal of Behavioural Medicine*, 29 (1): 95–124.

Jones, L., Othman, M., Dowswell, T., Alfirevic, Z., Gates, S., Newburn, M., Jordan, S., Lavender, T., Neilson, J.P. (2013) *Pain Management for Women in Labour: An Overview of Systematic Reviews (Review)*. The Cochrane Collaboration. UK: John Wiley

Kanji, N. (2000) Management of pain through autogenic training. *Complementary Therapies in Nursing and Midwifery*, 6: 143–148.

Kanji, N. and Ernst, E. (2000) Autogenic training for stress and anxiety: a systematic review. *Complementary Therapies in Medicine*, 8: 106–110.

Kanji, N., White, A.R and Ernst, E. (2006) Autogenic training for tension type headaches: a systematic review of controlled trials. *Complementary Therapies in Medicine*, 14: 144–150.

Kolb, B. and Whishaw, I.Q. (2011) *An Introduction to Brain and Behaviour* (3rd edn). New York: Worth.

Kwekkeboom. K.L. and Gretarsdottir, E. (2006) Systematic review of relaxation interventions for pain. *Journal of NursingScholarship*, 38 (3): 269–277.

Lazarus, R.S. (1966) *Psychological Stress and the Coping Process*. New York: McGraw-Hill.

Lazarus, R.S. (1991) *Emotion and Adaptation*. Oxford: Oxford University Press.

Lazarus, R.S. and Folkman, S. (1984) *Stress, Appraisal and Coping*. New York: Springer.

Lee, M.S. and Ernst, E. (2011) Acupuncture for pain: an overview of Cochrane reviews. *The Chinese Journal of Integrated Traditional and Western Medicine*, 17 (3): 187–189.

Linde, K., Witt, C.M., Streng, A., Weidenhammer, W., Wagenpfeil, S., Brinkhaus, B., Willich, S.N. and Melchart, D. (2007) The impact of patient expectations on outcomes in four randomised controlled trials of acupuncture in patients with chronic pain. *Pain*, 128: 264–271.

Linden, W. (1990) *Autogenic Training: A Clinical Guide*. New York: Guilford Press.

Liossi, C. and Hatira, P. (2003) Clinical hypnosis in the alleviation of procedure-related pain in pediatric oncology patients. *International Journal of Clinical and Experimental Hypnosis*, 51 (1): 4–28.

Liossi, C., White, P. and Hatira, P. (2009) A randomised clinical trial of a brief hypnosis intervention to control venepuncture-related pain of pediatric cancer patients. *Pain*, 142: 255–263.

Luthe, W. and Schultz, H. (1969) *Autogenic Therapy. 1: Autogenic Methods*. New York: Grune and Stratton.

Marc, I., Toureche, N., Ernst, E., Hodnett, E.D., Blanchet, C., Dodin, S. and Njoya, M.M. (2011) Mind–body interventions during pregnancy for preventing or treating women's anxiety. *Cochrane Database of Systematic Reviews*, 6 (7): CD007559.

McKee, D., Kligler, B. Fletcher, J., Biryukov, F., Casalaina, W., Anderson, B. and Blank, A. (2013) Outcomes of acupuncture for chronic pain in urban primary care. *Journal of the American Board of Family Medicine*, 26 (6): 692–700.

Melzack, R. and Wall, P.D. (1965) Pain mechanisms: a new theory. *Science*, 150: 971–979.

Melzack, R. and Wall, P.D. (1982/1988) *The Challenge of Pain* (2nd edn). Harmondsworth: Penguin.

Nestoriuc, Y., Martin, A., Rief, W. and Andrasik, F. (2008) Biofeedback treatment for headache disorders: a comprehensive efficacy review. *Applied Psychophysiology and Biofeedback*, 33: 125–140.

Patterson, D.P. and Jensen, M.P. (2003) Hypnosis and clinical pain. *Psychological Bulletin*, 129: 495–521.

Rankin-Box, D. (2001) Hypnosis. In D. Rankin-Box (ed.), *The Nurses' Handbook of Complementary Therapies* (2nd edn). London: Baillière Tindall/Royal College of Nursing.

Rice, P.L. (1999) *Stress and Health* (3rd edn). Pacific Grove, CA: Brooks-Cole.

Rosenbaum, M. (1993) The three functions of self-control behaviour: redressive, reformative and experiential. *Work and Stress*, 7: 33–46.

Selye, H. (1956) *The Stress of Life*. New York: McGraw-Hill.

Shinozaki, M., Kanazawa, M., Kano, M., Endo, Y., Nakaya, N., Hongo, M. and Fukudo, S. (2010) Effect of autogenic training on general improvement in patients with irritable bowel syndrome: a randomised controlled trial. *Applied Psychophysiology and Biofeedback*, 35: 189–198.

Sloman, R. (1995) Relaxation and the relief of cancer pain. *Nursing Clinics of North America*, 30: 697–709.

Stetter, F. and Kupper, S. (2002) Autogenic training: a meta-analysis of clinical outcome studies. *Applied Psychophysiology and Biofeedback*, 27 (1): 45–98.

Welford, A.T. (1974) *Man under Stress: Proceedings of the Ninth Annual Conference of the Ergonomics Society of Australia and New Zealand, 1972.* London: Taylor and Francis.

Willich, S.N., Reinhold, T., Selim, D., Jena, S., Brinkhaous, B. and Witt, C.M. (2006) Cost-effectiveness of acupuncture treatments in patients with chronic neck pain. *Pain*, 125: 107–113.

Zsombok, T., Juhasz, G., Budavari, A., Vitrai, J. and Bagdy, G. (2003) Effect of autogenic training on drug consumption in patients with primary headache: an 8-month follow-up study. *Headache*, 43: 251–257.

# 13

# Quality, safety and organizational issues in pain management

## Learning objectives

The learning objectives of this chapter are to:

- recognize the types of barrier to achieving quality and safety in pain management
- recognize the importance of pain education of all healthcare professionals
- understand that patient education is an essential aspect of nursing care of the person with pain
- consider risk factors and the clinical decision making for each patient requiring pain treatment and management

## Introduction

Barriers to optimal pain management are multifactorial. Each barrier constitutes a problem and is not of itself the entire problem, so achieving quality and safety in pain management requires identifying multiple barriers and addressing each one. This chapter explores governmental and professional projects which aim to identify barriers and challenges to optimal pain management and suggest how these might be resolved through education and performance improvement.

# Defining quality and safety in pain management

The mission of Joint Commission Resources is 'to continuously improve the safety and quality of care in the United States and in the international community through the provision of education and consultation services and international accreditation' (Joint Commission Resources, 2012). The Joint Commission Resources (2010) conducted a survey of its consumer consultants in the USA, who identified the following 10 challenges in the healthcare setting to optimal pain management:

- fear of addiction;
- lack of planning across transitions of care;
- lack of coordination among providers;
- actual practice patterns versus documented action;
- nurses in general having inadequate knowledge of pain medications;
- nurses' opinions about chronic pain influencing the care they provide;
- short length of stay for inpatients, meaning there is little time available to effectively assess and address pain needs;
- ineffectiveness of some physicians in managing pain;
- physicians' variable receptiveness to additional education on pain management;
- physician challenges, including time management, lack of expertise and lack of clarity about who is responsible for pain management.

The JCR (2010) survey also found that pain was poorly managed across the care continuum and that nurses and physicians would benefit from education and performance improvement tools.

The top three challenges to effective pain management were identified by the Joint Commission Resources (2010) respondents as:

1. Resistance to collaborative, interdisciplinary approaches.
2. Limitations on necessary resources (for example, staff and budget).
3. Lack of measurement instruments.

# Educational barriers to quality and safety in pain management

Research estimates that about 75–150 million Americans have pain and only 3 million people seek help from a pain specialist. Many people live and suffer with needless pain which is treatable. The medical knowledge and treatments exist. The need for education and training for healthcare professionals in pain medicine at all stages of their development is a recurring theme in studies identifying issues relevant to the under-treatment of pain (for example, McGee et al., 2011).

Inadequate pain management knowledge and practice is a reality and an ongoing serious professional concern. Education has been identified as a vital step in improving the quality of pain management. However, pain management has until very recently not been viewed as an essential requirement of the undergraduate or post-graduate core curriculum for healthcare professionals of any speciality, and the vast majority of graduating nursing and medical students lack basic pain knowledge. These views are changing, and there is an increasing professional, global conversation about the need for both undergraduate and postgraduate education in pain management for all healthcare specialities.

Pain expertise is core for a few postgraduate specialty areas (for example, anaesthetics, surgery, oncology, dentistry), with nurses, physiotherapists, psychiatrists and other healthcare professional specialists working in these pain specialities also becoming experts in relevant pain knowledge for their professional work as part of the interdisciplinary team. Pain management is highly complex and professionals need to work as a team to meet patients' care needs for pain management. Each professional must respect the expert contribution of the other healthcare team members – no single team member can have all the knowledge required to adequately care for the patient with pain (Watt-Watson et al., 2004).

The Institute of Medicine's *Relieving Pain in America: A Blueprint for Transforming Prevention, Care, Education and Research* (2011), in a chapter on education challenges, states that all specialities have strong reasons to engage in pain medicine as most professionals treat patients in pain and this is true for both nurses and doctors. For example, studies show that 'psychiatric disorders are commonly associated with alterations in pain processing' and that 'chronic pain may impair both neurocognitive and emotional functioning' (Elman et al., 2011: 201). Psychiatrists trained in pain medicine have a more informed and indepth insight of the link between pain syndromes and psychiatric conditions. The American College of Emergency Physicians, the American Pain Society, the Emergency Nurse Association and the American Society for Pain Management have enunciated 14 core principles regarding pain management, two of which are educational issues:

- clinician education and resources (should support optimal pain management);
- research and education are encouraged to support widespread dissemination of evidence-based analgesic practices;

Specific to nurse education, the American Association of Colleges of Nursing (2008), citing an Institute of Medicine (2003) report, stated that Baccalaureate-prepared nurses should provide patient-centered care that identifies, respects and addresses patients' differences, values, preferences and expressed needs (Institute of Medicine, 2003). Patient-centered care also involves the coordination of continuous care, listening to, communicating with and educating patients and caregivers regarding health, wellness and disease management and prevention. The generalist nurse provides the human link between the healthcare system and the patient by translating the plan of care to the patient. A broad skill set is required to fill this human interface role (American Association of Colleges of Nursing, 2008, citing Institute of Medicine, 2003). The Institute of Medicine (2011) report states that nursing leaders emphasize their profession's focus on the whole patient, which is a helpful perspective, considering the complex interplay of factors involved in caring for people with acute and chronic pain.

A major intervarsity project, 'Pain Management Core Competencies for PreLicensure Clinical Education' (Fishman et al., 2013), began in 2011 between universities in America, Canada and the United Kingdom across multiple health professions. Senior Nurses comprised more than one-third of a 29-person project team of university representatives. The project's aim was to develop core competencies in pain management for prelicensure clinical education as a basis for delivering comprehensive and high-quality pain care across four domains relevant to pain management for all healthcare professionals. The project core values state:

> To deliver the highest quality of care, health professionals must be able to determine and address the needs of patients from a variety of cultures and socio-economic backgrounds; advocate for patients on individual, system and policy levels; and communicate effectively with patients, families and professionals. These principles transcend any single domain and reflect the need for evidence-based comprehensive pain care that is patient-centered and is delivered in a collaborative, team-based environment:

| | |
|---|---|
| Advocacy | Empathy |
| Collaboration | Ethical Treatment |
| Communication | Evidence-Based Practice |
| Compassion | Health Disparities Reduction |
| Comprehensive Care | Interprofessional Teamwork |
| Cultural Inclusiveness | Patient-Centered Care |

(Fishman et al., 2013:1)

The Fishman et al. project aligned domains of the multidimensional nature of pain, pain assessment and measurement, management of pain and clinical pain conditions with categories of the International Association for the Study of Pain curriculae to meet relevant learning outcomes. The four domains and learning outcomes are set out in Figure 13.1.

These domains are intended as the learning starting point in pain management for undergraduates of all healthcare professions, and may also be relevant to postgraduates. They represent a minimum standard. Topics may vary in emphasis depending on professional, institutional and educational requirements. These domains can be incorporated into diverse professional curricula (Fishman et al., 2013).

A survey of pain management knowledge and attitudes of Baccalaureate Nursing students and Faculty, by Duke et al. (2013), showed that simply teaching nursing curriculum pain management content does not equate with students having related knowledge. The authors advise that a longitudinal approach is required to assess

Domain one
Multidimensional nature of pain: What is pain?
This domain focuses on the fundamental concepts of pain including the science, nomenclature, and experience of pain, and pain's impact on the individual and society.

1. Explain the complex, multidimensional, and individual-specific nature of pain.
2. Present theories and science for understanding pain.
3. Define terminology for describing pain and associated conditions.
4. Describe the impact of pain on society.
5. Explain how cultural, institutional, societal, and regulatory influences affect assessment and management of pain.

Domain two
Pain assessment and measurement: How is pain recognized?
This domain relates to how pain is assessed, quantified, and communicated, in addition to how the individual, the health system, and society affect these activities.

1. Use valid and reliable tools for measuring pain and associated symptoms to assess and reassess related outcomes as appropriate for the clinical context and population.
2. Describe patient, provider, and system factors that can facilitate or interfere with effective pain assessment and management.
3. Assess patient preferences and values to determine pain-related goals and priorities.
4. Demonstrate empathic and compassionate communication during pain assessment.

Domain three
Management of pain: How is pain relieved?
This domain focuses on collaborative approaches to decision-making, diversity of treatment options, the importance of patient agency, risk management, flexibility in care, and treatment based on appropriate understanding of the clinical condition.

1. Demonstrate the inclusion of patient and others, as appropriate, in the education and shared decision-making process for pain care.
2. Identify pain treatment options that can be accessed in a comprehensive pain management plan.
3. Explain how health promotion and self-management strategies are important to the management of pain.
4. Develop a pain treatment plan based on benefits and risks of available treatments.
5. Monitor effects of pain management approaches to adjust the plan of care as needed.
6. Differentiate physical dependence, substance use disorder, misuse, tolerance, addiction, and nonadherence.
7. Develop a treatment plan that takes into account the differences between acute pain, acute-on-chronic pain, chronic/persistent pain, and pain at the end of life.

Domain four
Clinical conditions: How does context influence pain management?
This domain focuses on the role of the clinician in the application of the competencies developed in domains 1–3 and in the context of varied patient populations, settings, and care teams.

1. Describe the unique pain assessment and management needs of special populations.
2. Explain how to assess and manage pain across settings and transitions of care.
3. Describe the role, scope of practice, and contribution of the different professions within a pain management care team.
4. Implement an individualized pain management plan that integrates the perspectives of patients, their social support systems, and health care providers in the context of available resources.
5. Describe the role of the clinician as an advocate in assisting patients to meet treatment goals.

**Figure 13.1**   Pain management domains and core competencies

Source: Fishman et al. (2013) Core competencies for pain management: results of an interprofessional consensus summit. *Pain Medicine*, 14: 971–981. Copyright (2013). Republished with permission of John Wiley and Sons.

under- and postgraduate nurses' pain-related knowledge and attitudes over time and, critically, that nurses work with other professions and disciplines in studying and facilitating effective pain management, combining learning and application to clinical practice. The Institute of Medicine, in *The Future of Nursing: Leading Change, Advancing Health* (2010), emphasizes the role of nurses as leaders who should practise to the full extent of their education and training and be full partners, with physicians and other healthcare professionals, in redesigning healthcare.

## Personal and attitudinal barriers to pain management

It is clear that some of these identified barriers reflect healthcare personnel and organizational attitudes, long known to be factors in barriers to optimal pain management. The theme 'who is responsible for …' is recurrent, leaving the patient with a vital care need unmet through a lack of interdisciplinary communication, staff commitment and sense of responsibility for patient care.

Another theme is a challenging 'block' in mental approach to measurement in patient care. Chapter 5 on pain measurement outlines the difference between the concepts of pain threshold and pain tolerance. Sometimes these concepts are erroneously viewed as 'scientific psychological measurement' that is more relevant to the research setting and of little relevance to patient care. In fact, the concepts of pain threshold and pain tolerance are at the very core of pain measurement in patient care. Educators of all healthcare professionals, including nurses, need to fully understand these concepts and be able to explain them clearly.

Pain tolerance is closely related to emotional experience. It is widely recognized that the subjective experience of pain is aversive and impacts on the pain sufferer's mood. However, unless teaching on pain reflects this affective component of the patient's pain experience, the pain practitioner may disregard the patient's feeling and be far more influenced in their attitudes to patients and patient care by the attitudes demonstrated by peers, colleagues and influential others in the organizational environment as well as the ethos of a given environment. For example, whether the care provided by a given organization is really patient-centred or whether the primary focus is on saving time at the expense of patient-centred care because it takes time to listen to the patient's narrative.

In the past, nursing was viewed as task-orientated, and talking to the patient about his or her illness experience, especially sitting down to really listen to the patient, was viewed as wasting time. Therefore, the way healthcare professionals are taught about pain impacts strongly on their ability to empathize with patients. Healthcare professional communication skills training programmes, especially in the oncology setting, have demonstrated that role-play is a powerful method of improving empathy with another person (Bylind et al., 2010). Studies have shown that, prior to communication skills training, nurses and doctors may not have good communications skills. However, following brief communications skills training, their ability to relate to patients is very much improved (McCarthy et al., 2008; Maguire and Pitceathly, 2010).

## The need for emotional development in doctors and nurses as part of professional education

A study by Murinson et al. (2011) implemented a four-day programme in pain medicine for 118 medical students to address the affective and cognitive dimension of the patients' pain experience. The programme comprised four lectures, three learning laboratories, three team-based learning exercises, three small groups and an assessment block. Many Faculty members and topic experts took part in the teaching. A principle aim of the programme was to help foster positive emotional development in the participants and build awareness of the affective dimensions of pain.

Emotional development was defined as emotional strength (e.g. empathy, compassion, caring), emotional intelligence (e.g. awareness of the impact of pain on mood, perception of emotion in others), emotional resilience (e.g. capacity for emotional self-repair, ability to tolerate frustration) and emotional regulation (e.g. tolerance of difficulties, sense of professional duty). Students were required to complete a written portfolio about exercises demonstrating the link between pain and emotion. For example, they were asked to write a brief pain narrative or describe a painting depicting a painful scene. The students were asked to give feedback on their personal views of pain in expert panel discussions. The following are brief excepts from portfolio comments:

> '... acknowledging that doctors need to work with staff, repeatedly check on patients and follow up on the status of pain management is refreshing'

> 'the nurse manager ... seemed personally invested in the care of her patients and consistently advocated sitting down and getting to know your patients'

> 'I really liked how much emphasis was put on team work'

> '... emphasized the need to listen to patients and address their anxiety, especially before surgery'

> (Murinson et al., 2011)

## Patient-related barriers to effective pain management

Patient-related barriers to effective pain management include fear of addiction and tolerance, fatalism (fear that pain cannot be managed), concerns about treatment side-effects, the desire to be considered a good patient, fear of distracting the physician from treating the disease, and fear that increased pain signifies increase in disease progression. Patient-related barriers have several potentially serious consequences. They prevent the patient disclosing accurate information about their pain experience to the nurse, doctor, other healthcare professional or caregiver, and may lead to less than adequate analgesic use or incorrect analgesic use. Fears of opioid side-effects, especially if associated with previous experience, can limit a patient's willingness to follow prescribed treatment. All community-living patients should be educated to keep a pain diary. This is especially necessary if they are taking opioid medications. They should be encouraged to note the type and frequency of side-effects, and strongly encouraged to obtain advice early on from the Community Health Nurse, with referral to the General Practitioner/ Primary Health Physician if required. Patient education programmes facilitated by nurses using educational booklets and leaflets as support material help to identify individual concerns and misconceptions, especially erroneous beliefs which may impede adherence to pain treatment regimens.

Patient-related barriers to pain management can be measured with the Barriers Questionnaire (Ward et al., 1993). Providing accurate information and correcting misinformation can help patients have better a understanding about pain relief, reduce fears of addiction, be more informed and educated to seek help early with medication side-effects, change beliefs and improve patient–nurse communication, leading to improved coping and adherence to pain medication regimens. Patients should be empowered and encouraged to seek help early about any problems with medication side-effects so that treatment regimens have minimal disruption.

Table 13.1 shows the essential topics of patient education sessions or programmes and the rational for the topic. Sensitive discussion helps to identify and clarify the patient's concerns, beliefs and misconceptions. Carers' behaviours can also have an impact and carers may benefit from educational interventions. Patient education programmes for patients with cancer and patients with low back pain have shown significant benefits (Bennett et al., 2009; Insitute of Medicine, 2011; Ward et al., 2000).

For patients living in long-term care, caregiver, patient and organizational barriers may interfere with optimal pain management. Caregiver barriers are often related to knowledge deficits, lack of pain assessment and poor attitudes to both the need for pain assessment and for pain relief. Patient-related barriers are as outlined above, as well as cognitive impairment, not wanting to bother the nurses, stoic attitudes of residents and thinking that pain is an inevitable aspect of older age. Organizational barriers are related to lack of or deficient pain policies, which is a recurring problem throughout many organizations and healthcare systems, as well as inadequate continuing education in pain management. Poor staffing levels, leading to a lack of time, and poor nurse–patient and inter-healthcare professional communication, andsimilar scenarios are found across other healthcare settings. Insufficient time spent with the patient means there is a greater risk of poor patient care (Egan and Cornally, 2013; Institute of Medicine, 2004).

**Table 13.1** Patient education – essential topics

| Essential patient education topic | Reason why the topic is essential |
|---|---|
| Steps people can take on their own – such as relaxation strategies, exercises, or weight loss – to prevent or obtain relief, help prevent acute pain from progressing to chronic pain, and help prevent chronic pain conditions from worsening | To prevent pain from progressing (that is, secondary prevention), to provide quick relief, to empower people to manage their own care as appropriate, and to avoid unnecessary healthcare expenditures |
| Differences between pain that is protective (adaptive) and pain that is not protective (maladaptive) | To advise people why pain that is not protective should be treated |
| Reasons why the need for relief is important, especially the possibility that poorly managed acute pain will progress to chronic pain | To persuade people to obtain early treatment when necessary |
| When and how emergency or urgent care should be obtained | To encourage seeking immediate intervention, which sometimes can prevent pain from severely worsening |
| Treatment-related pain (such as post-operative pain) and major categories of available pain therapies, along with the main advantages and disadvantages of each (such as potential benefits and risks of opioids) | To enable patients to be informed consumers |
| Different types of health professionals who may be able to help, and how they may help | To provide information about a full range of available services, to promote individual choice |
| Treatments health insurers may or may not reimburse or may reimburse only partially | To equip people to make choices that are cost-effective for them and prepare them for reimbursement problems |
| Ways in which family, employer, colleagues, friends, school, and other contacts can help prevent the pain from progressing or becoming prolonged | To empower patients to marshal support from those who are willing and able to help them |
| How pain is measured, including the difference between numeric ('subjective', or intensity) scales and functional ('objective', or disability) assessments | To enable patients to place their pain in a context health professionals will recognize and serve as an informed member of their own healthcare team |
| The fact that pain involves a complex mind–body interaction, rather than being strictly physical (biological) or strictly emotional (psychological) | To provide patients with an understanding of the need to address both dimensions of their pain and with appropriate, rather than unrealistically high, expectations |
| The right to pain care, including access to medications that are medically necessary and properly used | To alert patients to the possible need to advocate on their own behalf |
| Self-management techniques (surveyed in Chapter 3) | To furnish patients with enough information to obtain some relief on their own and contribute meaningfully to their own care |

# Medical and institutional barriers to access to opioid analgesia

The International Narcotics Control Board (INCB) was established in 1968 as an independent monitoring body to implement UN international drug control conventions. The INCB recognizes that 'one of the objectives of the Single Convention on Narcotic Drugs (1961) … is to ensure the availability of opiates, such as codeine and morphine, that are indispensible for the relief of pain and suffering, while minimizing the possibility of their abuse or diversion' (INCB Annual Report, 1999: 1). Two specific mechanisms are intended to ensure adequate availability of opioid analgesics in countries while preventing non-medical use. First, governments must provide an annual estimate of the amount of opioids required for medical and scientific purposes for the coming year. Second, governments must report the amounts of each narcotic drug consumed, that is, the amount distributed to the retail level in a country: to institutions and programme licensed to dispense to patients, such as hospitals, nursing homes, pharmacies, hospices and palliative care programmes. In 1995, the INCB surveyed government drug control authorities about barriers in their respective countries. Their findings are still relevant today.

The barriers to the availability and use of opioid analgesics, as identified by the 1995 INCB survey were as follows:

- fear of addiction to opioids;
- lack of training of healthcare professional about the use of opioids;
- laws or regulations that restrict the manufacturing, distribution, prescribing or dispensing of opioids;
- reluctance to prescribe or stock opioids stemming from fear of legal consequences;
- overly burdensome administrative requirements related to opioids;
- insufficient amount of opioids imported or manufactured in the country;
- fear of diversion;
- cost of opioids;
- inadequate healthcare resources, such as facilities and healthcare professionals;
- lack of national policy or guidelines related to opioids. (INCB and WHO, 2012: 35)

Professionals who have responsibility for drug regulation in a given country may be ill-informed about addiction and not re-examine and update regulatory policies regarding barriers to opioid access, thereby imposing barriers on opioid access. Outdated knowledge and attitudes, and fear of addiction can impact negatively on opioid access from government regulators to prescribers potentially resulting in undertreatment of patients' pain (INCB and WHO, 2012).

The 1999 Annual Report of the INCB states that the INCB Board 'recognizes that medicines can be of great benefit in relieving pain and suffering, but pharmacotherapy is not a panacea. In addition to pharmacotherapy, there is a wide variety of complementary and/or alternative treatment modalities available in different parts of the world, including counselling and psychotherapy, which may often be more culturally relevant and more effective in relieving many types of human pain and suffering. Such alternative treatment modalities, if proven to be effective, deserve to be promoted, taking into account the cultural and social environment' (INCB Annual Report, 1999: 9).

The International Association for Pain and Chemical Dependency fosters communication and cooperation among healthcare professionals, particularly regarding healthcare and law enforcement policy and regulation, to try to improve pain management for all patients, including patients with a current or previous addictive disorder. The website www.opioidrisk.com/node/1397 offers several tools for assessing risks of providing opioids to patients in different pain situations – for example, to patients who are recently diagnosed with chronic pain, or to patients who have chronic long-term pain – by assessing their family and personal substance abuse history and other risk factors for potential opioid abuse.

The Opioid Risk Tool (Figure 13.2; also available at: www.partnersagainstpain. com/printouts/Opioid_Risk_Tool.pdf) checks the history of family and personal substance abuse, preadolescent sexual abuse and any history of psychological disorder, with items scores and scores risk rates.

The benefits of using the Opioid Risk Tool (ORT) are as follows:

- **Estimated time:** it takes less than a minute to administer and score.
- **Length:** it contains only five items.
- **Administration:** it is administered by self-report.
- **Intended settings:** primary care.
- **Scoring and interpretation:** the risk assessment can be scored by hand, either by the patient or the health professional. Each item that the patient answers positively on the ORT is awarded a certain point value. The points of the entire assessment add up to a patient opioid risk score. Total score risk categories are: low risk 0–3; moderate risk 4–7; high risk 8+. (www.opiodrisk.com/node/1397; Webster, 2005)

## Understanding the potential side-effects of opioid analgesia

**Physical dependence, tolerance and addiction** are the potential side-effects of opioid analgesia (see Chapter 7). **Physical dependence** is a state which develops due to the body's adaptation to ongoing opioid use because of the process of resetting of various homoestatic mechanisms to a different set point (known as allostasis). Ongoing use of opioids puts various body systems into a new balance which requires continued opioid use to maintain normal function. **Withdrawal syndrome** occurs when the opioid drug is stopped suddenly, producing dilated pupils and tachycardia (in contrast

Date _____

Patient name _____

## OPIOID RISK TOOL

| | | Mark each box that applies | Item score if female | Item score if male |
|---|---|---|---|---|
| **1. Family history of substance abuse** | Alcohol | [ ] | 1 | 3 |
| | Illegal drugs | [ ] | 2 | 3 |
| | Prescription drugs | [ ] | 4 | 4 |
| **2. Personal history of Substance Abuse** | Alcohol | [ ] | 3 | 3 |
| | Illegal drugs | [ ] | 4 | 4 |
| | Prescription drugs | [ ] | 5 | 5 |
| **3. Age** (mark box if 16–45) | | [ ] | 1 | 1 |
| **4. History of preadolescent sexual abuse** | | [ ] | 3 | 0 |
| **5. Psychological disease** | Attention deficit disorder, obsessive compulsive disorder, bipolar, schizophrenia | [ ] | 2 | 2 |
| | Depression | [ ] | 1 | 1 |
| | **TOTAL** | | _____ | _____ |

**Total score risk category**

Low risk 0–3

Moderate risk 4–7

High risk ≥ 8

**Figure 13.2** Opioid Risk Tool

Source: Webster, L.R (2005) Predicting aberrant behaviours in opioid-treated patients: preliminary validation of the Opioid Risk Tool. *Pain Medicine*, 6 (6): 432–442. Copyright (2005). Republished with permission of John Wiley and Sons.

to opioid sedation or overdose which produces miotic (constricted) pupils and slow heart rate). **Tolerance** (requiring a higher dose of the drug to maintain the same analgesic effect), **physical dependence** and **withdrawal** are natural consequences of drug use. For **addiction** to occur there needs to be an aberrant behaviour pattern in taking the drug over time, or a psycho-behavioural syndrome, which is defined as a compulsive, irresistible need to consume the drug, despite the harm caused. The drug is craved and the person loses control over their behaviour, being unable to control the initiation, quantity or termination of drug intake. This behavioural syndrome is now termed **substance dependence** (Mitra, 2011).

The terminology requires clarification because it is very important for patient care. **Opioid dependence** can mean two different things. The **first meaning** is if a person is taking ongoing opioid medication which is abruptly stopped, then their body will react with a biologically natural withdrawal syndrome. The **second meaning** is a clinical syndrome which may include tolerance and, if the drug is stopped, withdrawal, but also includes a second, clinical, psycho-behavioural syndrome, defined as a compulsive, irresistible need to consume the drug, despite the harm caused. These two types of opioid dependencies need to be distinguished from each other to avoid undermedication of each type according to pain requirement situation (Mitra, 2011).

## Substance use disorders

Substance use disorders include substance dependence and substance abuse. **Substance dependence** is a cluster of cognitive behavioural and physiological symptoms indicating continued use despite tolerance, withdrawal and compulsive drug-taking behaviours. The substance is often taken in larger amounts than intended, with a persistent but unsuccessful desire to control the substance use. Much time is spent trying to obtain the substance, which takes the place of other social, occupational or recreational activities – the substance use continues despite awareness of physiological and/or psychological harm (American Psychiatric Association, 2000).

**Substance abuse** is a maladaptive pattern of substance use manifested by recurrent and significant adverse consequences related to the repeated use of the substances. The behaviour may lead to a failure to fulfil major role obligations, repeated use in physically hazardous situations, multiple legal problems and recurrent social and interpersonal problems (American Psychiatric Association, 2000).

**Adherence** describes the extent to which a patient correctly takes medication or follows medical advice.

The attitudes and knowledge of nurses are crucial in ensuring that each individual patient's pain medication and management needs are met through the judicious use of the combination of opioid and non-opioid drugs and nonpharmacological methods. Ongoing research and constant leadership and education endeavours are required to ensure the appropriate, optimal use of opioids for pain relief and to improve the standards and quality of pain management in nursing practice.

## Chapter summary

- A recent study by the Joint Commission Resources (2010) indicated that there are 10 challenges in the healthcare setting to optimal pain management and that pain was poorly managed across the care continuum.

- While medical knowledge and treatments exist, the need for pain education and training for healthcare professionals at all stages of their development is a recurring theme in studies identifying issues relevant to the under-treatment of pain.
- The Institute of Medicine's *Relieving Pain in America: A Blueprint for Transforming Prevention, Care, Education and Research* (2011), in a chapter on education challenges, states that all specialties have strong reasons to engage in pain medicine as most professionals treat patients in pain and this is true for both nurses and doctors.
- The project core values of an international intervarsity pain education project for all healthcare professional state: 'To deliver the highest quality of care, health professionals must be able to determine and address the needs of patients from a variety of cultures and socio-economic backgrounds; advocate for patients on individual, system and policy levels; and communicate effectively with patients, families and professionals'.
- The concepts of pain threshold and pain tolerance are at the very core of pain measurement in patient care. Educators of all healthcare professionals, including nurses, need to fully understand these concepts and be able to explain them clearly. Pain tolerance is closely related to emotional experience.
- Patient-related barriers to effective pain management prevent the patient disclosing accurate information about their pain experience to the nurse, doctor, other healthcare professional or caregivers, and may lead to less than adequate analgesic use or incorrect analgesic use.
- Organizational barriers are related to a lack of or deficient pain policies, as well as inadequate continuing education in pain management, poor staffing levels and poor nurse–patient and inter-healthcare professional communication.
- Professionals who have responsibility for drug regulation in a given country may be ill-informed about addiction. Outdated knowledge and attitudes and fear of addiction can negatively impact on opioid access from government regulators to prescribers, and by nurses giving inadequate opioid medication to patients.

## Reflective exercise

A 25-year-old male with a history of (non-opioid) substance abuse and depression presents to the emergency department having undergone emergency abdominal surgery within the past two months for appendicitis. You are assigned to this patient, who tells you the pain medicine-acetaminophen PRN no longer works and he is feeling very sick. You take his vital signs and pain score and find he has a high temperature, rapid pulse and low blood pressure, clammy skin and is in severe pain. The emergency department physician, on examination of the patient, finds an extended abdomen and

*(Continued)*

*(Continued)*

reduced bowel sounds, indicating possible severe abdominal infection or bowel perforation. Consider how the emergency team will approach the immediate patient-centred care of this patient in terms of optimizing analgesic requirement and patient comfort.

If the patient undergoes surgery on this occasion, consider the implications for meeting the patient's post-operative analgesic needs in the immediate and longer term. Consider the roles of the patient's Community Health Nurse, General Practitioner, local pharmacist and family or social support network, and the precautions to be put in place to help reduce risk and prevent this patient's possible further substance abuse or dependence.

## Recommended reading

Fishman, S.M., Arwood, E.L., Chou, R., Herr, K., Murinson, BB., Watt-Watson, J., Carr, D.B., Gordon, D.B., Stevens, B.J., Bakerjian, D., Ballantyne, J. C. Courtenay, M., Djukic, M., Koebner, I.J., Mongoven, J.M., Paice, J.A., Prasad, R., Singh, N.,Sluka, K.A., St Marie, B. and Strassels, S.A. (2013) Core competencies for pain management: results of an interprofessional consensus summit. *Pain Medicine*, 14: 971–981.

Institute of Medicine (2004) *Keeping Patients Safe: Transforming the Work Environment of Nurses*. Quality Chasm Series. Washington, DC: The National Academies Press.

Institute of Medicine (2011) *Relieving Pain in America*: *A Blueprint for Transforming Prevention, Care, Education and Research*. Washington, DC: The National Academies Press.

Joint Commission Resources (2012) *Pain Management: A Systems Approach to Improving Quality and Safety. Joint Commission on Accreditation of Healthcare Organizations*. Washington, DC. Available at: www.jcrinc.com/pain-management-a-systems-approach-to-improving-quality-and-safety/

## Websites relevant to this chapter

Interprofessional Pain Management Competency Programme:
www.aacn.nche.edu/ccne-accreditation/Pain-Management.pdf
International Association for Pain and Chemical Dependency (IAPCD):
www.opioidrisk.com/node/1397
Tools for checking opoid risk rates:
www.partnersagainstpain.com/printouts/Opioid_Risk_Tool.pdf

# References

American Association of Colleges of Nursing (2008) *The Essentials of Baccalaureate Education for Professional Nursing Practice*. Washington, DC: American Association of Colleges of Nursing.

American Psychiatric Association (2000) *Diagnostic and Statistical Manual of Mental Disorders* (Text Revision DSM-IV-TR) (4th edn). Washington, DC: American Psychiatric Association.

Bennett, M.I., Bagnall, A. and José Closs, S. (2009) How effective are patient-based educational interventions in the management of cancer pain? Systematic review and meta-analysis. *Pain*, 143: 192–199.

Bylind, C.L., Brown, R., Lubrano di Ciccone, B. and Konopasek, L. (2010) Facilitating skills practice in communication role-play sessions: essential elements and training facilitators. In D.W. Kissane, B.D. Bultz, P.N. Butow and I.G. Finlay (eds) *Handbook of Communication in Oncology and Palliative Care*. Oxford: Oxford University Press.

Duke, G., Haas, B.K., Yarbrough, S. and Northam, S. (2013) Pain management: knowledge and attitudes of Baccalaureate Nursing students and Faculty. *Pain Management Nursing*, 14: 11–19.

Egan, M. and Cornally, N. (2013) Identifying barriers to pain management in long-term care. *Nursing Older People*, 25: 25–31.

Elman, I., Zubieta, J-K., and Borsook, D. (2011) The missing P in psychiatric training: why it is important to teach pain to psychiatrists. *Archives of General Psychiatry*, 68 (1): 12–20.

Fishman, S. et al. (2013) *Pain Management Core Competencies for Prelicensure Clinical Education*. Available at: www.aacn.nche.edu/ccne-accreditation/Pain-Management.pdf (accessed 26 June 2014).

Fishman, S.M., Arwood, E.L., Chou, R., Herr, K., Murinson, B.B., Watt-Watson, J., Carr, D.B., Gordon, D.B., Stevens, B.J., Bakerjian, D., Ballantyne, J.C., Courtenay, M., Djukic, M., Koebner, I.J., Mongoven, J.M., Paice, J.A., Prasad, R., Singh, N., Sluka, K.A., St Marie, B. and Strassels, S.A. (2013) Core competencies for pain management: results of an interprofessional consensus summit. *Pain Medicine*, 14: 971–981.

INCB and WHO (2012) *Guide on Estimating Requirements for Substances under International Control Developed by the International Narcotics Control Board and the World Health Organization for use by Competent National Authorities*. New York: United Nations.

INCB Annual Report (1999) Available at: http://incb.org/documents/Publications/ AnnualReports/AR1999/Annual_Report_1999_ENGLISH.pdf (accessed 9 July 2014).

Institute of Medicine (2003) *The Future of the Public's Health in the 21st Century*. Washington, DC: The National Academies Press.

Institute of Medicine (2004) *Keeping Patients Safe: Transforming the Work Environment of Nurses*. Quality Chasm Series. Washington, DC: The National Academies Press.

Institute of Medicine (2010) *The Future of Nursing: Leading Change, Advancing Health*. Washington, DC: The National Academies Press.

Institute of Medicine (2011) *Relieving Pain in America: A Blueprint for Transforming Prevention, Care, Education and Research*. Washington, DC: The National Academies Press.

Joint Commission Resources (2010) *Voice of the Customer Survey*. Cited in Joint Commission Resources (2012) *Pain Management: A Systems Approach to Improving Quality and Safety. The Joint Commission on Accreditation of Healthcare Organizations*. Washington, DC. Available at: www.jcrinc.com/pain-management-a-systems-approach-to-improving-quality-and-safety/.

Joint Commission Resources (2012) *Pain Management: A Systems Approach to Improving Quality and Safety. Joint Commission on Accreditation of Healthcare Organizations.* Washington, DC. Available at: www.jcrinc.com/pain-management-a-systems-approach-to-improving-quality-and-safety/.

Maguire, P. and Pitceathly, C. (2002) Key communication skills and how to acquire them. *British Medical Journal*, 325 (7366): 697–700.

McCarthy, B., O'Donovan, M. and Twomey, A. (2008) Person-centered communication: design, implementation and evaluation of a communication skills module for under-graduate nursing students – an Irish Context. *Contemporary Nurse* 27: 207–222.

McGee, S.J., Kaylor, B.D., Emmott, H. and Christopher, M.J. (2011) Defining chronic pain ethics. *Pain Medicine*, 12: 1376–1384.

Mitra, S. (2011) Opioid tolerance and dependence. In R.S. Sinatra, J.S. Jahr and J.M. Watkins-Pitchford (eds), *The Essence of Analgesia and Analgesics*. Cambridge: Cambridge University Press.

Murinson, B.B., Nenortas, E., Mayer, R.S., Mezei, L., Kozachik, S., Nesbit, S. and Haythornthwaite, J.A. (2011) A new program in pain medicine for medical students: integrating core curriculum knowledge with emotional and reflective development. *Pain Medicine*, 12: 186–195.

Ward, S., Goldberg, N., Miller-McCauley, B., Mueller, C., Nolan, A., Pawlik-Plank, D., Robbins, A., Stormoen, D. and Weissman, D. (1993) Patient-related barriers to management of cancer pain. *Pain*, 52: 319–324.

Ward, S., Scharf Donovan, H., Owen, B., Grosen, E. and Serlin, R. (2000) An individualised intervention to overcome patient-related barriers to pain management in women with gynaecologic cancers. *Research in Nursing and Health*, 23: 393–405.

Watt-Watson, J., Hunter, J., Pennefeather, P., Librach, L., Raman-Wilms, L., Schreiber, M., Lax, L., Stinson, J., Dao, T., Gordon, A., Mock, D. and Salter, M. (2004) An integrated under-graduate curriculum based on IASP curricula for six Health Science Faculties. *Pain*, 110: 140–148.

Webster, L.R. (2005) Predicting aberrant behaviors in opioid-treated patients: preliminary validation of the Opioid Risk Tool. *Pain Medicine*, 6 (6): 432–442.

# 14

# Pain and human rights

## Learning objectives

The learning objectives of this chapter are to:

- recognize that the alleviation of pain is a fundamental human right
- view governments, healthcare professionals and patients as synergistic in improving access to pain treatment and care
- be aware of the rationale for national pain strategies and local policies, standards and guidelines
- recognize the need for pain education for healthcare professionals, patients and the general public

## Introduction

This chapter gives an overview of recent progress regarding the development of national pain strategies and addresses the issues of pain and human rights.

Significant barriers to effective pain treatment, which include failures to provide essential medicines and to relieve suffering, as well as human rights abuses, include:

- the failure of many governments to put in place functioning drug supply systems;
- the failure to enact policies on pain treatment and palliative care;
- poor training of healthcare workers;
- the existence of unnecessarily restrictive drug control regulations and practices;

- fear among healthcare workers of legal sanctions for legitimate medical practice;
- the inflated cost of pain treatment. (Lohman et al., 2010: 8)

These factors need to be addressed individually and collectively to effectively tackle the problem of pain. To comprehensively address the problem in each country, the starting point is strategy development and government endorsement, followed by the establishment of pain services and the implementation of systems and policies, and optimal healthcare professional training and education.

## Access to pain treatment as a human right

The 1961 Single Convention on Narcotic Drugs addressed the control of illicit narcotics and obligated countries to work towards universal access to narcotic drugs necessary to alleviate pain and suffering. While effective analgesic medicines are available and continue to be developed, tens of millions of people around the world continue to suffer from moderate to severe pain each year without treatment. As described earlier, chronic pain is acknowledged to be one of the most significant causes of suffering and disability globally. Studies show that up to 70% of patients with cancer have pain, while people with HIV/AIDS have wide prevalence of pain across all stages of the infection. Pain is both under-recognized and under-treated. Pain has a profound negative impact on quality of life, leading to reduced mobility and or strength, and reduced immune system function as part of the overall physical, psychological and social consequences of the pain experience. People who have chronic pain are much more likely to suffer from depression and anxiety (Lohman et al., 2010).

According to international human rights law, countries must provide pain treatment medications as part of their core obligations under the right to health. Failure to take reasonable steps to ensure that people who suffer pain have access to adequate pain treatment may result in the violation of the obligation to protect against cruel, inhuman and degrading treatment (Lohman et al., 2010):

> Studies show that analgesic medications have an internationally uneven distribution, with North America and Europe consuming about 89% of the morphine used worldwide, while low- and middle-income countries with much higher cancer and HIV rates consume about 6% of the morphine used worldwide. However, poor availability of pain medication in pharmacies, fear of addiction, fear of criminal sanction are problems contributing to pain under-treatment in the USA, while in Europe pain is often underestimated and under-treated. In some countries laws require reforming. In many countries policies need to be reviewed and implemented. A compelling response is required to mobilize attention.

A human rights framework is viewed as a potentially powerful mechanism to demand greater access to pain relief medications and to obligate government accountability to respect, protect and fulfil the rights of people with pain. (Lohman et al., 2010: 8)

## 2010: National pain strategies to meet human rights

Professor Michael Cousins, considered to be the 'Father of Chronic Pain' because he has worked in the field of persistent pain for more than 40 years, leading major pain education and service development projects, led the organization of the first International Pain Summit in Montréal, Canada, in 2010. Two important documents released by the International Association for the Study of Pain (IASP) at the International Pain Summit in Montréal in September, 2010, were the 'Declaration of Montréal' (see this page) and 'A Statement of Desirable Characteristics of National Pain Strategies' (see pp.265–266).

---

### The Declaration of Montréal

We, as delegates to the International Pain Summit (IPS) of the International Association for the Study of Pain (IASP) (comprising IASP representatives from Chapters in 64 countries plus members in 130 countries, as well as members of the community), have given in-depth attention to the unrelieved pain in the world.

Findings were that pain management is inadequate in most of the world because:

- There is inadequate access to treatment for acute pain caused by trauma, disease, and terminal illness and failure to recognize that chronic pain is a serious chronic health problem requiring access to management akin to other chronic diseases such as diabetes or chronic heart disease.
- There are major deficits in the knowledge of health care professionals regarding the mechanisms and management of pain.
- Chronic pain with or without diagnosis is highly stigmatized.
- Most countries have no national policy at all or very inadequate policies regarding the management of pain as a health problem, including an inadequate level of research and education.
- Pain Medicine is not recognized as a distinct specialty with a unique body of knowledge and a defined scope of practice founded on research and comprehensive training programs.

*(Continued)*

---

*(Continued)*

- The World Health Organization (WHO) estimates that 5 billion people live in countries with low or no access to controlled medicines and have no or insufficient access to treatment for moderate to severe pain.
- There are severe restrictions on the availability of opioids and other essential medications, critical to the management of pain.

And, recognizing the intrinsic dignity of all persons and that withholding of pain treatment is profoundly wrong, leading to unnecessary suffering which is harmful, we declare that the following human rights must be recognized throughout the world:

*Article 1.* The right of all people to have access to pain management without discrimination (Footnotes 1–4).

*Article 2.* The right of people in pain to acknowledgment of their pain and to be informed about how it can be assessed and managed (Footnote 5).

*Article 3.* The right of all people with pain to have access to appropriate assessment and treatment of the pain by adequately trained health care professionals (Footnotes 6–8).

In order to assure these rights, we recognize the following obligations:

1.  The obligation of governments and all health care institutions, within the scope of the legal limits of their authority and taking into account the health care resources reasonably available, to establish laws, policies, and systems that will help to promote, and will certainly not inhibit, the access of people in pain to fully adequate pain management. Failure to establish such laws, policies, and systems is unethical and a breach of the human rights of people harmed as a result.
2.  The obligation of all health care professionals in a treatment relationship with a patient, within the scope of the legal limits of their professional practice and taking into account the treatment resources reasonably available, to offer to a patient in pain the management that would be offered by a reasonably careful and competent health care professional in that field of practice. Failure to offer such management is a breach of the patient's human rights.

*Note:* This Declaration has been prepared having due regard to current general circumstances and modes of health care delivery in the developed and developing world. Nevertheless, it is the responsibility of: governments, of those involved at every level of health care administration, and of health professionals to update the modes of implementation of the Articles of this Declaration as new frameworks for pain management are developed.

*Source:* IASP (2010a)
www.iasp-pain.org/Advocacy/Content.aspx?ItemNumber=1821)

# A Statement of Desirable Characteristics of National Pain Strategies: Recommendations (IASP, 2010b)

| Characteristics | Examples | Responsible Parties |
|---|---|---|
| **Pain Education** | | |
| Undergraduate | At an early stage in training to equip trainees with both the knowledge and skills to address all types of pain. The IASP core curriculum sets out standards for education in pain. | Centers of learning, regulatory bodies |
| Postgraduate | All clinicians required to have ongoing education in the relief of pain; clinicians trained to a specialist level in pain medicine. | Centers of learning, regulatory bodies |
| Public awareness | To understand pain and its management, empower consumers, and reduce the stigma of having ongoing pain, access to information on pain should be available to the general public. | Providers of health care, patient organizations, and health educator programs |
| **Patient Access and Care Coordination** | | |
| Care in differing settings | Rapid access to expert pain care. All hospitals should have staff with expert training in pain assessment and management to call upon. All primary care practitioners should be able to perform a basic assessment of need with regard to pain that includes determination of relief of pain and suffering. | Health care policy makers, providers and commissioners of health care |
| Medicines | The World Health Organization's list of essential medicines should be available in preparations suitable for all ages. Support from the pharmaceutical industry will be needed to achieve this goal. | Government regulatory agencies, drug enforcement agencies, and key clinical staff |
| Informed choice | Coordination of the system so that access to the right help is available as early as possible with a fully informed choice on options. | |
| Care pathways | Care pathways agreed on by consensus are a useful way to achieve this goal. | Providers and commissioners of health care |
| Expert care | Establish pain care networks to ensure excellent relationships between providers. | Commissioners and providers of health care |
| | Where secondary care exists, there should be a vertical system for escalation of referrals of difficult problems from primary, through secondary, to tertiary care centers. | |
| Interdisciplinary approach | A biopsychosocial approach to assessment and management that involves a team of health care professionals working closely together within a non-hierarchical framework. | Providers of health care |

*(Continued)*

*(Continued)*

| Characteristics | Examples | Responsible Parties |
|---|---|---|
| Family and caregiver involvement | Families and caregivers should be actively included in the management of a person in pain. | |
| Self-care | Adoption of approaches and systems that support self-care. Any pain management program must engage the community both in advocacy and in use of trained volunteers in the care program. Development of patient-led support networks. | |
| Special populations | Special populations include the very young and very old, victims of torture and natural calamities, those with learning difficulties, those with mental health and addiction disorders, ethnic minorities, and impaired persons. Their needs should be recognized and provided for. | Providers and commissioners of health care |
| **Monitoring-Quality** Improvement | | |
| Time to care | Standards for access times and activity planning that allow sufficient time to assess and care for people in pain. | |
| Quality of service | Improvements in patient experience should be routinely sought, including reduction in waiting times for care. | |
| Quality of life | Improvements in individual patients' quality of life (pain relief if possible and improvement in function) using both generic and disease-specific measures. | |
| Economic burden | Monitoring should include work loss and school absence due to pain, prescription costs, urgent care, and use of other services. | |
| Outcomes | Outcomes from care should be routinely measured including patient safety, patient experience, and clinical effectiveness, drawing upon IMMPACTs recommendations. | |
| **Pain Research** | | |
| Epidemiologic | A national health survey to determine population needs for pain care and monitor progress both in the general population and within institutions. | Public health services, health economists |
| Science | Prioritization of pain for funding opportunities that target gaps in pain treatment, implementation science, knowledge transfer, education, and policy development. | Federal health research funding bodies |

# First National Pain Strategy (Pain Australia) (2010)

Australia was the first country in the world to develop a national framework for the treatment and management of pain. It was the major outcome of the National Pain Summit held at Parliament House, Canberra, in March 2010, chaired by Professor Michael Cousins. The key goals of the Strategy are as follows:

- people in pain should be a national priority;
- knowledgeable, empowered and supported consumers;
- skilled professionals and best-practice evidence-based care;
- access to interdisciplinary care at all levels;
- quality improvement and evaluation;
- research. (National Pain Strategy (Pain Australia), 2010: 4–6)

The mission of the Strategy is 'To improve quality of life for people with pain and their families, and to minimise the burden of pain on individuals and the community'. Indeed, the burden of pain is huge in humanitarian, health care and financial terms. Pain is Australia's third most costly health problem and arguably the developed world's largest 'undiscovered' health priority (National Pain Strategy (Pain Australia), 2010: 5).

The executive summary to the Australian National Pain Strategy states that:

One in five Australians, including children and adolescents, will suffer chronic pain in their lifetime and up to 80 per cent of people living with chronic pain are missing out on treatment that could improve their health and quality of life ... chronic pain costs the Australian economy $34 billion per annum and is the nation's third most costly health problem. Yet a person with chronic pain, that is, constant daily pain for a period of three months or more in the past six months faces the following:

- their condition is not officially recognised as a disease or a public health issue;
- their family, friends, employers, schools and health professionals will often not believe they are in pain;
- many health professionals will have received little or no training in how to treat their condition;
- they may have to wait more than a year for an appointment at a service that can help them;
- they have little access to community based support;
- their productivity at work may be lowered, which frequently leads to unemployment and impoverishment;
- they are personally likely to carry more than half the total economic cost.

People with chronic pain are at substantially increased risk of depression, anxiety, physical deconditioning, poor self-esteem, social isolation and relationship breakdown. Children and adolescents with chronic pain are absent from school more often than

*(Continued)*

*(Continued)*

their peers, and participate in fewer sporting activities. They may never reach their full academic or vocational potential. Their reduced physical function and mobility can lead to loss of independence, and they may not be diagnosed and treated for social anxieties that may have contributed to, or result from, their condition. People with cancer-related pain have their own particular needs which are often not well met, despite effective techniques being known to relieve their burden. Acute pain, a normal, time limited response to trauma, surgery or other 'noxious' experience also continues to be poorly managed.

*Source*: National Pain Strategy (Pain Australia) (2010), p. 1

# 2010: The Prague Charter

The Prague Charter (2010) urges governments to relieve suffering and recognize palliative care as a human right. The European Association for Palliative Care (EAPC), The International Association for Palliative Care (IAHPC), the World Wide Palliative Care Alliance (WPCA) and the Human Rights Watch (HRW) are working together to advocate access to palliative care as a human right.

**A right to palliative care**: access to palliative care is a legal obligation, as acknowledged by United Nations conventions, and has been advocated as a human right by international associations, based on the right to the highest attainable standard of physical and mental health. In cases where patients face severe pain, government failure to provide palliative care can also constitute cruel, inhuman and degrading treatment. Palliative care can effectively relieve or even prevent this suffering and can be provided at comparably low cost. Yet the governments of many countries throughout the world have not taken adequate steps to ensure patients with incurable illnesses can realise the right to access palliative care. The EAPC, IAHPC, WPCA and HRW call on governments to:

- Develop health policies that address the needs of patients with life-limiting or terminal illnesses.
- Ensure access to essential medicines, including controlled medications, to all need them.
- Ensure that Healthcare workers receive adequate training on palliative care in pain management at undergraduate and subsequent levels.
- Ensure the integration of palliative care into healthcare systems at all levels.

The signatories and the representatives of the regional and international organisations **urge**:

Governments worldwide to ensure that patients and their families can realise the right to access palliative care by integrating such care into healthcare policies, as well as ensuring access to essential medicines, including opioid analgesics, is assured.

Major international organisations and forums such as the Council of Europe, the European Union, the World Health Organisation, the World Health Assembly, the World Medical Association and the International Council of Nurses (in order) to promote the right to palliative care, **invite:**

- Regional and national palliative care associations to support a palliative care philosophy that includes not only the development of specialist services but is centered around a public health approach.
- Academic institutions, teaching hospitals universities in developing and developed countries to train and motivate healthcare professionals working in primary care to integrate palliative care into their services.

**Express the hope**: that the general public recognises the need for access to palliative care for all and supports the Prague Charter through participation of social and media activities and in signing the petition.

*Source*: The Prague Charter (2010)

## May 2011: European Road Map Monitor for the Development of Pain Services for all European Countries

A meeting of the European Chapters of the International Association for the Study of Pain, in Brussels, May 2011 endorsed a **European Road Map Monitor for the Development of Pain Services for all European Countries**. The European Road Map Monitor outlines **seven concrete steps** on how national governments and EU institutions can effectively address the societal impact of pain in Europe: The 'Societal Impact of Pain' (SIP) is an international platform created in 2010 which aims for:

- raising awareness of the relevance of the impact that pain has on societies, health and economic systems;
- exchanging information and sharing best-practices across all member states of the European Union;
- developing and fostering European-wide policy strategies and activities for an improved pain care in Europe (Pain Policy). (SIP, 2014)

---

## The SIP Road Map for Action calls on European governments and the EU Institutions to:

1. Acknowledge that pain is an important factor limiting the quality of life and should be put on the top of the priority list of the national health care system.
2. Activate patients, their family, relatives and care-givers through the availability of information and access to pain diagnosis and management.
3. Raise awareness of the medical, financial and social impact that pain and its management has on the patients, their family, care-givers, employers, and the healthcare system.
4. Raise awareness of the importance of prevention, diagnosis and management of pain amongst all healthcare professionals, notably through further education.
5. Strengthen pain research (basic science, clinical, epidemiological) as a priority in EU framework programme and in equivalent research road maps at national and EU level, addressing the societal impact of pain and the burden of chronic pain on the health, social, and employment sectors.
6. Establish an EU platform for the exchange, comparison and benchmarking of best practices between member states on pain management and its impact on society.
7. Use the EU platform to monitor trends in pain management, services, and outcomes and provide guidelines to harmonize effective levels of pain management to improve the quality of life of European Citizens.

*Source*: Treed et al. (2011)

---

Preliminary data from a survey of 27 participating countries in 2011, showed that the majority of countries are in the process of establishing a platform representing the societal impact of pain. However, there are major discrepancies and gaps across Europe regarding policy implementation, particularly regarding pain care outcomes.

## 2011: *Relieving Pain in America: A Blueprint for Transforming Prevention, Care, Education, and Research* (Institute of Medicine, USA)

According to the report *Relieving Pain in America: A Blueprint for Transforming Prevention, Care, Education, and Research*, published by the US Institute of Medicine of the National Academy of Sciences (Institute of Medicine, 2011):

Chronic pain conditions affect approximately 100 million U.S. adults at a cost of $560–635 billion annually in direct medical treatment costs and lost productivity. Pain's occurrence, severity, duration, response to treatment, and disabling consequences vary from person to person because pain, like other severe chronic conditions, is much more than a biological phenomenon and has profound emotional and cognitive effects.

The report provides recommendations for improving the care of people who experience pain, the training of pain clinicians and the collection of data on pain in the United States. The important principles underpinning the report are:

- **A moral imperative.** Effective pain management is a moral imperative, a professional responsibility, and the duty of people in the healing professions.
- **Chronic pain can be a disease in itself.** Chronic pain has a distinct pathology, causing changes throughout the nervous system that often worsen over time. It has significant psychological and cognitive correlates and can constitute a serious, separate disease entity.
- **Value of comprehensive treatment.** Pain results from a combination of biological, psychological, and social factors and often requires comprehensive approaches to prevention and management.
- **Need for interdisciplinary approaches.** Given chronic pain's diverse effects, interdisciplinary assessment and treatment may produce the best results for people with the most severe and persistent pain problems.
- **Importance of prevention.** Chronic pain has such severe impacts on all aspects of the lives of its sufferers that every effort should be made to achieve both primary prevention (e.g., in surgery for a broken hip) and secondary prevention (of the transition from the acute to the chronic state) through early intervention.
- **Wider use of existing knowledge.** While there is much more to be learned about pain and its treatment, even existing knowledge is not always used effectively, and thus substantial numbers of people suffer unnecessarily.
- **The conundrum of opioids.** The committee recognizes the serious problem of diversion and abuse of opioid drugs, as well as questions about their long-term usefulness. However, the committee believes that when opioids are used as prescribed and appropriately monitored, they can be safe and effective, especially for acute, post-operative, and procedural pain, as well as for patients near the end of life who desire more pain relief.
- **Roles for patients and clinicians.** The effectiveness of pain treatments depends greatly on the strength of the clinician–patient relationship; pain treatment is never about the clinician's intervention alone, but about the clinician and patient (and family) working together.
- **Value of a public health and community-based approach.** Many features of the problem of pain lend themselves to public health approaches: concern about the

*(Continued)*

*(Continued)*

large number of people affected, disparities in occurrence and treatment, and the goal of prevention cited above. Public health education can help counter the myths, misunderstandings, stereotypes, and stigma that hinder better care.

The IOM report concludes that: Chronic pain alone affects the lives of approximately 100 million Americans, making its control of enormous value to individuals and society. To reduce the impact of pain and the resultant suffering will require a transformation in how pain is perceived and judged both by people with pain and by the health care providers who help care for them. The overarching goal of this transformation should be gaining a better understanding of pain of all types and improving efforts to prevent, assess, and treat pain.

*Source*: Institute of Medicine (2011)

# October 2011: World Medical Association resolution

In the resolution adopted by the **World Medical Association** at its 62nd General Assembly in Montevideo, Uruguay, in October 2011, the following principles were laid down:

- The right to access to pain treatment for all people without discrimination, as laid down in professional standards and guidelines and an international law, should be respected and effectively implemented.
- Physicians and other health care professionals have an ethical duty to offer proper clinical assessment to patients with pain and to offer appropriate treatment, which may require prescribing medications-including opioid analgesics-as medically indicated. This also applies to children and other patients who cannot always adequately express their pain.
- Instruction on pain management, including clinical training lectures and practical classes, should be included in mandatory curricula and continuing education for physicians and other health care professionals. Such education should include evidence-based therapies effective for pain, both pharmacological and non-pharmacological. Education about opioid therapy for pain should include the benefits and risks of the therapy. Safety concerns regarding opioid therapy should be emphasised to allow the use of adequate doses of analgesia while mitigating detrimental effects of the therapy. Training should also include recognition of pain in those who may not be able to adequately express their pain including children and cognitively impaired and mentally challenged individuals.

- Governments must ensure the adequate availability of controlled medicines, including opioids, for the relief of pain and suffering. Governmental drug control agencies should recognise severe and/or chronic pain as a serious and common healthcare issue and appropriately balance the need to relieve suffering with the potential for the illegal use of analgesic drugs. Under the right to health, people facing pain have a right to appropriate pain management, including effective medications such as morphine. Denial of pain treatment violates the right health and may be medically unethical.
- Many countries lack necessary economic, human and logistic resources to provide optimal pain treatment to the population. The reasons for not providing adequate pain relief must therefore be fully clarified and made public before accusations of violating the right to health are made.
- International and national drug control policy should balance need for adequate availability and accessibility of controlled medicines like morphine and other opioids for the relief of pain and suffering with efforts to prevent the misuse of these controlled substances. Countries should review their drug control policies and regulations to ensure they do not contain provisions that unnecessarily restrict the availability and accessibility of controlled medicines for the treatment of pain. Where unnecessary or disproportionately restrictive policies exist, they should be revised to ensure the adequate availability of controlled medicines. Each government should provide the necessary resources for the development and implementation of a national pain treatment plan, including a responsive monitoring mechanism and process for receiving complaints when pain is inadequately treated.

*Source*: Resolution adopted by the 62nd WMA General Assembly (2011)

## 2011: Health Survey for England

The 2011 Health Survey for England has revealed significant data about chronic pain. The headline finding was that over 14 million people live with chronic pain in England. Certain groups are more likely to experience chronic pain:

- 37% of women, in comparison to 31% of men, reported chronic pain;
- 42% in the lowest income households had chronic pain, compared with 27% in the highest;
- although chronic pain was most prevalent in older people, one in six 16–34 year olds were affected. (Health Survey for England, 2011)

## November 2011: First English Pain Summit

In November 2011: the first **English Pain Summit** took place at Central Hall, Westminster, with the Report of the first English Pain Summit '**Putting Pain on the Agenda**' launched on 4 July 2012.

The key recommendations of the English Pain Summit are:

---

A.  Clear standards and criteria must be agreed and implemented nationally for the identification, assessment, and initial management of problematic pain
B.  An awareness campaign should be run to explain the nature, extent, impact, prevention and treatment of chronic pain to the wider general and NHS community
C.  Nationally-agreed commissioning guidance must be developed and agreed,describing best value care in chronic pain to reduce unwarranted variation
D.  A data strategy for chronic pain should be agreed through creation of an epidemiology of chronic pain working group

---

The 'Putting Pain on the Agenda' report states: 'Over recent years, multiple national reports have described the extent and impact of chronic pain, and highlighting necessary areas for improvement.'

Several consistent major themes have emerged over time:

---

- Chronic pain is a major public health problem, affecting large numbers of people with great impact on those affected, their families, the health service and the wider national economy;
- Pain, including chronic pain is one of the key reasons that people seek healthcare, yet pain is often overlooked by health professionals and those providing care in clinics, hospitals and care homes and documentation is poor;
- Chronic pain education for most healthcare professionals is weak at both undergraduate and postgraduate levels with the exception of pain medicine training in anaesthesia;
- People with chronic pain would often benefit from early intervention to prevent disability, but those in need are not consistently referred for specialist treatment, and waiting times are often long;
- Services for people with chronic pain are of inconsistent standard and quality and are not always available for those who need them. This is particularly true for centres specialising in treating children with chronic pain.

*Source*: English Pain Summit (2012)

---

## 2012: Canadian Pain Summit

In April 2012: the **Canadian Pain Summit** took place, endorsing the Canadian draft National Pain Strategy (2011), which outlines core values of:

- Access to the treatment of pain without discrimination is a fundamental human right
- The treatment of pain requires an inter-professional approach to care
- The treatment of pain must be patient and family centered
- Pain is a continuum (from acute to chronic and from birth to death)
- Pain is a biological, psychosocial as well as a spiritual problem
- People in pain must be part of the solution

The Canadian draft National Pain Strategy (2011) states that:

- Pain is often poorly managed in Canada. This includes both acute pain caused by ongoing tissue damage, trauma or surgery and chronic pain persisting beyond normal healing. Poor management of pain has a major impact on quality of life and the ability to function. The management of cancer pain has improved over the past decade, but the majority of Canadians still do not have access to adequate pain and palliative care at the end of life and increasingly, survivors of cancer and HIV suffer with chronic pain.
- The economic costs of pain are significant. Extrapolating from US figures, just released, the cost of pain in Canada is estimated to be approximately $60 Billion dollars.
- The economic cost to people waiting for pain treatment at multidisciplinary pain treatment facilities in Canada is $17,544 per year.
- The personal cost of pain is the toll it takes on the lives of those suffering pain as well as their families and caregivers. We have the knowledge and the tools to treat the majority of pain, however these tools are not being used and Canadians are suffering needlessly.
- Chronic pain sufferers report the lowest health related quality of life when compared to others with chronic health conditions including advanced heart disease.
- Chronic pain is associated with high rates of depression, anxiety and suicidal thoughts. The risk of suicide compared to people without chronic pain is double.
- A recent survey of health science and veterinary training programs across Canada discovered that veterinarians receive five times more education about pain than people doctors.

Inadequate pain assessment and treatment is a growing problem in Canada. The incidence of pain increases as we grow older. Necessary actions are not being taken to address the gaps that exist in prevention, pain assessment and management, timely access to care, the lack of education for healthcare professionals, and inadequate private and public funding for pain research.

*Source*: Canadian Pain Strategy (2012)

## 2013: First publication of the *Civic Survey on the Respect of Unnecessary Pain: Patients' Rights in Europe. Report on Patients' Rights to Avoid Unnecessary Suffering and Pain*

The European Charter of Patients' Rights, drawn up in 2002, is based on the experience of the Tribunal for Patients' Rights and in particular on previous national, regional and local Italian Charters for Patients' Rights and on the Charter of Fundamental Rights of the European Union. The European Charter brings together the inalienable rights of the patient which each EU country should protect and guarantee. All of the following rights under the Charter of Fundamental Rights of the European Union are fundamental for European citizens and health services:

---

**1 Right to Preventive Measures**

Every individual has the right to a proper service in order to prevent illnesses.

**2 Right of Access**

Every individual has the right of access to the health services that his or her health needs require. The health services must guarantee equal access to everyone, without discriminating on the basis of financial resources, place of residence, kind of illness or time of access to services.

**3 Right to Information**

Every individual has the right to access all information regarding his/her state of health, the health services and how to use them, and all the scientific research and technological innovation available.

**4 Right to Consent**

Every individual has the right of access to all information that might enable him/her to actively participate in the decisions regarding his/her health; this information is a prerequisite for any procedure and treatment, including the participation in scientific research.

**5 Right to Free Choice**

Each individual has the right to freely choose among different treatment procedures and providers on the basis of adequate information.

**6 Right to Privacy and Confidentiality**

Every individual has the right to the confidentiality of personal information, including that regarding his/her state of health and potential diagnostic or therapeutic

---

procedures, as well as the protection of his/her privacy during the performance of diagnostic exams, specialist visits, and medical/surgical treatment in general.

## 7 Right to Respect of Patients' Time

Each individual has the right to receive necessary treatment within a swift and predetermined period of time. This right applies at each phase of the treatment.

## 8 Right to the Observance of Quality Standards

Each individual has the right of access to high quality health services on the basis of the specification and observance of precise standards.

## 9 Right to Safety

Each individual has the right to be free from harm caused by the poor functioning of health services, medical malpractice and errors, and the right of access to health services and treatments that meet high safety standards.

## 10 Right to Innovation

Each individual has the right of access to innovative procedures, including diagnostic procedures, according to international standards and independently of economic or financial considerations.

## 11 Right to Avoid Unnecessary Suffering and Pain

Each individual has the right to avoid as much suffering and pain as possible, in each phase of his/her illness.

## 12 Right to Personalized Treatment

Each individual has the right to diagnostic or therapeutic programmes tailored as much as possible to his/her personal needs.

## 13 Right to Complain

Each individual has the right to complain whenever he/she has suffered harmful treatment and the right to receive a response or other feedback.

## 14 Right to Compensation

Each individual has the right to receive sufficient compensation within a reasonably short time whenever he/she has suffered physical or moral and psychological harm caused by a health service treatment.

*Source*: Pain Alliance Europe (2013)

In the First Report on the Patient's Right to avoid unnecessary suffering and pain in Europe civic organizations were involved in collecting information through interviews with institutions, professionals and patients, helping to put into practice the right to participate in the evaluation of services and policies. The starting point of the present civic survey was the listing of five evaluation factors emphasised by the Irish and Italian patient charters of rights for people with chronic/unnecessary pain:

1. The patient's right to be believed.
2. The patient's right to have pain treated and managed at the earliest possible stage.
3. The patient's right of access to the best possible technologies and therapies in pain treatment and management.
4. The patient's right to be informed about all the pain management options available so that he/she can make the best decisions and choices for his/her wellbeing.
5. The patient's right to live with the least amount of pain possible. (Plain Alliance Europe, 2013: 20; Ireland, 2009; Italy, 2005)

Results from this survey underpin the need for national pain management strategies, law reform and policy implementation through reinforcing alliance building between organizations and groups, enlarging participation in the assessment procedures and producing civic information for policy input (Pain Alliance Europe, 2013: 87).

## Chapter summary

- Barriers to achieving effective pain prevention and treatment need to be addressed individually and collectively to tackle the problem of pain. This requires recognition by governments, pain strategy and service developments, together with healthcare professional education and training. Patient and caregiver pain management education is essential for optimal patient outcomes.
- The 2010 Declaration of Montréal, released in response to an international high-level professional finding that pain management is inadequate in most of the world, addresses three human rights regarding pain and requires these rights to be recognized throughout the world.
- The 2010 IASP 'Statement of Desirable Characteristics of National Pain Strategies' centres on multidisciplinary pain education for undergraduates, postgraduates and the general public, patient access and care coordination, monitoring, quality improvement, and pain research.
- Australia was the first country to develop a national framework for the treatment and management of pain, an outcome of the National Pain Summit in Canberra in March 2010. Canada, the USA and the United Kingdom are in the process of developing and/or having their national pain strategies endorsed by government. In some other countries, for example Ireland, pain medicine has been recognised as a medical speciality in its own right.

- The 2010 Prague Charter urges governments to relieve suffering and recognize palliative care as a human right. The European Association of Palliative Care, the International Association for Palliative Care, the World Wide Palliative Care Alliance and Human Rights Watch are working together to advocate access to palliative care as a human right.
- The European Societal Impact of Pain (SIP) (2010) international platform aims to foster European-wide policies and strategies for improved pain care. In the USA, the Institute of Medicine (2011) report, *Relieving Pain in America: A Blueprint for Transforming Prevention,Care, Education and Research*, provides recommendations for improving the care of people experiencing pain, the training of pain clinicians and the collection of data on pain in the USA.
- At the 62nd General Assembly of the World Medical Association in 2011, one of a set of principles regarding the adequate pain treatment as a human right was laid down. It states 'the right to access to pain treatment for all people without discrimination, as laid down in professional standards and guidelines and international law, should be respected and effectively implemented'.
- The 2013 publication of the *Civic Survey on the Respect of Unnecessary Pain: Patients Rights in Europe*, report found wide discrepancies in the treatment and management of chronic pain, underpinning a major need for a national pain management strategy, policy implementation and law reform across Europe.

## Reflective exercise

In this chapter reread 'Detailed Desirable Characteristics of National Pain Strategies, IASP'. You will note this book aligns with **Pain Education** on p.265. Reflect on the characteristics outlined under the four categories of Pain Education, Patient Access and Care Co-ordination, Monitoring and Quality Improvement and Pain Research, and consider those characteristics which resonate most strongly with you. How can you aim to improve your patient-centred nursing practice in accordance with these characteristics? Reread the Declaration of Montréal and consider the importance of interdisciplinary teamwork and personal qualities and skills in achieving your aims.

## References

Australian and New Zealand College of Anaesthetists (ANZCA) (2001) Statement on patients' rights to pain management and associated responsibilities. ANZCA PS45. Available at: www.anzca.edu.au/resources/professional-documents/pdfs/ps45–2010-statement-on-patients-rights-to-pain-management-and-associated-responsibilities.pdf (accessed 8 July, 2014).

Brennan, F., Carr, D.B. and Cousins, M.J. (2007) Pain management: a fundamental human right. *Anesthesia and Analgesia*, 105: 205–221.

Canadian Pain Summit (2012) *Rise Up Against Pain*. Available at: http://canadian painstrategy.ca/en/home/about-the-2012-summit.aspx (accessed 9 February 2014).

Cousins, M.J., Brennan, F., Carr, D.B. (2004) Pain relief: a universal human right. *Pain*, 112: 1–4.

Cousins, M.J. and Lynch M.E. (2011) The Declaration of Montréal: access to pain management is a fundamental human right. *Pain*, 152: 2673–2674.

English Pain Summit (2012) *Putting Pain on the Agenda: The Report of the First English Pain Summit*. London: English Pain Summit. p. 4.

European Federation of the IASP Chapters (EFIC), www.efic.org (accessed 9 February 2014).

FEDELAT (2008) *Proclamation of Pain Treatment and the Application of Palliative Care as Human Rights*, 22 May.

Health Survey for England (2011) Available at: www.policyconnect.org.uk/cppc/news/health-survey-england-14-millon-people-live-pain (accessed 9 February 2014).

International Association for the Study of Pain (IASP) (2010a) *Declaration of Montréal*. Available at: www.iasp-pain.org/Advocacy/Content.aspx?Item Number=1821.

International Association for the Study of Pain (IASP) (2010b) *A Statement of Desirable Characteristics of National Pain Strategies: Recommendations by the International Association for the Study of Pain*. Washington, DC: International Association for the Study of Pain.

Institute of Medicine (2011) *Relieving Pain in America: A Blueprint for Transforming Prevention, Care, Education and Research*. Summary of Report. Washington, DC: The National Academies Press.

International Association for Hospice and Palliative Care (IAHPC) and the Worldwide Palliative Care Alliance (WPCA) (2009) *Joint Declaration and Statement of Commitment on Palliative Care and Pain Treatment as Human Rights*. Houston, TX: IAHPC. Available at: www.hospicecare.com (accessed 26 June 2014).

Ireland (2009) *Charter of Rights for People Living in Chronic Pain*. Available at: www.chronicpain.ie/about-us/charter-rights.

Italy (2005) *Charter of Rights against Unnecessary Pain*. Available at: www.citta-dinanzattira.it/corporate/salute/1954-carte-dei-diritti-sul-dolore-inutile.html.

Lohman, D., Schleifer, R. and Amon, J.L. (2010) Access to pain treatment as a human right. *BMC Medicine*, 8: 8.

National Pain Strategy (Pain Australia) (2010) Available at: www.painaustralia.org.au/images/pain_australia/NPS/National%20Pain%20Strategy%202011.pdf (accessed 9 February 2014).

Pain Alliance Europe and Active Citizenship Network (2013) *Civic Survey on the Respect of Unnecessary Pain*. Available at: www.sip-platform.eu/tl_files/redakteur-bereich/National%20Initiatives/Europe/Report%20Civic%20Survey,%20 Pain%20Patient%20Pathway%20Recommendations.pdf.

Resolution adopted by the 62nd WMA General Assembly, Montevideo, Uraguay, October 2011. Available at: www.pipain.com/4/post/2012/08/world-medical-association-wma.html (accessed 9 February).

Scholten, W., Nygren-Krug, H. and Zucker, H.A. (2007) The World Health Organization paves the way for action to free people from the shackles of pain. *Anesthesia and Analgesia*, 105: 1–4.

Societal Impact of Pain (SIP) (2014) *Societal Impact of Pain* Available at: www.sip-platform.eu/home.html (accessed 9 February 2014).

Somerville, M. (1994) Death of pain: pain, suffering, and ethics. In G.F. Gebhart, D.L. Hammond and T.S. Jensen (eds), *Proceedings of the 7th World Congress on Pain: Progress in Pain Research and Management* (Vol. 2). Seattle, WA: International Association for the Study of Pain. pp. 41–58.

The Prague Charter (2010) Available at: www.eapcnet.eu/Themes/Policy/PragueCharter.aspx (accessed 9 February 2014).

Treede, R.D. and van Rooij, N., with Alon, E., Kress, H.G., Langford, R., Krcevski Skvarc, N., Varrassi, G., Vissers, K.C.P. and Wells, J.C.D. (2011) *The Societal Impact of Pain: A Road Map for Action*. The European Federation of the IASP Chapters (EFIC)/Societal Impact of Pain (SIP).

Treede, RD., Van Rooij, N. (2011) *The Societal impact of Pain – A Road Map for Action: European Road Map Monitor*. Available at: www.sip-platform.eu/home.html.

# Glossary

**Acute pain** unpleasant sensory and emotional experience associated with tissue damage and with activation of nociceptor transducers at the site of local tissue damage.

**Addiction** a behavioural pattern of craving for and compulsive use of a substance despite harm.

**Afferent neurons** neurons (nerve fibres) which conduct nerve impulses from the body periphery to the central nervous system via the spinal cord.

**Agonist** a chemical (drug) substance capable of combining with a cell receptor and initiating the same action or response typically produced by the binding of an endogenous substance.

**Allodynia** pain due to a stimulus which does not normally provoke pain.

**Analgesia** absence of pain in response to stimulation which would normally be painful.

**Antagonist** a chemical that opposes the action of a drug or an endogenous substance by combining with and blocking its receptor.

**Assessment** the act of making a judgment; in pain management a clinical judgement about the nature of the range of pain characteristics and their impact on the patient's health and well being.

**Autonomy** quality or state of being self-governing.

**Aversive stimulus** stimulus which causes avoidance behaviour because of its noxious or punishing nature; chronic pain is an aversive stimulus which may result in reduced physical activity in order to avoid the associated pain.

**Avoidance behaviour** response to avoid an (anticipated) aversive stimulus.

**Bereavement** the death of a family or close friend; the state of being bereaved (deprived) of someone close.

**Biopsychosocial** regarding a person's personal context, comprised of any computation of biological, genetic, racial, sex and age (bio), emotional, cognitive and spiritual (psycho) and cultural, environmental and ethnic (social) factors.

**Cancer pain** a compilation of acute and chronic pain associated with any aspects of the person's experience of cancer including disease progression and associated treatments (e.g. consequences of chemotherapy, radiotherapy and/or surgery) the term 'cancer pain' does not distinguish between acute and chronic pain in the context of cancer.

**Cardiac syncope** a temporary reduction of blood flow to the brain causing faintness due to abnormalities of the heart such as abnormal heartbeat, valve or muscle structure or function.

**Care** responsibility for or attention to health, well-being and safety of another person or persons.

**Catastrophising** magnification of pain-related stimuli accompanied by negative outlook and sense of loss of control.

**Central neuropathic pain** pain caused by a lesion or disease of the central somatosensory nervous system.

**Central sensitisation** increased responsiveness of nociceptive neurons in the central nervous system to normal or subthreshold afferent input.

**Chronic pain** unpleasant sensory and emotional experience which may be elicited by injury or disease, usually perpetuated by factors that are removed from the original cause of pain and extending beyond the expected period of healing.

**Compassion** sympathetic awareness of another's distress with a desire to alleviate it.

**Competency** having the required qualities of abilities and skills.

**Component** a constituent part.

**Congruence** quality or state of agreeing; in communication, accepting the person's perspective.

**Context** interrelated conditions in which something exists or occurs.

**Culture** beliefs, customs, behaviours and attitudes of a particular society or group.

**Curative** a course of treatment (for example, pharmacological, surgical or other type of appropriate therapy) which results in remission of signs and/or symptoms of a disease especially during a prolonged period of observation.

**Delirium** a cognitive disorder characterised by a confusional state with varying psychomotor agitation, illusions and hallucinations.

**Dermatomes** segmental fields of sensation on the skin, each innervated by a spinal nerve.

**Determinant** a thing that controls or influences future events in a given context, e.g. socio-economic determinants of health.

**Diagnosis** The identification of a disease by examination of the patient, their signs and symptoms and relevant tests.

**Disability** inability to function socially or pursue an occupation because of physical or mental impairment causing loss of capacity; refers to optimal functionality obtained after full rehabilitation.

**Disease** a condition which impairs normal functioning and is typically manifested by distinguishing signs and symptoms.

**Distress (NCCN definition)** a multifactorial unpleasant emotional experience of a psychological (cognitive, behavioral, emotional), social, and/or spiritual nature that may interfere with the ability to cope effectively with cancer, its physical symptoms and its treatment. Distress extends along a continuum, ranging from common normal feelings of vulnerability, sadness, and fears to problems that can become disabling, such as depression, anxiety, panic, social isolation, and existential and spiritual crisis; the term equally applies to people with pain and is chosen to avoid stigmatization.

**Dynorphins** one of three kinds of endogenous opioids.

**Efferent neurons** neurons which conduct nerve impulses from the central nervous system towards internal organs, tissues or the body periphery.

**Empathy** the ability to be sensitive to (*putting oneself in another's shoes*) and to try to understand the thoughts and feelings of another person, while recognising separateness from the other and acknowledging the uniqueness of their experience (*without losing the 'as if' quality*).

**Empower** to give power to a person or people; in the healthcare context to afford the patient/close other status to facilitate him or her to proactively engage in their own healthcare/that of a close other.

**Endogenous opioids** family of peptide neurotransmitters.

**Enkephalins** one of three kinds of endogenous opioids.

**Endorphins** one of three kinds of endogenous opioids.

**Epidemiology** the study of the incidence, prevalence and control of diseases in populations.

**Ethnic** a particular kindred affiliation or group with shared traditions and customs.

**Ethos** the distinguishing guiding beliefs of a person, group, or institution.

**Ethics** a theory or system of moral values referring to and defining good or bad behaviour.

**Etiology** the cause of a disease or abnormal condition.

**Forebrain** *Prosencephalon* the front division of the neural tube containing the cerebral hemispheres, thalamus and hypothalamus.

**Genetic** relating to or caused by genes.

**Grief** major distress usually associated with severe loss and/or suffering.

**Hind brain** *Rhombencephalon* the rear division of the brain containing the cerebellum pons and medulla.

**Humanism** philosophy which stresses an individual's value, dignity, and capacity for self-actualization through reason.

**Hyperalgesia** an increased pain response to a stimulus that is normally painful.

**Hypoalgesia** a diminished pain response to a stimulus that is normally pain.

**Illness** the subjective biopsychosocial experience of a disease or condition.

**Incidence** the rate of occurrence of new cases of a particular disease in a given population.

**Integrated care** patient care which is coordinated among and between different disciplines; represents the ideal of interdisciplinary care and may be based on formulated care pathways.

**Interdisciplinary team (see also multidisciplinary team)** the dynamic interaction of the multidisciplinary team implying optimal communication and cooperation between and among the healthcare professional team members, including the patient.

**Measurement: in pain** a quantified subjective pain experience.

**Mesmerism** a type of induced hypnotic trance based on the principle of Animal Magnetism promulgated by Anton Mesmer in the 18th century.

**Metabolite** drug constituent following metabolism. For example, the liver metabolizes about two-thirds of a dose of oral morphine to inactive M3G metabolites and one-third to active M6G metabolites.

**Metastases** spread of a primary cancer tumour to another site in the body by the spread of cancer cells through the body's circulatory systems.

**Midbrain** *Mesencephalon* the area of the brain situated below the hypothalamus and above the pons.

**Modulation** a reversible change in histological structure due to physiological factors.

**Mourning** a time of sadness following a bereavement when grief is experienced.

**Multidisciplinary team** concept first formulated by Professor John Bonica, anaesthetist and founder of the Internal Association for the Study of Pain, to have a team of healthcare professionals with different professional skills and competencies to facilitate the patient's optimal functional recovery in all spheres of quality of life.

**Neural tube** embryonic structural divisions corresponding to the undeveloped fore-, mid- and hindbrain.

**Neuropathic pain** pain caused by a lesion or disease of the somatosensory nervous system.

**Neuropathy** a disturbance of function or pathological change in a nerve.

**Neuroplasticity** nociceptive input to the nervous system as changed responses to stimuli, leading to structural and functional neuronal change.

**Neurovegetative** particularly relevant to chronic, especially visceral pain, related to the autonomic nervous system and limbic system; the patient may show signs of emotional distress, nausea, vomiting, anxiety and changes in vital signs.

**Nocebo effects** the adverse treatment effects induced by a dummy medicine or intervention which contains no detrimental or toxic substance.

**Nociception** the neural process of encoding noxious stimuli.

**Nociceptive neuron** a central or peripheral neuron of the somatosensory nervous system that is capable of encoding noxious stimuli.

**Nociceptive pain** pain that arises from actual or threatened damage to non-neural tissue and is due to the activation of nociceptors.

**Nociceptive stimulus** an actual or potentially damaging event transduced and encoded by nociceptors.

**Nociceptor** a high-threshold sensory receptor of the peripheral somatosensory nervous system that is capable of transducing and encoding noxious stimuli.

**Noxious stimulus** a stimulus that is damaging or threatens damage to normal tissues.

**Pain** an unpleasant sensory and emotional experience associated with *actual or potential* tissue damage or described in terms of such damage.

**Pain behaviour** observable verbal and non-verbal actions which indicate that a person may be experiencing pain and suffering.

**Pain threshold** the minimum intensity of a stimulus that is perceived as painful.

**Pain tolerance level** the maximum intensity of a pain-producing stimulus a person is willing to tolerate.

**Palliative** treatments and management interventions which aim to control the signs and symptoms of a malignant (especially metastatic cancer) or non-malignant (for example, multiple sclerosis) incurable disease to improve the patient's quality of life; (from Latin *palliare*: to cloak).

**Perception** awareness of elements of the environment through the five senses; also implies additional cognitive awareness through organisation and interpretation of information.

**Peripheral sensitization** increased responsiveness and reduced threshold of nociceptive neurons in the periphery to the stimulation of their receptive fields.

**Person-centered medicine** practice of holistic care in which the patient is a person at the centre of their care.

**Placebo** a dummy medicine, surgical procedure or therapeutic intervention, which, in the context of a clinical trial (the only situation in which giving a dummy intervention for pain is ethical) the patient believes could be the real thing; frequently used to control patients' expectations about the efficacy of an intervention.

**Placebo effect** the positive benefits experienced by the recipient of the placebo intervention, which are generally only achieved with an active treatment intervention.

**Prognosis** predication about the likelihood of duration of and recovery from a disease/illness.

**Prevalence** percentage of a specific population with a particular disease at a given time.

**Race** a person's unchangeable genetic and biological characteristics such as eye and skin colour.

**Rehabilitation** restoration of maximum physiological and psychosocial functioning from a state of impairment.

**Reliability** in pain measurement: the extent to which a measuring tool yields the same results on repeated trials.

**Sign** objective evidence of disease.

**Stimulus** an event that prompts a change or a reaction.

**Substrate** a substance acted upon; base, underlayer.

**Suffering** subjective perceived threat to the integrity of the person (in response to unrelieved pain) associated with feelings of helplessness, hopelessness and lack of controllability.

**Symptom** subjective evidence of disease or physical disturbance.

**Synapse** the junction point from one neuron to the next and the point of information transmission.

**Systems theory** theory with broad applicability to all types of sciences; in the context of health care: complex, adaptable and self-regulating relationships between the person and his or her environment; recognising health services as potentially adaptive systems with many interacting elements and computations, with the service user as the actively participating patient experiencing illness influenced by social, psychological and cultural factors.

**Transduction** action or process of converting something (especially energy) into another form.

**Utility** the quality or extent of usefulness.

**Validity** relevant and meaningful; in pain measurement: that a scale measures what it purports to measure.

**Variable** characterised by changes or variations; in pain measurement, measurable characteristics of pain which may vary such as intensity, temporality, location and quality.

**Wind-up** temporal summation of pain mediated by repetitive noxious stimulation of C-fibres.

# Appendix

The following table is a general guide only for non-opioid and weak opioid medications for Steps 1 and 2 of the WHO Analgesic Ladder. Please check the relevant, up-to-date National Formulary for all drug dosages, routes and schedules of administration, adverse effects (many of which are not listed on this table) and contraindications, especially in pregnancy, pre-term infants and lactating mothers, for which many drugs are contraindicated. Drugs can usually be given through a number of different routes, in varying formats and dosages, which must be pre-checked. Time to analgesic onset is highly variable and half-life is often the dose and route taken. Many drugs interact with alcohol and may also impair driving ability.

| Drug | WHO Ladder Step | Mechanism of analgesic action | Indication | Time to plasma peak concentration | Plasma half-life | Metabolism CYP subset and excretion | Suitable for child pediatric format | Adverse effects in patients | Risk factor/ interaction CAUTION: |
|---|---|---|---|---|---|---|---|---|---|
| Acetaminophen (paracetamol – often not classed as NSAID as not anti-inflammatory) Adult starting dose po: 0.5–1g q4–6h; max in 24 h 4 g  **Bio-availability** 60% after 500 mg PO;  **Onset of action** 15–30 min PO; **Duration of action** 4–6 h PO | 1 | May work in CNS and periphery to inhibit COX and prostaglandin synthesis | Mild to moderate nociceptive pain of dental, ENT musculoskeletal-origin; post-immunization fever; substitute for aspirin | Widely variable | 1.5–3h | M: liver E: urine | Yes * Infant suspension | Hepatotoxicity in large/ overdoses; caution in renal, hepatic and cardiac impairments; possibly safer than NSAIDs with anticoagulants with careful monitoring; CYP3A4 substrate may have altered pharmacokinetics in patients lacking enzyme | • Pregnancy • Alcohol (potentially lethal) • Anticoagulants |
| Aspirin NSAID (higher risks overall than newer NSAIDs)  Adult starting dose po: 300–900 mg q4–6h Max in 24 h 4 g Duration of action 4 h | 1 | Action on hypothalamus; inhibition of COX; decrease in prostaglandin synthesis; anti-inflammatory; antipyretic; anti-platelet | Dental (temporary) musculoskeletal; inflammatory conditions; Acute rheumatic fever; as adjunct for neuropathic pain | rapid | 15–20 min | M: liver E: renal | No | Increased risk of gastric bleeding; peptic ulcers; newer NSAIDs preferred to treat inflammatory conditions | • 3rd trimester pregnancy • Warfarin and other anticoagulants • Methotrexate • Gout • Liver disease • Haemophilia • Alcohol (may increase risk of bleeding) |

| Drug | WHO Ladder Step | Mechanism of analgesic action | Indication | Time to plasma peak concentration | Plasma half-life | Metabolism CYP subset and excretion | Suitable for child pediatric format | Adverse effects in patients | Risk factor/ interaction CAUTION: |
|---|---|---|---|---|---|---|---|---|---|
| Ibuprofen NSAID Adult starting dose po: 300–400 mg q6h max in 24h: 2.4 g **Bio-availability** 90% PO; **Onset of action** 20–30 min; **Duration of action** 4–6 h | 1 | Mostly peripheral; interrupts arachidonic cascade; inhibits COX and prostaglandins formation in inflamed tissue | Mild to moderate nociceptive pain; dysmenorrhea fever; headaches musculoskeletal; post-operative analgesia; post-immunisation pyrexia | 1–2 h | 2–3 h | M: liver E: urine | Yes* | Dermatitis; hypersensitivity to aspirin NSAIDs; potential for gastric bleeding/toxicity; caution in renal hepatic impairment; older persons; safe at low dose for GI; high doses risk for CVD events; not suitable for acute gout | • Pregnancy<br>• Anticoagulants<br><br>Methotrexate, lithium, digoxin, clofarabine, SSRIs<br><br>• Furusemide<br>• Do not give with other NSAIDs |
| Naproxen NSAID Adult starting dose po: 500 mg initially, then 250 mg q6–8h; max dose 1st day: 1.25 g **Bioavailability** 95% PO; **Onset of action** 20–30 min; **Duration of action** 6–8 h single dose; >12 h multiple doses | 1 | Mostly peripheral; interrupts arachidonic cascade; inhibits COX and prostaglandins formation in inflamed tissue | Pain and inflammation in rheumatic disease; musculoskeletal orders; dysmenorrhea; gout; juvenile idiopathic arthritis | 1.5–4 h | 12–15 h | M: liver E: rapid urinary; mostly | Yes* | Dermatitis; hypersensitivity to aspirin NSAIDs; potential for gastric bleeding/toxicity; caution in cardiac, renal hepatic impairment; older persons; high adverse GI effects; at low dose safest NSAID in CVD | Pregnancy Anticoagulants; Methotrexate, lithium, digoxin, clofarabine, SSRIs; Possible fatal interactions with:<br>• Methotrexate<br>• Probenecid High doses not recommended |

*(Continued)*

(Continued)

| Drug | WHO Ladder Step | Mechanism of analgesic action | Indication | Time to plasma peak concentration | Plasma half-life | Metabolism CYP subset and excretion | Suitable for child pediatric format | Adverse effects in patients | Risk factor/ interaction CAUTION: |
|---|---|---|---|---|---|---|---|---|---|
| Diclofenac NSAID Adult starting dose po: 75 mg bd; **Bioavailability** 50% PO; suppositories about 33%; **Plasma half-life** 1–2h. **Duration of action** 8h. | 1 | Mostly peripheral; interrupts arachidonic cascade; inhibits COX and prostaglandins formation in inflamed tissue | Mild to moderate pain and inflammation in rheumatic disease; musculoskeletal orders; dysmenorrhea; gout; juvenile idiopathic arthritis; opthalmic post-operative pain | 2.5h PO; 1h: PR | 1–2h | M: liver E: kidneys | Yes* | Hypersensitivity to aspirin NSAIDs; potential for gastric bleeding/toxicity; caution in cardiac, renal hepatic impairment; older persons; avoid in acute porphyria; low risk of adverse GI events; high risk of CVD events | Caution in post-operative ophthalmic use, may cause ocular side-effects; Contraindicated in wearers of soft contact lenses; Risk of haemorrhage with anticoagulants; Methotrexate, lithium, digoxin, clofarabine, SSRIs |
| Celecoxib Selective COX 2 Inhibitor Adult starting dose po: 100 mg bd; max in 24h: 200 mg bd; **Bioavailability:** Not known in humans; 22–40% in dogs; onset of action 60 min **Duration of action** 5 h | 1 | Mostly peripheral; interrupts arachidonic cascade; inhibits COX and prostaglandins formation in inflamed tissue | Pain and inflammation in osteoarthritis; rheumatoid arthritis; post-operative pain; dysmenorrhoea | 3h | 11h | M: almost exclusively hepatic | No (16+) | As above with NSAIDS; similar profile to Diclofenac; only prescribe if pt has serious risk of/ may be safer for gastric/hepatic events; no cardio-protection | Pregnancy and breastfeeding; Inflammatory bowel disease; Anticoagulants; Methotrexate, lithium, digoxin, clofarabine, SSRIs; Not for patients with CVD |

| Drug | WHO Ladder Step | Mechanism of analgesic action | Indication | Time to plasma peak concentration | Plasma half-life | Metabolism CYP subset and excretion | Suitable for child* <12yrs | Adverse/effects in patients | Risk factor/ interaction CAUTION: |
|---|---|---|---|---|---|---|---|---|---|
| Tramacet: (tramadol hydrochloride 37.5 mg; paracetamol 325 mg) Weak opioid agonist tramadol Adult starting dose po: 2 tablets q6h Max in 24 h; **Bioavailability** 75%; Rapid onset of action; **Duration of action** 4–6 h; with paracetamol (information as above) (Step 2 of WHO ladder recommended add weak opioid to non-opioid) | 2 | Tramadol acts on CNS, high affinity for μ receptor; inhibits noradrenaline (norepinephrine) (norepinephrine) uptake (Paracetamol may act on CNS and periphery) Synergistic analgesic effect of combined T and P may be more than each separately | Moderate to severe post-operative, dental and chronic pain | 2 h | T: 6–7 h | M: liver via CYP2D6 E: kidneys; | No | Not for patients with renal, hepatic and cardiac impairment less constipating than codeine dizziness and vomiting | Hypersensitivity to product constituents Reduced effect/ potential for altered pharmacokinetics in poor metabolisers about 10% of population lacks CYP2D6 enzyme Opioid toxicity Many: see literature |

*(Continued)*

(Continued)

| Drug | WHO Ladder Step | Mechanism of analgesic action | Indication | Time to plasma peak concentration | Plasma half-life | Metabolism CYP subset and excretion | Suitable for child* <12yrs | Adverse/effects in patients | Risk factor/ interaction CAUTION: |
|---|---|---|---|---|---|---|---|---|---|
| Tylex: (Codeine phosphate 30 mg; paracetamol 500 mg) Adult starting dose po: 1–2 tablets q4h; max in 24h: 8 capsules **Bioavailability** 40% **Onset of action** 15–30 min **Duration of action** 4–6 h with paracetamol (information as above) (Step 2 of WHO ladder recommended add weak opioid to non-opioid) | 2 | Codeine affinity for µ receptor Weak opioid agonist Metabolised by CYP2D6 enzyme to morphine; acts on CNS and bowel Synergistic analgesic effect of combined T and P may be more than each separately | Mild to moderate to severe pain | C: 1–2 h prodrug | C: 3–4 h | C: M: liver via CYP2D6; E: kidneys | No | Caution in patients with hepatic and renal impairment; very constipating | Hypersensitivity to product constituents reduced effect/ potential for altered pharmacokinetics in poor metabolisers: about 10% of population lacks CYP2D6 enzyme Opioid toxicity Many: see literature |

Commonly used adjuvant medications for Steps 1, 2 and 3 of the WHO Analgesic Ladder; all doses (based on BNF Formularies) are approximate only, and need to be adjusted according to patient response. Please check the relevant up-to-date National Formulary for all drug dosages, routes and schedules of administration, adverse effects (many of which are not listed on this table), contraindications especially in pregnancy, pre-term infants and lactating mothers, for which many drugs are contra-indicated. Drugs can usually be given through a number of different routes, in varying formats and dosages which must be prechecked; time to analgesic onset is highly variable and half-life is often dependent on dose and route. Many drugs interact with alcohol and may also impair driving ability.

| Drug type | Drug | WHO Ladder Step | Mechanisms of action | Indication | Time to plasma peak concent | Plasma half-life | Metabolism and excretion | Suitable for child in pediatric *format | Adverse effects in patients | Risk factor/ interaction CAUTION: |
|---|---|---|---|---|---|---|---|---|---|---|
| Tricyclic Antidepressant (TCA) | Amitriptyline Adult starting dose po: 25 mg Bioavailability 45% Onset of action 7 days in neuropathic pain Duration of action 24 h | 1,2,3 | Increases CNS synaptic concentration of noradrenaline (norepinephrine) and serotonin through re-uptake inhibition; may act on multiple receptors; may be NMDA antagonist or sodium channel blocker; possibly acts on descending pain inhibitory systems | Chronic pain, especially neuropathic; fibromyalgia Headache (migraine, tension-type) | 6 h PO; 24–48 h IM | 13–36 h | M: mainly by CYP2D6 in liver E: renal | No | Dangerous in acute overdose: increased risk of (a) sudden cardiac death; (b) delirium; lower doses required for older persons; high risk of femoral fractures; may impair alertness; multiple potential adverse effects | Possible serious anticholinergic, sedative and orthostatic side-effects; interaction with MAOIs, TCAs and other drugs; potential for reduced effect/altered pharmacokinetics in poor metabolisers; about 10% of population lacks CYP2D6 enzyme |
| Tricyclic Antidepressant (TCA) | Nortriptyline (primary active metabolite of and secondary amino side chain to amitriptyline) adult starting dose po:10–50 mg Bioavailability60% Onset of action 2–6 weeks Duration of action variable 24+h | 1,2,3 | Increases CNS synaptic concentration of noradrenaline (norepinephrine) and serotonin through re-uptake inhibition; may act on multiple receptors; may be NMDA antagonist/ sodium channel blocker; possibly acts on descending pain inhibitory systems | Chronic pain, especially neuropathic | 7–8 h highly variable impacted by 3–10% of population having reduced isoenzyme poor metabolisers | 15–40 h Prolonged and highly variable | M: liver by CYP2D6 enzyme; P450IID6 isoenzyme; E: renal | No | Dangerous in acute overdose: increased risk of (a) sudden cardiac death; (b) delirium; lower doses required for older persons; may impair alertness; multiple potential adverse effects | Fewer sedative and orthostatic side-effects than amitriptyline multiple effects: interaction with MAOIs and other drugs; potential for reduced effect/altered pharmacokinetics in poor metabolisers; about 10% of population lacks CYP2D6 enzyme |
| Tricyclic Antidepressant (TCA) | Imipramine Adult starting dose po: up to 150 mg Bioavailability 45% Onset of action 2–4 weeks Duration of action variable | 1,2,3 | Increases CNS synaptic concentration of noradrenaline (norepinephrine) and serotonin through re-uptake inhibition; may act on multiple receptors; may be NMDA antagonist or sodium channel blocker; possibly acts on descending pain inhibitory systems | Chronic pain; especially neuropathic | 2–6 h | 11–25 h | M: liver – extensively by several CYP enzymes inc CYP2D6/ CYP3A4 E: 80% renal; 20% faeces | No | Dangerous in acute overdose: increased risk of (a) sudden cardiac death; (b) delirium; lower doses required for older persons; may impair alertness; multiple potential adverse effects | Potential for less anticholinergic and sedative effect but greater orthostatic side-effects than amitriptyline: interaction with MAOIs and many other drugs; potential for reduced effect/altered pharmacokinetics in poor metabolisers; about 10% of population lacks CYP2D6 enzyme |

| Drug type | Drug | WHO Ladder Step | Mechanisms of action | Indication | Time to plasma peak concentr | Plasma half-life | Metabolism and excretion | Suitable for child in pediatric *format | Adverse effects in patients | Risk factor/ interaction CAUTION: |
|---|---|---|---|---|---|---|---|---|---|---|
| Tricyclic Antidepressant (TCA) | Desipramine (secondary amino side chain metabolite of imipramine) Bioavailability 75–90% Onset and duration of action delayed | 1,2,3 | Increases CNS synaptic concentration of noradrenaline (norepinephrine) and serotonin through uptake inhibition; may act on multiple receptors; may be NMDA or sodium channel blockers; possibly acts on descending pain inhibitory systems | Chronic pain; especially neuropathic | 4–6h | 7–60+h | M: liver by CYP enzymes especially CYP2D6 E: 70% renal | No | Dangerous in acute overdose: increased risk of (a) sudden cardiac death; (b) delirium; lower doses required for older persons; may impair alertness | As nortriptyline but fewer anticholinergic effects; interaction with MAOIs and other drugs; reduced effect/altered pharmacodynamics in poor metabolisers; about 10% of population lacks CYP2D6 enzyme |
| Combined serotonin-noradrenaline (norepinephrine) re-uptake inhibitor (SNRI) | Duloxetine Adult starting dose 60mg Bioavailability >50% Duration of action >24h situation dependent | 1,2,3 | Increases CNS synaptic concentration of noradrenaline (norepinephrine) and serotonin through re-uptake inhibition; possibly acts on descending pain inhibitory systems | Diabetic neuropathy; fibromyalgia (not 1st line treatment see Finnerup et al 2005) | 6–10h | 8–17h | M: liver by CYP2D6 enzyme E: renal | no | Data limited in/not recommended for patients with moderate liver or renal impairment; possible sexual dysfunction; nausea, vomiting; sedation; light-headedness; serotonin toxicity; not for use in patients taking MAOIs | Potential for raised BP; caution with anticoagulants and NSAIDS; interacts with other antidepressants; concurrent use not recommended; reduced effect/altered pharmacodynamics in poor metabolisers; about 10% of population lacks CYP2D6 enzyme |
| Combined serotonin-noradrenaline (norepinephrine) re-uptake inhibitor (SNRI) | Venlafaxine Adult starting dose 37.5 mg daily Bioavailability 45% Duration of action 12–24h; situation dependent | 1,2,3 | Increases CNS synaptic concentration of noradrenaline (norepinephrine) and serotonin through re-uptake inhibition; possibly acts on descending pain inhibitory systems | Diabetic/painful neuropathy; fibromyalgia (not first-line treatment, see Finnerup et al. 2005) Headache/ migraine | 2.5h | 5h | M: liver by CYP2D6 enzyme E: renal | no | Data limited in/not recommended for patients with moderate liver or renal impairment; possible sexual dysfunction; nausea, vomiting; sedation; lightheadedness; not for use in patients taking MAOIs | Used advisedly for patients with history of MI or unstable heart disease; bipolar disorder; higher plasma concentrations in CYP2D6 metabolisers; may interact with other drugs in CYP2D6 poor metabolisers |

*(Continued)*

Finnerup, N. B., Otto, M., McQuay, H. J., Jensen, T. S. and Sindrup, S. H. (2005) Algorithm for neuropathic pain treatment: an evidence-based proposal. *Pain*, 118: 289–305.

| Drug type | Drug | WHO Ladder Step | Mechanisms of action | Indication | Time to plasma peak concentr | Plasma half-life | Metabolism and excretion | Suitable for child in pediatric *format | Adverse effects in patients | Risk factor/ interaction CAUTION: |
|---|---|---|---|---|---|---|---|---|---|---|
| Selective serotonin re-uptake inhibitor (SSRI) | Fluoxetine Adult starting dose 20 mg PO Bioavailability 90% Onset and duration of action: highly variable | 1,2,3 | Increases CNS synaptic concentration of serotonin through re-uptake inhibition; (both N and S reuptake inhibition favours analgesic effectiveness when used as single approach) | Chronic pain, rheumatic pain conditions; arthritis fibromyalgia | 4–8 h | 4–6 days | M: liver Inhibits CYP2D6* E: renal | No | SSRIs less sedating with fewer antimuscarinic and cardiotoxic side-effects than TCAs; not for patients taking/recently stopped MAOIs – potential for fatal reactions; headache, nausea, insomnia, fatigue | Strong hepatic enzyme inhibitor – potential for serious interaction if used with other drugs metabolised by these enzymes; gastro-intestinal effects common; potential risk for: hypersensitivity reactions; seizures; *avoid during tamoxifen treatment |
| Selective serotonin re-uptake inhibitor (SSRI) | Paroxetine Adult starting dose 20 mg PO Bioavailability 50% Onset and duration of action: highly variable | 1,2,3 | Increases CNS synaptic concentration of serotonin through re-uptake inhibition; (both N and S re-uptake inhibition favours analgesic effectiveness when used as single approach) | Chronic pain, neuropathic; fibromyalgia | 5 h | 15–20 h | M: liver Inhibits CYP2D6* E: renal and faeces | No | SSRIs less sedating with fewer antimuscarinic and cardiotoxic side-effects than TCAs; not for patients taking /recently stopped MAOIs – potential for fatal reactions | Strong hepatic enzyme inhibitor -- Potential for serious interaction if used with other drugs metabolised by these enzymes; gastro-intestinal effects common; *avoid during tamoxifen treatment |
| Antiepileptic (neuromodulator) | Carbamazepine Adult starting dose po; 100 mg twice daily needs careful titration Bioavailability 85%; Onset of action 48 h Duration of action: no data | 1,2,3 | Blocks voltage-gated sodium channels; also acts at calcium channels; modulates neuronal excitability | Trigeminal neuralgia first-line | 4–8 h | 36 h | M: liver E: renal and faeces | Yes | Dizziness; drowsiness, unsteadiness, nausea and vomiting; leucopenia; fluid retention; avoid abrupt withdrawal | CNS adverse reactions; gastro-intestinal disturbances; ADH-like effects |

| Drug type | Drug | WHO Ladder Step | Mechanisms of action | Indication | Time to plasma peak concentr | Plasma half-life | Metabolism and excretion | Suitable for child in pediatric *format | Adverse effects in patients | Risk factor/ interaction CAUTION: |
|---|---|---|---|---|---|---|---|---|---|---|
| Antiepileptic (neuromodulator) | Gabapentin Adult starting dose po 300 mg Bioavailability 74% Onset of action 1–3 h Duration of action 8–12 h | 1,2,3 | Modulation of a₂δ subunits of calcium channels; reduction in release of neurotransmitters glutamate and substance P in spinal cord; modulates neuronal excitability | Trigeminal neuralgia; spinal cord injury/ neuropathic pain; postherpetic neuralgia; central neuropathic pain; post-operative pain prevention | 2–3 h | 5–7 h | Eliminated unchanged by renal excretion | No | Fatigue; fever; peripheral oedema; bmalaise; flu symptoms; impotence; avoid abrupt withdrawal | High dose can lead to CNS adverse reactions; somnolence; dizziness, Ataxia; fatigue; renal impairment impacts duration of action |
| Antiepileptic (neuromodulator) | Pregabalin Adult starting dose po; 75 mg bd; Bioavailability 90% Onset of action <30 min; Duration of action>12 h | 1,2,3 | Modulation of a₂δ subunits of calcium channels; reduction in release of neurotransmitters glutamate and substance P in spinal cord; modulates neuronal excitability | Trigeminal neuralgia; diabetic neuropathy; spinal cord injury neuropathic pain; postherpetic neuralgia, fibromyalgia; peripheral neuropathic pain; post-operative pain prevention | 1 h | 5–9 h | Eliminated unchanged by renal excretion | | Avoid abrupt withdrawal; Contraindicated in patients with severe congestive cardiac failure | Very high binding affinity; displaces gabapentin from a₂δ subunit; wide range of CNS adverse reactions possible; reduced dose may be required in older patients with compromised renal function |
| Benzodiazepine | Midazolam Adult starting dose PO Bioavailability 35–44% Onset of action 15 min Duration of action: ultra-short < 4 h | 1,2,3 | Acts selectively on GABA receptors enhances GABA inhibitory synaptic transmission throughout the CNS; facilitates opening of GABA-activated chloride channels Peri-operative sedative; hypnotic; used as intravenous anaesthetic; range of applications for symptom control in terminal care | Reduces effect of emergence reactions following ketamine administration; often combined with ketamine or fentanyl as effective sedative-anxiolytic sedation | 60 min PO | 2–5 h (prolonged in critically ill) | M: liver Metabolised by CYP3A4 E: Renal | Over 1 mnth | Use with caution in patients with hepatic or renal impairment or history of alcohol or drug abuse | In patients with chronic respiratory insufficiency; interacts with alcohol and many drugs; may give symptoms of dependence-withdrawal on cessation; can be reversed by flumazenil; pharmaceutical interaction with CYP3A4 inhibitors or inducers more pronounced for oral midazolam – requires careful monitoring for CYP3A4 inhibitor |

(Continued)

(Continued)

| Drug type | Drug | WHO Ladder Step | Mechanisms of action | Indication | Time to plasma peak concentr | Plasma half-life | Metabolism and excretion | Suitable for child in pediatric *format | Adverse effects in patients | Risk factor/ interaction CAUTION: |
|---|---|---|---|---|---|---|---|---|---|---|
| NMDA receptor antagonist Abuse potential | Ketamine Adult starting dose depends on route and procedure time PO: Bioavailability: 20% Onset of action: 30 min Duration of action 4–6 h | 1,2,3 | Sedation, amnesia, marked analgesia; dissociative anaesthesia; may depress/interrupt older/newer CNS pain pathway associations; binds to NMDA receptor/ blockade of glutamate | Sedation/ anaesthesia prior to short/long diagnostic/painful procedures; procedure may require concomitant analgesia | 30 min Po | 2–3h | M: liver E: renal | Yes | Respiratory and CNS depression; respiratory overdose; incompatible with barbiturates and diazepam; range of possible physical and psychological adverse effects; delirium; hallucinations; intracranial pressure; ataxia | In patients with hypertension, psychiatric illness, URTI hyperthyroidism, cardiac disease; alcoholism; patients should be undisturbed during recovery (does not preclude vital sign monitoring); no reversible agent so should be used in settings where advanced airway skills available |
| Synthetic corticosteroid | Dexamethasone Long duration of action IV Intermediate dose dexamethasone 0.11 to 0.2 mg/kg is safe effective multimodal strategy after surgical procedures | 1,2,3 | Anti-inflammatory inhibits expression of COX 2; | Wide range of disorders; latest evidence advises that pre-operative administration provides greater effect on reduction of post-operative pain and opioid consumption; may reduce nausea and vomiting; bone/nerve compression pain relief in cancer; rheumatic disease | Wide inter-individual variation | 36–54 h | M: liver and kidney E: urine | Yes | Patients with any one of number of conditions require careful monitoring; possible growth retardation in children; Cushing's syndrome; avoid abrupt withdrawal | Many potential: check literature carefully; for possible undesirable effects in all systems; highly variable pharmacokinetics need monitoring on individual basis |

| Drug type | Drug | WHO Ladder Step | Mechanisms of action | Indication | Time to plasma peak concentr | Plasma half-life | Metabolism and excretion | Suitable for child in pediatric *format | Adverse effects in patients | Risk factor/interaction CAUTION: |
|---|---|---|---|---|---|---|---|---|---|---|
| Muscle relaxant | Baclofen Adult starting dose: 5 mg PO Bioavailability >90% PO Onset of action 3–4 days Duration of action: 6–8h | 1,2,3 | Acts on GABA receptor to depress monosynaptic and polysynaptic reflex transmission, in turn inhibiting release of glutamate and aspartate at the spinal and supraspinal sites, decreases skeletal muscle spasm | Relief of voluntary muscle spasticity of cerebral/CNS origin/associated with multiple sclerosis and other neurodegenerative chronic diseases and spinal cord lesions | 1–3h | 3–4 h | M: 15% in liver E: 80% excreted unchanged in urine | Yes with v. low dose | Most beneficial to patients whose spasticity restricts activities/ physiotherapy; low dose required in patients with renal impairment and spastic sates of cerebral origin | Careful titration required to achieve satisfactory control of symptoms to avoid side-effects; caution in patients with psychiatric disorders and active peptic ulceration; wide range of interactions with other drugs; withdraw treatment gradually; no antidote to overdose |
| Local anaesthetic | Lidocaine IV according to patient's age and weight; surface 2–4% | 1,2,3 | Causes nerve fibre conduction block; blocks voltage sensitive sodium channels and prevents injury induced hyperexcitability in the P/CNS | Anaesthesia for dental, surface and certain types of neuropathic pain | Dose and route dependent; IV 1–25 min | Short: 2h: (longer in reduced cardiac output) Dose and route dependent | M: liver-extensive: E: urine | Yes | High plasma concentrations caused by too rapid administration/ reduced cardiac output /inadvertent intravascular injection; myocardial depression; potential for serious CNS effects | Can lead to neurotoxicity in older patients; long acting preferred IV should be given slowly, special caution with children; contraindicated in children with complete heart block |
| Local anaesthetic | Capsaicin Absorption after topical application is unknown; pea-sized amount to skin at intervals of at least 4 h; max dose x 4 daily Wash hands immediately after use; avoid eyes | | Thought to: deplete and prevent reaccumulation of substance P in peripheral nervous system; induce nerve terminal degeneration | Osteoarthritis pain; post-herpetic neuralgia (PHN); peripheral neuropathic pain in non-diabetic patients | Depends on strength of cream (0.025% or 0.075% or patch 8%) | | | No | | Activates TRPV1 receptor; apply sparingly, may give transient burning sensation; PHN: apply when lesions have healed; peripheral neuropathic pain in non-diabetic patients apply under supervision; avoid skin of untreated areas and eyes |

Commonly used mu agonist (unless stated otherwise) strong opioids for Step 3 WHO Analgesic Ladder: initial doses for moderate to **severe pain.**

All doses (based on BNF Formularies) are approximate only, and need to be adjusted according to patient response! (NR = not recommended)

Please check the relevant up-to-date National Formulary for all drug dosages, routes and schedules of administration, adverse effects (many of which are not listed on this table), contraindications especially in pregnancy, pre-term infants and lactating mothers, for which many drugs are contra-indicated. Drugs can usually be given through a number of different routes, in varying formats and dosages which must be prechecked; time to analgesic onset is highly variable and half-life is often dose and route. Many drugs interact with alcohol and may also impair driving ability. NB all opioids can induce potentially fatal respiratory depression at therapeutic doses: Naloxone must be available to counter respiratory depression/coma.

GRAM: Milligrams= mg: 1 thousand
        Micrograms = mcg: 1 millionth

| Opioid | Half-life hours | Approx oral bio availability | Analgesic duration | Metabolism and elimination mode | Indications | Main/adverse effects | Adult oral initial dose | Adult initial dose parenteral | Child oral initial dose 12–18 years | Neonate initial dose intravenous injection | Child 1–12 months initial dose IV injection | Child 1–6 years oral initial dose | Child 6–12 years oral initial dose |
|---|---|---|---|---|---|---|---|---|---|---|---|---|---|
| Morphine Standard of comparison for opioid analgesics Rapid onset Switching from Morphine to Hydromorphone ratio 5:1 | 2–3.5 | 35% | approx 4 h orally administered plasma conjugated morphine levels peak at about 1–2h | Hepatic metabolism to active metabolite M6G which contributes to analgesia; renal elimination of M3G and M6G metabolites; renal impairment associated with M6G accumulation and potential for respiratory depression | Gold standard therapy for severe acute and cancer pain; data showing limited effectiveness for management of severe chronic pain | Sedation; respiratory depression; drowsiness; nausea and vomiting; cough suppression; miosis; constipation; itching; euphoria; hallucinations; tolerance; dependence | 5–10 mg+ q4 h titrate to response | 2.5–10 mg+ q4 h titrate to response | 5–10 mg q4 h titrate to pain need | 50 mcg/kg Over at least 5 mins | 100 mcg/kg Over at least 5 mins | 200–300 mcg/kg q4h | 200–300 mcg/kg q4h |
| Hydromorphone Highly Potent Semisynthetic opioid About 7.5 times potent as morphine; Rapid onset | 2–3 | 37–62% | 4–5h Peak plasma contr 1h PO | Hepatic metabolism; renal elimination; potential retention of neurotoxic metabolite in renal failure | Acute, chronic/ cancer pain; advantageous for opioid tolerant, cachectic patients | As morphine Potentially neurotoxic for patients with renal disease | 2–4 mg Q4h titrate to response | ---------- | 1.3 mg Q4h titrate to response | NR | NR | NR | NR |
| Oxycodone Semisynthetic derivative of thebaine; most used opioid world wide (major drug of abuse) Onset of action 20–30min Switching PO Oxycodone to morphine:ratio: 1:1.5 | 3.5 | 75% PO | 4–6 h | Hepatic metabolism; hepatic and renal elimination of metabolites Some metabolism by CYP2D6 which may increase CNS effects for ultra rapid metabolisers | Primarily used for pain control in palliative care; effective for acute, post-operative chronic especially neuropathic and visceral pain; may have kappa agonist activity | As morphine Possible lower hallucination and itch rates than morphine; slow-release combined with slow release naloxone shown to reduce constipation while maintaining analgesia CYP2D6 enzyme substrate may have altered pharmacokinetics in poor metabolisers | 5–7.5 mg Q4–6h titrate to response | intravenous 2 mg/hr titrate to response | 5 mg Q4–6h titrate to response | NR | NR | 200 mcg/kg q4–6 h titrate to response | 200 mcg/kg q4–6 h titrate to response |

*(Continued)*

(Continued)

| Opioid | Half-life hours | Approx oral bio availability | Analgesic duration | Metabolism and elimination mode | Indications | Main/adverse effects | Adult oral initial dose | Adult initial dose parenteral | Child oral initial dose 12–18 years | Neonate initial dose intravenous injection | Child 1–12 months initial dose IV injection | Child 1–6 years oral initial dose | Child 6–12 years oral initial dose |
|---|---|---|---|---|---|---|---|---|---|---|---|---|---|
| Buprenorphine synthetic derivative of thebaine Partial agonist at µ receptor and a k antagonist; Weak δ agonist | 3–16 IV 13–35 TD 24–69 SL | 15% PO 50% SL | 6–8h SL Rapid onset IV long duration of action; steady state after 1st patch;after patch removal concentration declines 50% in 12 h | Hepatic metabolism and elimination biliary, renal and faecal excretion; no accumulation in renal impairment | Induces less respiratory depression and constipation than other opioids; established role in cancer and chronic pain | Can antagonise effect of other opioids; may relieve withdrawal symptoms; less likely to cause physical or psychological dependence. not suitable for treatment of acute pain; hepatic necrosis, hepatitis, other physical effects observed | Sub lingual 200–400 mcgs Q6–8h | Patches Initially patch of 5mcgs/hr For 7 days when starting analgesia system should be evaluated after 72h to give time for increase in plasma buprenorphine concentration | Sublingual 200–400 mcgs Q8h | NR | NR | NR | Sub lingual 100–200 mcgs Q6–8 h See weight guidance |
| Diamorphine Banned in many countries --very lipid soluble, popular among abusers Bioavailability – Onset of action 5–10min; Duration of action 4hr | 2–3 min | ------- | Crosses blood brain barrier easily; rapidly absorbed | Rapid prodrug | Powerful opioid analgesic; no advantage over morphine in systemic routes; greater solubility allows effective doses in small volumes; advantageous for neuroaxial administration; generally reserved for parenteral use | More sedating than morphine | 5–10 mg Q4 h titrate to response | Subcut intramuscular injection 5–10 mg q4h | 5–10 mg Q4 h titrate to response | (non-ventilated) 2.5–7mcgs/kg/hr | 20 mcgs/kg Dose varies to age in months Q6 h titrate to response | 100–200 mcgs/kg q4 h titrate to response max 10 mg | 100–200 mcgs/kg q4 h titrate to response max 10 mg |

| Opioid | Half-life hours | Approx oral bio availability | Analgesic duration | Metabolism and elimination mode | Indications | Main/adverse effects | Adult oral initial dose | Adult initial dose parenteral | Child oral initial dose 12–18 years | Neonate initial dose intravenous injection | Child 1–12 months initial dose IV injection | Child 1–6 years oral initial dose | Child 6–12 years oral initial dose |
|---|---|---|---|---|---|---|---|---|---|---|---|---|---|
| Tramadol Non-selective pure agonist at µ,δ and K; High affinity for µ receptor receptors; onset of action 30–60mins; inhibits noradrenaline (norepinephrine) uptake; Has abuse potential; can be highly toxic when misused; Potency ratio with morphine 1:10 | 4–6 Longer in patients aged 75+ | 75%PO | 4–6h | Renal excretion Not recommended for patients with renal, hepatic or respiratory Impairment or if taking MAOIs; substrate for CYP2D6 enzyme in the liver; Potential for decreased response/ altered pharmaco kinetics by poor metabolisers | Moderate to severe pain; More useful in neuropathic/ chronic than acute pain widely used for post-operative pain; lowest effective does should be selected; anti tussive effect | Slow titration to minimise risk of lowering seizure threshold; can be highly toxic; may cause withdrawal symptoms; less likely to cause physical or psychological dependence; no respiratory depression; can cause nausea, vomiting and dizziness, headache | 50–100 mg Q4 h to max 400 mg | Intramuscular/ intravenous injection 50–100mg Q4h Post-operative 100 mg initially max 600 mg daily | 50–100 mg Q4 h to max 400 mg | NR | NR | NR | NR |
| Pentazocine Synthetic derivative of benzomorphan; methadone-like; K agonist and µ antagonist =weak partial agonist | 2–3 | 18+/–8% Highly variable Contributes to variation in patient analgesic response | 3–6 h Peak plasma concentration in 1–3h | Hepatic metabolism renal elimination diffuses across placenta; can cause opioid effects in foetus caution with patients with hepatic and renal impairment | Used orally for severe pain | As morphine sedation and drowsiness; nausea and vomiting; can cause dysphoria; psychotomimetic symptoms; can precipitate opioid withdrawal; not for MI pain caution with patients on MAOIs; less likely to cause physical or psychological dependence | 50 mg 3–4 h After food max 600 mg | Subcut/ intramuscular/ Iv injection 45–60 mg 3–4 h | 25 mg 3–4 h | NR | 500 mcg/kg | NR | 25 mg 3–4h |

(Continued)

(Continued)

| Opioid | Half-life hours | Approx oral bio availability | Analgesic duration | Metabolism and elimination mode | Indications | Main/adverse effects | Adult oral initial dose | Adult initial dose parenteral | Child oral initial dose 12–18 years | Neonate initial dose intravenous injection | Child 1–12 months initial dose IV injection | Child 1–6 years oral initial oral dose | Child 6–12 years oral initial oral dose |
|---|---|---|---|---|---|---|---|---|---|---|---|---|---|
| Methadone synthetic derivative: Methadone series; highly potent orally; high affinity for µ and lower affinity for K and δ receptors | 13–50 | 80% | 4–6h initially, increasing after steady state; Peak plasma concentration 1–4h; long duration of action; steady state plasma concentration may take 10 days | Risk of accumulation of metabolites with repetitive dosing; extensive binding to tissue proteins; high concentrations in lung, liver and kidneys; acid urine increases renal clearance | Neuropathic pain, opioid induced allodynia and hyperalgesia; opioid rotation; may relieve withdrawal symptoms | As morphine Risk of excessive sedation unpredictable variation in half life; contraindicated with MAO inhibitors; substrate for CYP3A4 may cause altered pharmacokinetics in patients lacking enzyme | 5–10 mg 6–8h titrate to response | Subcut/ Intramuscular injection 5–10 mg 6–8h titrate to response | NR | NR | NR | NR | NR |
| Fentanyl (synthetic derivative, phenylpiperidine series) | 3.7 Prolonged in neonate | 50% | 1–2 rapidly absorbed from buccal mucosa; peak plasma concentration within 60 min; DTrans removal 17h + pl. concentrat to decrease 50% potent; short acting | Extreme caution with patients with intracranial pressure, renal or hepatic impairment; hepatic metabolism may induce neurotoxic side-effects; hepatic and renal elimination | Rapid onset, short duration of action; post-operative, acute cancer / breakthrough and chronic pain; preferred over sustained release morphine for fewer side-effects | As morphine Highly potent; care required regarding transdermal patches with residual depot and delay in peak plasma concentration and offset with patch removal; should only be used in opioid tolerant patients due to risk of fatal respiratory depression | 100mcgs buccal; repeat x1 if required after 15–30min | Transdermal patches 12–100mcg/hr for 72h  Child 12 mcg or 25 mcg/h over 72h *see table for Conversion values | Trans mucosal 200mcgs Over 15 min | NR | NR | NR | NR |

| Opioid | Half-life hours | Approx oral bio availability | Analgesic duration | Metabolism and elimination mode | Indications | Main/adverse effects | Adult oral initial dose | Adult initial dose parenteral | Child oral initial dose 12–18 years | Neonate initial dose intravenous injection | Child 1–12 months initial dose IV injection | Child 1–6 years oral initial dose | Child 6–12 years oral initial dose |
|---|---|---|---|---|---|---|---|---|---|---|---|---|---|
| Alfentanil (synthetic derivative, phenylpiperidin series) High intra- and inter-patient variability in pharmacokinetics | Sequential half lives, 1, 14 Prolonged in neonate | | Immediate onset of action; potent; short acting | Hepatic biotransformation; urinary excretion of metabolites | Analgesic supplement for use before and during anaesthesia | Low toxic potential at therapeutic doses; potential for apnoea, respiratory and CNS suppression; bradycardia, muscle rigidity; substrate for CYP3A4 may cause altered pharmacokinetics in patients lacking enzyme | | Assisted ventilation Intravenous injection 30–50mcgs/kg | | 5–20mcgs/kg | 1 month– 18 years 10–20mcgs/kg | | |
| Pethidine Synthetic derivative phenylpiperidine series Complex drug with additional anticholinergic effects | 3–4 | 30% increased in cirrhosis | 2–3 h After IV injection rapid decline in plasma concentration followed by slower phase | Hepatic metabolism Hepatic and renal elimination | Obstetric analgesia Extreme caution in neonates, children; Kinetic properties altered in cirrhosis | As morphine May cause respiratory depression in adults and new born! Hypotension with tachycardia Excreted in breast milk Contraindicated in patients with renal impairment or on MAOIs | 50–150mg q4h max in 24h 400mg | 25–100mg Subcut or IM injection 25–100mg for obstetric pain Repeat 1–3h if required; Child 12–18yrs 0.5–1mg/kg Intramuscular Max in 24h 400mg | NR | NR | NR | NR | NR |
| Tapentadol Potent μ agonist and a noradrenaline (norepinephrine) re-uptake inhibitor; has abuse potential | 4 | 32% | 4–6h | Renal elimination; Caution in patients with respiratory and hepatic impairment; reduce dose and extend length between doses; consider alternative medication; dr interactions increase risk of respiratory depression | Moderate to severe pain which requires opioid analgesia | Dual mechanism of action appears to result in reduced adverse gastro-intestinal effects of nausea, vomiting constipation compared to conventional opioids; may be more effective for neuropathic pain; contraindicated in patients taking MAOIs | 50–100mg q4–6 h according to pain intensity, if not currently taking opioids max in 24h: 600mg | ---------------- | NR | NR | NR | NR | NR |

# Index

Figures and Tables are indicated by page numbers in bold. The abreviation 'bib' after a page number refers to bibliographical information in the 'Recommended reading' sections.